Minimally Invasive Surgery in Orthopedics

T0094323

Giles R. Scuderi • Alfred J. Tria
Editors

Minimally Invasive Surgery in Orthopedics

Foot and Ankle Handbook

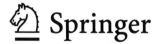 Springer

Editors
Giles R. Scuderi, MD
Insall Scott Kelly Institute
  for Orthopaedics and Sports Medicine
New York, NY, USA
grscuderi@aol.com

Alfred J. Tria, MD
Department of Orthopedic Surgery
Robert Wood Johnson Medical School
Piscataway, NJ, USA
atriajrmd@aol.com

ISBN 978-1-4614-0892-5   e-ISBN 978-1-4614-0893-2
DOI 10.1007/978-1-4614-0893-2
Springer New York Dordrecht Heidelberg London

Library of Congress Control Number: 2011936743

Printed on acid-free paper

Springer is part of Springer Science+Business Media (www.springer.com)

Contents

Contributors

Jamal Ahmad, MD Assistant Professor, Department of Orthopaedic Surgery, Rothman Institute and Thomas Jefferson University Hospital, Philadelphia, PA, USA

Gregory C. Berlet, MD Chief, Foot and Ankle, Ohio State University, Orthopaedic Foot and Ankle Center, Columbus, OH, USA

Roberto Bevoni, MD Staff, Rizzoli Orthopedic Institute, University of Bologna, Bologna, Italy

Matteo Cadossi, MD Staff, Rizzoli Orthopedic Institute, University of Bologna, Bologna, Italy

James B. Carr, MD Private Practice, Associate Clinical Professor, Lewis Gale Orthopedics, Salem, VA, USA

Department of Orthopedics, University of South Carolina, Columbia, SC, USA

Dominic S. Carreira, MD Private Practice, Broward Health Orthopedics, Fort Lauderdale, FL, USA

Michael P. Clare, MD Director of Fellowship Education, Division of Foot and Ankle Surgery, The Florida Orthopaedic Institute, Tampa, FL, USA

J. Chris Coetzee, MD, FRCSC Attending Physician, Surgeon, Fairview University Medical Center, Minneapolis, MN, USA

Minnesota Sports Medicine and Twin Cities Orthopedics, Eden Prairie, MN, USA

P.A.J. de Leeuw, MD Department of Orthopaedic Surgery, Academic Medical Centre, University of Amsterdam, Amsterdam, the Netherlands

Christopher W. DiGiovanni, MD Associate Professor and Chief, Division of Foot and Ankle, Department of Orthopedic Surgery, Brown University Medical School, Rhode Island Hospital, Providence, RI, USA

Sandro Giannini, MD Director, School of Orthopaedics,
Rizzoli Orthopedic Institute, Bologna University, Bologna, Italy

John E. Herzenberg, MD, FRCSC Director, Pediatric Orthopedics,
International Center for Limb Lengthening, Sinai Hospital of Baltimore,
Baltimore, MD, USA

Beat Hintermann, MD Associate Professor and Chairman,
Department of Orthopaedic Surgery, University of Basel, Basel, Switzerland

Juha Jaakkola, MD Staff Physician, Southeastern Orthopedic Center,
Savannah, GA, USA

Anish R. Kadakia, MD Clinical Lecturer, Department of Orthopedic
Surgery, University of Michigan, Ann Arbor, MI, USA

Bradley M. Lamm, DPM Head for Foot and Ankle Surgery,
International Center for Limb Lengthening, Rubin Institute for Advanced
Orthopedics, Sinai Hospital of Baltimore, Baltimore, MD, USA

Nicola Maffulli, MD, MS, PhD, FRCS (Orth) Centre Lead
and Professor of Sports and Exercise Medicine, Consultant Trauma
and Orthopaedic Surgeon, Centre for Sports and Exercise Medicine,
Barts and the London School of Medicine and Dentistry, Queen Mary
University of London, London, UK

Peter B. Maurus, MD Orthopedic Surgeon, Steindler Orthopedic Clinic,
Iowa City, IA, USA

Mark S. Myerson, MD Director, Foot and Ankle Institute,
Mercy Medical Center, Baltimore, MD, USA

James A. Nunley, MD Chairman, Division of Orthopaedic Surgery,
Department of Surgery, Duke University Medical Center, Durham, NC, USA

Geert I. Pagenstert, MD Attending Physician, Department of Orthopaedic
Surgery, University of Basel, Basel, Switzerland

Dror Paley, MD, FRCSC Director, Paley Advanced Limb Lengthening
Institute, St. Mary's Hospital, West Palm Beach, FL, USA

Fernando A. Pena, MD Assistant Professor, Department of Orthopaedic
Surgery, University of Minnesota, Minneapolis, MN, USA

Steven M. Raikin, MD Director, Foot and Ankle Service,
Assistant Professor; Department of Orthopaedic Surgery, Rothman Institute
and Thomas Jefferson University Hospital, Philadelphia, PA, USA

Martinus Richter, MD Professor, Chirurgische Klinik, Klinikum Coburg,
Coburg, Germany

Michael M. Romash, MD Private Practice, Orthopedic Foot and Ankle
Center of Hampton Roads, Chesapeake Regional Medical Center,
Chesapeake, VA, USA

S. Robert Rozbruch, MD Director and Chief, Associate Professor
of Clinical Orthopaedic Surgery, Limb Lengthening and Deformity Service,
Hospital for Special Surgery, Weill Medical College of Cornell University,
New York, NY, USA

Nicholas Savva, MBBS, BMedSci, FRCS (Tr & Orth) Staff,
Foot and Ankle Surgery, Brisbane Private Hospital, Brisbane, Australia

Jonathan R. Saluta, MD Private Practice, Los Angeles Orthopedic Center,
Los Angeles, CA, USA

Roy W. Sanders, MD Director, Orthopaedic Trauma Service,
Tampa General Hospital, The Florida Orthopaedic Institute, Tampa, FL, USA

Terry Saxby, MBBS, FRACS Staff, Foot and Ankle Surgery,
Brisbane Private Hospital, Brisbane, Australia

Amol Saxena, DPM, FACFAS Section Chief, Podiatric Surgery,
Department of Sports Medicine, Palo Alto Medical Foundation, Palo Alto,
CA, USA

Murali K. Sayana, MB, ChB, AFRCSI, FRCS Senior Specalist Registrar,
Department of Trauma and Orthopaedics, Royal College of Surgeons
in Ireland, Dublin, Ireland

Pierce Scranton, MD Associate Clinical Professor,
Department of Orthopedics, University of Washington, Seattle, WA, USA

Steven L. Shapiro, MD Director, Savannah Orthopaedic Foot
and Ankle Center, Savannah, GA, USA

A.C. Stroïnk, MD Department of Orthopaedic Surgery,
Academic Medical Center, University of Amsterdam, Amsterdam,
The Netherlands

C. Christopher Stroud, MD Attending Physician, Department of Surgery,
William Beaumont Hospital-Troy, Troy, MI, USA

Victor Valderrabano, MD, PhD Associate Professor,
Department of Orthopaedics, University Hospital, University of Basel,
Basel, Switzerland

C.N. van Dijk, MD, PhD Department of Orthopaedic Surgery,
Academic Medical Centre, University of Amsterdam, Amsterdam,
The Netherlands

Francesca Vannini, MD, PhD Assistant Professor,
Department of Orthopaedics and Traumatology, Rizzoli Orthopedic
Institute, University of Bologna, Bologna, Italy

Jonathan Young, MB, ChB, MRCS (Edin) Specialist Registrar,
Department of Orthopaedics and Trauma, University Hospitals Coventry
and Warwickshire, Coventry, UK

Percutaneous Repair of Acute Rupture of the Achilles Tendon

Jonathan Young, Murali K. Sayana, and Nicola Maffulli

The Achilles tendon is the strongest tendon in the human body, with a tensile strength on the order of 50–100 N/mm^2 [1]. Despite this, the Achilles tendon is the most commonly ruptured tendon in the human body [2, 3]. Rupture commonly occurs in middle-aged men who play sports occasionally. There is possibly a link with a sedentary lifestyle [3]. The aetiopathogenesis of Achilles tendon ruptures is still unknown, but histological evidence of degeneration is relatively common [2].

Anatomy

The tendinous portions of the gastrocnemius and soleus muscles merge to form the Achilles tendon [2]. The gastrocnemius tendon emerges as a broad aponeurosis at the distal margin of the muscle bellies, whereas the soleus tendon begins as a band proximally on the posterior surface of the soleus muscle. Distally, the Achilles tendon

J. Young
Department of Orthopaedics and Trauma, University Hospitals Coventry and Warwickshire, Coventry, UK

M.K. Sayana
Department of Trauma and Orthopaedics, Royal College of Surgeons in Ireland, Dublin, Ireland

N. Maffulli (✉)
Centre Lead and Professor of Sports and Exercise Medicine, Consultant Trauma and Orthopaedic Surgeon, Centre for Sports and Exercise Medicine, Barts and the London School of Medicine and Dentistry, Queen Mary University of London, London, UK
e-mail: n.maffulli@qmul.ac.uk

becomes progressively rounded in cross section until approximately 4 cm from its calcaneus insertion, where it flattens out prior to inserting into the proximal calcaneal tuberosity [4].

The calcaneal insertion is specialised. It is composed of an attachment of the tendon, a layer of hyaline cartilage, and an area of bone not covered by periosteum. There is a subcutaneous bursa between the tendon and the skin and a retrocalcaneal bursa between the tendon and the calcaneus [5].

Diagnosis

There is often a history of an audible snap at the back of the heel followed by pain and an inability to weight bear on the affected side. A palpable gap is often present (Fig. 1.1). The diagnosis is also aided with the Simmonds and Matles clinical tests [6, 7]. For the Simmonds test, the examiner gently squeezes the patient's calf muscles with the palm of the examiner's hand. If the Achilles tendon is intact, the ankle plantarflexes (Fig. 1.2). If the Achilles tendon is torn, the ankle remains still, or plantarflexes minimally (Fig. 1.3). The Matles' test involves asking patients to lie prone, and to flex both knees to 90°. If the injured foot falls into neutral or dorsiflexion, a ruptured Achilles tendon is diagnosed (Fig. 1.4).

Both tests are performed on the injured and uninjured sides for comparison. If there is uncertainty about the diagnosis, imaging can be considered, although it is not routine in our practice,

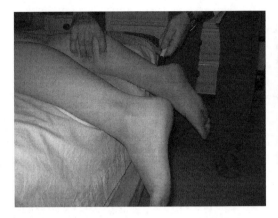

Fig. 1.1 Simmond's test: plantar flexion of the left foot with an intact Achilleser

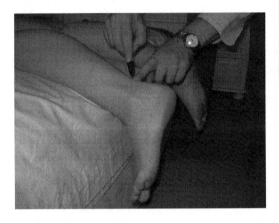

Fig. 1.2 Palpable gap, illustrated with finger

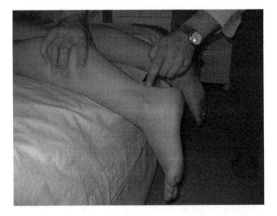

Fig. 1.3 Simmond's test: no plantar flexion on calf squeeze of the right foot due to a ruptured Achilles tendon

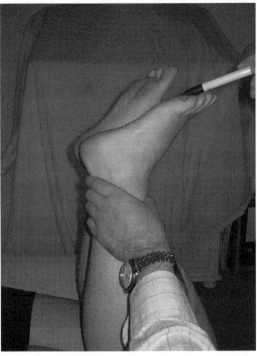

Fig. 1.4 Matles test, showing a ruptured right Achilles tendon

because the imaging does not add to the management of the injury. Ultrasound [8] or magnetic resonance imaging (MRI) scans [9] help confirm the diagnosis. Ultrasonography will reveal an acoustic vacuum between the tendon edges. Magnetic resonance imaging will reveal generalised high signal intensity on T2-weighted images. On T1-weighted images, the rupture will appear as a disruption of the signal within the tendon substance.

Management

The management options of acute ruptures of the Achilles tendon can be divided into two broad categories: conservative or operative. Operative methods can be divided into open or percutaneous techniques. There is still ongoing debate regarding what type of management is best [2]. This depends on the patient' condition, age, and level of fitness.

Conservative Management

Wallace et al. [10] reported excellent results with conservative management using a hard cast for 1 month before switching to a functional brace for 1 further month. In contrast, Persson and Wredmark [11] showed that 7 of 27 patients had a re-rupture, and a further seven patients were not satisfied with the result of conservative management. Moller et al. [12] in a prospective, randomised, multicentre study of 112 patients with acute rupture of the Achilles tendon demonstrated a re-rupture rate of 20.8% after non-surgical and 1.7% after surgical treatment ($P<0.001$).

Conservative management may lengthen the tendon, altering its function [13]. This may need surgical correction [14], and can be avoided in the first place if surgery is performed [2]. Many authors think that, aside from the functional problems of conservative management, there is also a higher re-rupture rate. Wong et al. [15] reported a re-rupture rate of 10.7% for conservative management of rupture. Lo et al. [16] reported an overall re-rupture rate of 2.8% for operatively managed and 11.7% for non-operatively managed patients ($P<0.001$).

Open Repair

Surgical management significantly reduces the risk of Achilles tendon re-rupture, but can increase the risk of infection when compared with conservative management [17]. Arner and Lindholm [18] reported a 24% complication rate in 86 operative repairs including one death from pulmonary embolism. Lo et al. [16] reported that open repair induces 20 times more minor to moderate complications than conservative management, but there were no significant differences between open surgical and conservative management regarding major complications.

Open repair can be performed in a variety of ways using simple end to end repairs (Bunnell/Kessler), or more complex techniques with fascial reinforcement or tendon grafts [19, 20]. There is no evidence that, in fresh ruptures, one suture method is superior to others. There is some evidence that primary augmentation with local reinforcement or tendon grafts prolongs operating times, and induces a greater rate of complications. There is no significant evidence to support more complex primary repairs in acute Achilles tendon ruptures [21]. The results of open repair vary markedly [18, 22]. These differences are likely to be multifactorial, and may well result from subtle variations in technique, degree of experience of the operating surgeon, the type of suture material used, and the location of incision.

Percutaneous Repair

Percutaneous repair [23] is a compromise between open surgery and conservative management. The aim of this procedure is to provide a better functional outcome than conservative treatment, with a similar functional outcome to that of open repair. Percutaneous repair also aims to decrease the problems of wound healing and skin breakdown associated with open repair. The early reports outlined an increased risk of re-rupture and of damage to the sural nerve, a potential downside to the procedure. Ma and Griffith [23] pioneered the technique with an excellent success rate with no re-ruptures and two minor complications. Some studies have demonstrated that the rate of re-rupture after percutaneous repair is higher than that after open operative procedures [24, 25], although these studies are now dated, and do not compare like with like.

More recent studies comparing open and percutaneous repair show that the two repair techniques produce similar outcomes. For example, Lim et al. [26] advocate percutaneous repair when comparing it with open techniques, concluding that percutaneous repair had a lower infection rate and was more cosmetically acceptable. The functional results comparing the open technique with the percutaneous technique showed no significant difference. Cretnik at al [27]. further expanded on the benefits of percutaneous repair and the controversy regarding the optimal treatment of fresh total Achilles tendon ruptures. A cohort study compared the results of percutaneous and open Achilles tendon repair. The results of 132 consecutive patients with acute complete Achilles tendon rupture who were operated on exclusively with modified percutaneous repair under local anaesthesia and followed up for at least 2 years were compared with the results of 105 consecutive patients who underwent open repair under general or spinal anesthesia in the same period. There were significantly fewer major complications in the group of percutaneous repairs in comparison with the group of open repairs ($P=0.03$), and a lower total number of complications ($P=0.013$). The study did report slightly more re-ruptures and sural nerve complications following percutaneous repairs, but no statistically significant difference. Functional assessment with the American Orthopaedic Foot and Ankle Society scale and the Holz score did not show any statistically significant difference.

Several percutaneous repair techniques have been described [23, 28–31]. Ma and Griffith [23] described a technique of percutaneous repair of the Achilles tendon using six stab incisions over the tendon in 18 patients. The suture was passed through the stab incisions, and crisscrossed through the tendon. They reported one incidence of sensory disturbance and one patient with sural nerve entrapment.

Webb and Bannister [28] described a percutaneous technique that reduced the potential risk to the sural nerve by placing the proximal of the incisions to the medial side, away from the sural nerve. McClelland and Maffulli [31] described a percutaneous technique of repair of ruptured Achilles tendons similar to that described by Webb and Bannister [28], but using a Kessler-type suture. We now perform percutaneous repair of Achilles tendon rupture using a minimally invasive procedure with five small incisions, four of which are 1-cm long, and the fifth, 2-cm long.

Pre-operative Planning

Once the diagnosis is made, the patient needs a full assessment regarding their general health and co-morbidities, their pre-operative functional status should also be noted.

The affected limb should be examined with regard to skin quality and also neurovascular status. Particular attention should be made to the possible pre-operative involvement of the sural nerve. Appropriate blood tests, electrocardiography (ECG) and chest X-ray (CXR) may also be required if the patient has a relevant co-morbidity. Deep vein thrombosis (DVT) prophylaxis may be necessary. An equinus backslab may be used pre-operatively for comfort. Once assessed and surgically worked up for the operating theatre, the patient will require valid written consent, ideally obtained by the operating surgeon. Sural nerve damage, re-rupture, infection, and impaired function should be discussed with the patient.

Operative Technique

Local anaesthetic infiltration is used. A 50:50 mixture of 20 ml of 1% lignocaine hydrochloride (Antigen Pharmaceuticals Ltd, Roscrea, Ireland) and 5 mg/ml of Chirocaine (Abbot Laboratories Ltd, Berkshire, England) is instilled into an area of between 8 and 10 cm around the ruptured Achilles tendon. The patient is placed prone, and a pillow is placed beneath the anterior aspect of the ankles to allow the feet to hang free. The operating table is angled down 20° cranially to reduce venous pooling in the feet and ankles. The affected leg is prepped. A calf tourniquet is used and inflated to 250 mmHg.

Five stab incisions are made over the Achilles tendon (Fig. 1.5). The first is directly over the

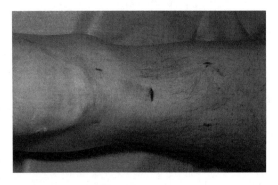

Fig. 1.5 The five stab incisions over the ruptured Achilles tendon

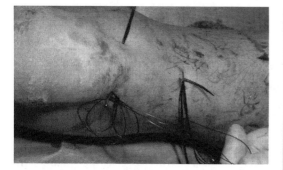

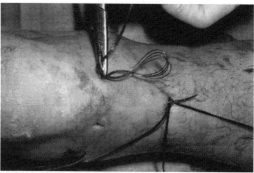

Fig. 1.6 Needle reintroduced into the medial distal stab incision through a different entry point in the tendon and passed longitudinally and proximally through the tendon, directed towards the middle incision and out through the ruptured tendon end

Fig. 1.7 The suture protruding from the lateral distal stab incision is rethreaded onto the needle and reintroduced via the lateral distal stab incision into the tendon substance. It is passed longitudinally and proximally through the tendon to exit from the middle incision

palpable defect, and is approximately 2 cm in a transverse direction. A small piece of tendon from the rupture site is removed and sent for histological examination. The other incisions are approximately 4 cm proximal and 4 cm distal to the first incision. The proximal incisions are vertical 1-cm stab incisions on the medial and lateral aspect of the Achilles tendon. We advocate blunt dissection with a small haemostat directly onto the Achilles tendon, and therefore avoid damaging the sural nerve, which crosses the lateral border of the Achilles tendon approximately 10 cm proximal to its insertion into the calcaneus [32].

A small haemostat is used to free the tendon sheath from the overlying subcutaneous tissue. A 1 Maxon (Tyco Healthcare UK Ltd) double-strand suture on a long curved needle is passed transversely through the lateral distal stab incision passing through the substance of the tendon and out through the medial distal stab incision. The needle is then reintroduced into the medial distal stab incision through a different entry point in the tendon and passed longitudinally and proximally through the tendon, to lock the tendon, and is directed towards the middle incision and out through the ruptured tendon end (Fig. 1.6).

The suture that is still protruding from the lateral distal stab incision is rethreaded onto the needle and reintroduced via the lateral distal stab incision into the tendon substance. It is passed

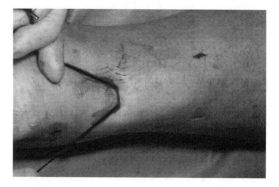

Fig. 1.8 Traction is applied to the suture to ensure a satisfactory grip within the tendon

longitudinally and proximally through the tendon to exit from the middle incision (Fig. 1.7). Traction is applied to the suture to ensure a satisfactory grip within the tendon (Fig. 1.8). If the suture pulls through, the procedure is repeated. The same procedure is carried out for the proximal half of the ruptured tendon. The sutures are then tied with the ankle in maximum plantar flexion (Fig. 1.9). The transverse skin wound is closed with subcuticular 3/0 Biosyn (Tyco Healthcare UK Ltd) sutures. The longitudinal stab wounds are juxtaposed, and closed with Steri-Strips. A non-adherent dressing is applied. A full Plaster of Paris cast is applied in the operating theatre with the ankle in maximum equinus. The cast is split on both the medial and lateral sides to allow for swelling (Fig. 1.10).

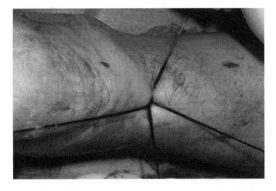

Fig. 1.9 The sutures are tied with the ankle in maximum plantar flexion

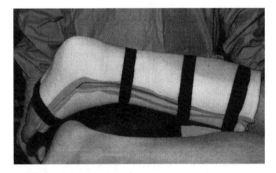

Fig. 1.10 A full plaster of Paris cast is applied in the operating theatre with the ankle in maximum equinus. The cast is split on both the medial and lateral sides to allow for swelling

Complications

Haematomas can lead to infection and wound breakdown especially in light of the tenuous blood supply to the Achilles tendon [31]. This is very infrequent given the small incisions used. Sural nerve damage can cause altered dermatomal sensation or a painful neuroma. Patients can experience anaesthesia of the lateral aspect of the foot, and some report difficulty with shoes as a result of this [33]. This can be avoided with blunt dissection directly onto the Achilles tendon using a blunt haemostat. The placement of the skin incision is such, however, that the sutures are distant from the sural nerve. The tenuous blood supply of the Achilles tendon increases the chance of wound infection. This is a recognised complication

of the open approach, and is reduced with percutaneous techniques [26, 31].

Re-rupture is a documented complication [24, 25]. The use of modern suture materials with a number of intratendinous threads comparable to that used in open repairs minimises this complication. More recent studies comparing the two repair techniques show similar results, with no difference in re-rupture rate between percutaneous and open repair [26], but a significantly higher rate of infective wound complications using open repair [26]. DVT should also be considered because the patient will be in a plaster cast. DVT should therefore be looked for when the patient is re-examined routinely out of the cast, and appropriate management administered if suspected [33]. Early post-operative rehabilitation aims to reduce this risk.

Post-operative Management

The operated leg is elevated immediately post-op. If the neurovascular status of the limb is acceptable, and after assessment by a physiotherapist making sure the patient is safe and the patient is comfortable in their cast, patients can be discharged. The full cast is retained for 2 weeks, and the patient is able to weight bear as comfort allows. During the period in the cast, patients are advised to perform gentle isometric contractions of the gastro-soleus complex, and elevate the limb when at rest.

At this time, patients are reviewed in outpatient clinic where the wounds are inspected. An anterior splint is worn with the foot plantar-flexed for a further 4 weeks. During this period, patients are advised to mobilise partial weight bearing initially, increasing to weight bearing as able by 4 weeks. In addition, patients are encouraged to invert and evert the foot and to plantar flex it against resistance on a regular basis. The splint is then removed, and physiotherapy follow-up for gentle mobilisation is arranged. Light exercise can be started 2 weeks after cast removal. Patients should be fully weight bearing by that time.

References

1. Viidik A. Tensile strength properties of Achilles tendon systems in trained and untrained rabbits. Acta Orthop Scand 1962;10:261–272
2. Maffulli N. Rupture of the Achilles tendon. J Bone Joint Surg Am 1999;81:1019–1036
3. Jozsa L, Kvist M, Balint BJ, Reffy A, Jarvinen M, Lehto M, Barzo M. The role of recreational sport activity in Achilles tendon rupture. A clinical, patho-anatomical, and sociological study of 292 cases. Am J Sports Med 1989;17(3):338–343
4. Cummins EJ, Anson BJ, Carr BW, Wright RR. The structure of the calcaneal tendon (of Achilles) in relation to orthopaedic surgery. With additional observations on the planatris muscle. Surg Gynecol Obstet 1946;83:107–116
5. Rufai A, Ralphs JR, Benjamin M. Structure and histopathology of the insertional region of the human Achilles tendon. J Orthop Res 1995;13(4):585–593
6. Simmonds FA. The diagnosis of the ruptured Achilles tendon. Practitioner 1957;179:56–58
7. Matles AL. Rupture of the tendo Achilles. Another diagnostic test. Bull Hosp Joint Dis 1975;36:48–51
8. Maffulli N, Dymond NP, Capasso G. Ultrasonographic findings in subcutaneous rupture of Achilles tendon. J Sports Med Phys Fitness 1989;29(4):365–368
9. Kabbani YM, Mayer DP. Magnetic resonance imaging of tendon pathology about the foot and ankle. Part I. Achilles tendon. J Am Podiatr Med Ass 1993;83:418–420
10. Wallace RG, Traynor IE, Kernohan WG, Eames MH. Combined conservative and orthotic management of acute ruptures of the Achilles tendon. J Bone Joint Surg Am 2004;86:1198–1202
11. Persson A, Wredmark T. The treatment of total ruptures of the Achilles tendon by plaster immobilisation. Int Orthop 1979;3:149–152
12. Moller M, Movin T, Granhed H, Lind K, Faxen E, Karlsson J. Acute rupture of tendon Achillis. A prospective randomised study of comparison between surgical and non-surgical treatment. J Bone Joint Surg Br 2001;83(6):843–848
13. Bohnsack M, Ruhmann O, Kirsch L, Wirth CJ. Surgical shortening of the Achilles tendon for correction of elongation following healed conservatively treated Achilles tendon rupture. Z Orthop Ihre Grenzgeb 2000;138:501–505
14. Soma C, Mandelbaum B. Repair of acute Achilles tendon ruptures. Orthop Clin North Am 1976;7:241–246
15. Wong J, Barrass V, Maffulli N. Quantitative review of operative and nonoperative management of Achilles tendon ruptures. Am J Sports Med 2002;30:565–575
16. Lo IK, Kirkley A, Nonweiler B, Kumbhare DA. Operative versus nonoperative treatment of acute Achilles tendon ruptures: a quantitative review. Clin J Sport Med 1997;7:207–211
17. Bhandari M, Guyatt GH, Siddiqui F, Morrow F, Busse J, Leighton RK, Sprague S, Schemitsch EH. Treatment of acute Achilles tendon ruptures: a systematic overview and metaanalysis. Clin Orthop Relat Res 2002; Jul(400):190–200
18. Arner O, Lindholm A. Subcutaneous rupture of the Achilles tendon. A study of 92 cases. Acta Chir Scand 1959;116(239):1–5
19. Bosworth D. Repair of defects in the tendo Achilles. J Bone Joint Surg Am 1956;38:111–114
20. Lynn T. Repair of torn Achilles tendon, using the plantaris tendon as a reinforcing membrane. J Bone Joint Surg Am 1966;48:268–272
21. Jessing P, Hansen E. Surgical treatment of 102 tendo Achilles ruptures – suture or tenoplasty? Acta Chir Scand 1975;141:370–377
22. Soldatis J, Goodfellow D, Wilber J. End to end operative repair of Achilles tendon rupture. Am J Sports Med 1997;25:90–95
23. Ma GWC, Griffith TG. Percutaneous repair of acute closed ruptures Achilles tendon. A new technique. Clin Orthop Relat Res 1977; Oct(128):247–255
24. Aracil J, Lozano J, Torro V, Escriba I. Percutaneous suture of Achilles tendon ruptures. Foot Ankle 1992; 13:350–351
25. Bradley J, Tibone J. Percutaneous and open surgical repairs of Achilles tendon ruptures. A comparitive study. Am J Sports Med 1990;18:188–195
26. Lim J, Dalal R, Waseem M. Percutaneous vs. open repair of the ruptured Achilles tendon – a prospective randomized controlled study. Foot Ankle Int 2001; 22(7):559–568
27. Cretnik A, Kosanovic M, Smrkolj V. Percutaneous versus open repair of the ruptured Achilles tendon: a comparative study. Am J Sports Med 2005;33(9): 1369–1379
28. Webb JM, Bannister GC. Percutaneous repair of the ruptured tendo Achillis. J Bone Joint Surg Br 1999; 81(5):877–880
29. Gorschewsky O, Vogel U, Schweizer A, van Laar B. Percutaneous tenodesis of the Achilles tendon. A new surgical method for the treatment of acute Achilles tendon rupture through percutaneous tenodesis. Injury 1999;30(5):315–321
30. Cretnik A, Zlajpah L, Smrkolj V, Kosanovic M. The strength of percutaneous methods of repair of the Achilles tendon: a biomechanical study. Med Sci Sports Exerc 2000;32(1):16–20
31. McClelland D, Maffulli N. Percutaneous repair of ruptured Achilles tendon. J R Coll Surg Edinb 2002; 41:613–618
32. Webb J, Moorjani N, Radford M. Anatomy of the sural nerve and its relation to the Achilles tendon. Foot Ankle Int 2000;21(6):475–477
33. Young JS, Kumta SM, Maffulli N. Achilles tendon rupture and tendinopathy: management of complications. Foot Ankle Clin 2005;10(2):371–382

Endoscopic Gastrocnemius Recession

2

Amol Saxena and Christopher W. DiGiovanni

Percutaneous techniques are becoming popular for treating many musculoskeletal conditions. Those developed for endoscopic carpal tunnel and plantar fascial release are currently among the most common. The reported benefits of endoscopic surgery include smaller incisions and shorter postoperative recovery time [1–3]. Visualization with an endoscope may also decrease perioperative complications from scarring such as incisional irritation or neuritis, although the overall safety of these interventions has yet to be determined. An endoscopic means of gastrocnemius recession (EGR) has recently been popularized for correction of ankle equinus contracture as an alternative to formal open gastrocnemius release (OGR) or Achilles tendon lengthening [4–21]. The OGR remains today's gold standard for aponeurotic lengthening because of its proven record as a safe, rapid, and effective procedure. This open "slide," however, can involve a large unsightly incision, which is particularly unpopular with young women, and can be associated with sural nerve scarring and neuritis [11, 14, 15, 19, 22]. The EGR, an alternative percutaneous approach, has been sought in an effort to avoid those problems, but it has a significant learning

curve, can be associated with poor visualization, and is somewhat instrument dependent [14, 17]. In consideration of its potential advantages and drawbacks, the authors have tried over the last several years to develop a safe and reliable endoscopic technique for gastrocnemius recession.

Gastrocnemius recession has been used successfully for over a century to correct ankle contracture, originally described to treat neurologically impaired individuals [16]. More recent data suggesting the presence of isolated gastrocnemius tightness in otherwise healthy patients, however, has popularized more widespread use of OGR in the United States and Europe during the past decade. EGR was first introduced as a treatment alternative in 2002 [13, 21]. Its purported benefits over the standard open means of gastrocnemius release included a smaller incision, a potentially faster recovery, and the versatility of being performed in any patient position. While its recent interest has emerged primarily in response to complications from the open technique, to date, its advantages remain promising but incompletely substantiated [14].

Early results of the endoscopic procedure appear comparable to the open technique regarding improvement of ankle dorsiflexion [5, 10–12, 14, 20]. Using an endoscopic technique, Saxena and Widtfeldt obtained an average 15° immediate improvement in postoperative dorsiflexion, which remained at 12.6° after 1-year follow-up of 18 cases [14]. Pinney et al. reported an 18° dorsiflexion increase sustained 2 months after open Strayer procedure [11]. DiDomenico et al. reported

A. Saxena
Department of Sports Medicine, Palo Alto Medical Foundation, Palo Alto, CA, USA

C.W. DiGiovanni (✉)
Division of Foot and Ankle, Department of Orthopedic Surgery, Brown University Medical School, Rhode Island Hospital, Providence, RI, USA
e-mail: christopher_digiovanni@brown.edu

G.R. Scuderi and A.J. Tria (eds.), *Minimally Invasive Surgery in Orthopedics: Foot and Ankle Handbook*,
DOI 10.1007/978-1-4614-0893-2_2, © Springer Science+Business Media, LLC 2012

their results on 31 procedures of EGR and noted an improvement of 18° with the knee extended [5]. Trevino et al. did not report the amount of dorsiflexion achieved with their endoscopic results, noting only "significant improvement in ankle dorsiflexion." [20] All three of these studies dealt with nonspastic equinus. A recent European study reported on 18 procedures on patients with cerebral palsy who exhibited neurological equinus [12]. These authors were also able to achieve total dorsiflexion improvement of almost 20° after using the endoscopic technique. Interestingly, despite available data, the amount of equinus correction actually required for gastrocnemius recession to be successful in impacting long-term outcome in these patients remains unknown. In fact, although many (including these authors) think that such equinus correction remedies varying pathologies of the foot, even the relationship between isolated gastrocnemius release and functional improvement remains obscure. For example, as of today, the mere definition of pathological equinus has only recently been more closely studied.

Historically, functional ankle joint dorsiflexion has been defined as 10° with the knee extended and more than 10° with the knee flexed (the Silverskiold maneuver) [23]. Values below these have been somewhat arbitrarily defined as "equinus contracture." In 2002, DiGiovanni et al. studied ankle dorsiflexion in nonneurologically impaired populations of individuals who were either asymptomatic controls or patients with symptomatic midfoot and/or forefoot complaints [24]. They concluded that 5° of ankle dorsiflexion with the knee extended and 10° with the knee flexed represented reasonably normal values, and suggested that values less than these should be considered evidence of gastrocnemius or Achilles contracture, respectively. They also found a statistically significant association between those individuals who met the criteria for gastrocnemius equinus and an increased incidence of painful midfoot and forefoot pathology. Another study contended that 0° of ankle dorsiflexion with the knee in extension could be "normal" in asymptomatic, adolescent athletes [25]. Based on this data, we consider patients candidates for gastrocnemius

Table 2.1 Indications for endoscopic gastrocnemius recession

1. Gastrocnemius equinus/tightness: (ankle dorsiflexion <5° with the knee in extension)
2. Nonspastic and nonbony deformity and
   Asymmetric posttraumatic symptomatic contracture and/or
   Calcaneal osteotomy and/or Hindfoot realignment and/or
   Subtalar arthroereisis and/or
   Midfoot arthrodesis and/or
   Noninfected forefoot ulcers/derangement

recession when their ankle dorsiflexion is less than 5° with the knee extended and they exhibit signs or symptoms of chronic foot overload or inflammation. Common examples would be posterior tibial tendon insufficiency, diabetic forefoot ulceration or Charcot arthropathy, stress fractures, metatarsalgia, Morton's foot deformity, plantar fasciitis, and insertional Achilles tendonitis, although we think this contracture may potentially play a role in many other biomechanical and functional pathologies of the foot as well. Alternative potential indications for performing an open or endoscopic gastrocnemius recession include patients with symptomatic ankle contracture or those who necessitate midfoot (Lisfranc) reconstruction/arthrodesis, calcaneal osteotomy for hindfoot realignment, or subtalar arthroereisis (Table 2.1). Whether performed openly or endoscopically, however, the procedure is not meant to take the place of an Achilles lengthening when indicated based on the Silverskiold test. Gastrocnemius recession should also be used cautiously in athletes.

The EGR procedure is typically performed supine under general anesthesia. It can also be performed prone in the event the patient requires such positioning during their foot/ankle surgery. Spinal or local anesthesia may be considered an option for patients who are not good candidates for or do not desire general anesthesia, but we have less experience with this method under such circumstances. Incision placement has been clarified by a recent anatomic study by Tashjian et al. [22]. Ideal sites are determined by locating the inferior extension of the medial gastrocnemius

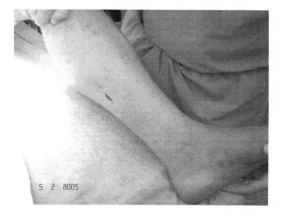

Fig. 2.1 Medial incision placement

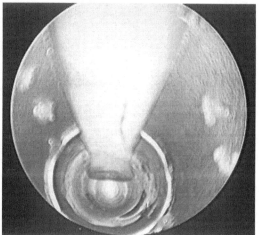

Fig. 2.2 Endoscopic view of gastrocnemius

muscle belly as well as identifying the midpole of the fibular shaft. These landmarks provide useful keys to optimal aponeurotic release. Knowledge of the neurovascular anatomy is mandatory, particularly the sural and saphenous structures. The great saphenous vein and the saphenous nerve should be anterior to a medially based incision, which is ideally placed in the midaxial line. This incision is made adjacent to edge of the medial gastrocnemius aponeurosis, typically 9–12 cm proximal to the medial malleolus, and is 1–1.5 cm long (Fig. 2.1). Once the superficial posterior compartment fascia is opened, a fascial elevator is used to create a pathway between subcutaneous fat and gastrocnemius fascia, in a medial to lateral direction. Care is taken to remain directly posterior to (on top of) the gastrocnemius aponeurosis, a characteristically glistening white structure. An endoscopic cannula with a blunt obturator is then placed through the medial incision and carefully advanced laterally. The obturator can then be removed for insertion of a 4.0-mm, 30° endoscope through the cannula. The gastrocnemius tendon (Fig. 2.2) is visualized anteriorly, and the endoscope subsequently advanced toward the lateral aspect of the leg where the subcutaneous tissue appears yellow. The endoscope and cannula are rotated posteriorly and then retrograded back medially approximately 1 cm to locate the sural nerve. Pinney et al. found that the sural nerve can lay directly behind this aponeurosis less than 25% of the time, but is more often outside of the field of view, and equally common interior and exterior

to the superficial posterior compartment fascia at this level. Regardless, care must be taken to ensure that the nerve does not exist between cannula and the site of aponeurotic release. Based on the findings of Tashjian et al., the sural nerve has been shown to course approximately 1.2 cm or 20% medial to the lateral gastrocnemius border at the myotendinous junction [19]. Their study did report one sural nerve transection with this EGR approach in the cadaveric setting, and the nerve was seen in only one third of the specimens evaluated endoscopically [19, 22]. Webb et al. also showed the sural nerve to cross the proximal portion of the Achilles tendon from the lateral side [26]. If possible, it is always advantageous to document that the nerve is located posterior to the cannula, and thereby protected by it (Fig. 2.3). Pinney et al. have also shown in their study on the Strayer technique that the nerve can often be adherent to the gastrocnemius aponeurosis [11]. Such situations may require modification or even abandonment of the endoscopic technique in lieu of a more formal, open procedure. Transillumination of the lateral aspect of the leg allows the surgeon to carefully make a cut-down incision over the cannula and insert a narrow-tipped suction device, which also helps avoid possible portal neuromas (Fig. 2.4). The use of suction improves visualization due to the moisture from the subcutaneous fat during transection of the gastrocnemius. Occasionally, serial swabbing with a cotton tip applicator is also helpful to clean the lens of the endoscope and its cannula.

Once anatomy has been properly and safely defined, the endoscope is temporarily removed and a cannulated knife is introduced as part of the camera, stabilized over the endoscope (Fig. 2.5). This assembly is designed to transect the tendon

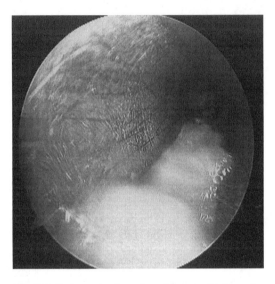

Fig. 2.3 Endoscopic view of sural nerve with the endoscope and cannula rotated posteriorly 180°

while pushing the blade located forward in its position immediately ahead of the camera, and can be done through only the medial portal. Alternatively, a separate independent "hook-blade" can be used, which is useful in cases when the sural nerve or numerous venous structures are located in the vicinity of the proposed transection. This latter technique requires two portals and a separate knife blade/handle, which is pulled from the far end toward itself during transaction, using the camera to follow the release. We have identified no specific advantage with either technique, and in either case the foot must remain forcibly dorsiflexed to tension the thick gastrocnemius aponeurosis and permit clean transection. Clamping the medial and lateral margins of the aponeurosis through each portal with a Kocher clamp may also facilitate this process, but requires slightly larger incisions. This adjunct technique can be useful because the gastrocnemius rests more curvilinear rather than straight when viewed in the coronal plane. Thus, the straight, rigid endoscope is sometimes ineffective at releasing the very medial and lateral edges of the tendon as they course more anteriorly away from the endoscope/cannula. As the gastrocnemius is transected with either blade construct, the soleus muscle

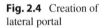
Fig. 2.4 Creation of lateral portal

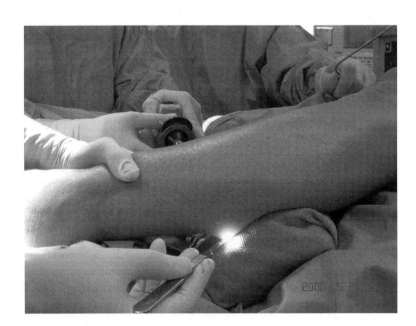

Fig. 2.5 Cannulated endoscopic blade applied to endoscope

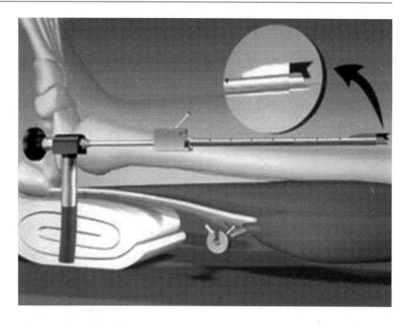

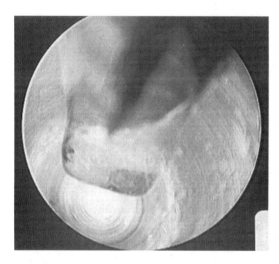

Fig. 2.6 Endoscopic view of gastrocnemius transection with soleus muscle above

belly should become visible anteriorly (Fig. 2.6). Ideally, the fascia of the soleus is not violated. If this occurs, the resultant bleeding can obscure visualization. Although typically only superficial, however, unfortunately this is sometimes unavoidable, and under such circumstances suction from the lateral portal can be helpful. While this inadvertent violation of the soleus fascia/muscle has not been of any identifiable clinical consequence in our experience, it still represents a potential risk and undesirable pitfall of this procedure. If the neurovascular structures limit advancement of the cannulated knife, one can transect the aponeurosis from either portal with various endoscopic blades. The hook blade can be used from the lateral portal to complete the transection.

After complete transaction of the tendon, ankle dorsiflexion improvement should be noted of at least 10–15°. Anything short of this suggests either the need for an Achilles lengthening or incomplete resection of the gastrocnemius. Recent research by Barouk et al. suggests that most if not almost all of the dorsiflexion correction is obtained by release of the medial as opposed to the lateral gastrocnemius aponeurosis [27]. This is in keeping with our own observations. Once instruments are removed, the medial incision is explored for the plantaris tendon, which is then also transected. In our experience, leaving this tendon behind intact can result in medial-sided discomfort as a result of its bowstringing while under dorsiflexion tension. Surgical sites are thereafter irrigated and 5 mL of 0.5% bupivacaine are introduced into the portals. Incisions are closed with one or two 3–0 nylon sutures, which remain for 2 weeks postoperatively. Oral muscle relaxants, along with dorsiflexion night splinting, can be useful in the postoperative setting to maintain release and minimize muscle cramping. If EGR is performed as an isolated procedure, patients are maintained in a below-knee walking boot for 4–6 weeks, during the latter half of which, it is only required at night and patients are allowed ambulation as tolerated during waking hours. When more extensive foot or ankle procedures are concomitantly performed, they generally dictate postoperative immobilization and weightbearing status. During the first few months of recovery, self-massage of the transection region and portals is recommended. Physical therapy after surgery is also encouraged, and can be helpful to improve gait and decrease fibrosis. The ability to single-leg "heel-raise" can occur as soon 6 weeks post-EGR [14].

The EGR procedure represents an evolving percutaneous technique that has the potential to minimize postoperative scar formation and maximize recovery after gastrocnemius recession. Caution must be exercised in recommending this technique, however, because its long-term outcome and relative complication rate as compared with the traditional open technique remain unknown. The most common adverse event noted postoperatively with this approach appears to be transient lateral foot dysesthesia. In our experience, this is most likely due to traction neuritis of the sural nerve, which we have also seen with the open procedure after obtaining an acute increase in ankle dorsiflexion [5, 15]. However, this is typically a benign and self-limiting problem. Based on cadaveric experimentation, sural nerve laceration and/or incomplete gastrocnemius release may prove to be significant risks of this procedure as compared with the open approach, primarily due to impaired visualization. Other potential complications of EGR yet to be fully defined include hematoma, adherence/tenting, push-off weakness, and calcaneus deformity (Fig. 2.7). The procedure is also highly equipment dependent, requiring significantly greater amounts of instrumentation as compared with the standard release. Unfortunately, this equipment is often not otherwise required for most foot/ankle

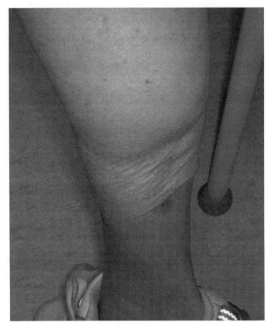

Fig. 2.7 "Tenting" or soleus adherence to subcutaneous tissue

procedures that might be required at the time of gastrocnemius recession, and thus this need represents an added burden to both surgeon and operating room personnel. With experience, the total time required for the EGR approaches that for the OGR.

Experience with the EGR technique remains in its infancy. Few studies have been published on any advantages, disadvantages, or comparative results of EGR. While the procedure may hold promise in terms of minimizing incisional issues and maximizing recovery times after isolated gastrocnemius recession, its use should be considered cautiously, and more thorough evaluation is mandatory before EGR can be safely advocated for general use (Table 2.2). With increased experience, however, we think the EGR may eventually become a safe and preferable means of gastrocnemius recession. To date, however, the open technique remains the gold standard and should still be considered the most efficient, reliable, and user-friendly means of gastrocnemius recession.

Table 2.2 Other authors' results of endoscopic gastrocnemius recession

Author	Comment	Net improvement in ankle dorsiflexion	Nerve transection	Lateral dysesthesia	Hematoma	Calcaneal gait	Poor cosmesis
Tashjian et al. [19, 22]	Cadaveric	NS	1	NA	NA	NA	NA
Saxena and Widtfeldt [14]	18 cases	12.6°	None	3	NS	NS	1
Trevino et al. [20]	31 cases	NS	None	NS	NS	NS	NS
DiDomenico et al. [5]	31 cases	18°	None	NS	1	3	NS
Poul et al. [12]	18 cases with cerebral palsy	20°	NS	NS	0	NS	NS
Saxena and Widtfeldt [15]	54 cases	14.8°	None	6/54 (11%)	1	1	6/54 (11%)

NS not studied, *NA* not applicable

References

1. Leversedge F, Casey P, Seiler J, Xerogeanes J. Endoscopically assisted fasciotomy: description of technique and in-vitro assessment of lower-leg compartment decompression. Am J Sports Med 30(2): 272–278, 2002
2. Mirza A, King E. Newer techniques of carpal tunnel release. Orthop Clin North Am 27:355–371, 1996
3. Saxena A. Uniportal endoscopic plantar fasciotomy: a prospective study on athletic patients. Foot Ankle Int 25(12):882–889, 2004
4. Armstrong D, Stacpoole-Shea S, Nguyen H, Harkless L. Lengthening of the achilles tendon in diabetic patients who are at high risk for ulceration of the foot. J Bone Joint Surg 81A(4):535–538, 1999
5. DiDomenico L, Adams H, Garehar, D. Endoscopic gastrocnemius recession for the treatment of gastrocnemius equinus. J Am Podiatr Med Assoc 95(4): 410–413, 2005
6. Hansen ST. Midfoot arthrodesis In: Wulker N, Stephens M, Cracchiolo A (eds.) Atlas of Foot and Ankle Surgery. St. Louis, MO, Mosby, p. 154, 1998
7. Hansen ST: Tendon transfers and muscle balancing techniques. Achilles tendon lengthening. In: Hansen S (ed.) Functional Reconstruction of the Foot and Ankle. Lippincott Williams & Wilkins, Baltimore, MD, pp. 415–421, 2000
8. Laborde J. Tendon lengthenings for forefoot ulcers. Wounds 17(5):122–130, 2005
9. Mueller M, Sinacore D, Hastings M, Johnson J. The effect of Achilles tendon lengthening on neuropathic plantar ulcers: a randomized clinical trial. J Bone Joint Surg 85-A(8):1436–45, 2003
10. Pinney S, Sangeorzan B, Hansen ST. Surgical anatomy of the gastrocnemius recession (Strayer procedure) Foot Ankle Int 25(4): 247–250, 2004
11. Pinney SJ, Hansen ST, Sangeorzan BJ. The effect on ankle dorsiflexion of gastrocnemius recession. Foot Ankle Int 23(1):26–29, 2002
12. Poul J, Tuma J, Bajerova J. Video-assisted tenotomy of the triceps muscle of the calf in cerebral palsy patients. Acta Chir Orthop Traumatol Cech 72(3): 170–172, 2005
13. Saxena A. Endoscopic gastrocnemius tenotomy. J Foot Ankle Surg 41(1):57–58, 2002
14. Saxena A, Widtfeldt A. Endoscopic gastrocnemius recession: a preliminary report on 18 cases. J Foot Ankle Surg 43(5):302–306, 2004
15. Saxena A, Gollwitzer H, DiDomenico L, Widtfeldt A, Die endoskopische Verlängerungsoperation des Musculus gastrocnemius zur Behandlung des Gastrocnemius equinus (German) Z Orthop Unfall 145:1–6, 2007
16. Saxena A, DiGiovanni C. Ankle equinus and the athlete. In: Maffulli N, Almekinders M (eds.) The Achilles Tendon. Springer, New York, 2006
17. Sgarlato TE. Medial gastrocnemius tenotomy to assist in body posture balancing. J Foot Ankle Surg 37(6):546–547, 1998
18. Takao M, Ochi M, Shu N, Uchio Y, Naito K, Tobita M, Matsusaki M, Kawasaki K. A case of superficial peroneal nerve injury during ankle arthroscopy. Arthroscopy 17(4):403–404, 2001
19. Tashjian RZ, Appel AJ, Banerjee R, DiGiovanni CW. Anatomic study of the gastrocnemius-soleus junction and its relationship to the sural nerve. Foot Ankle Int 24:473–476, 2003
20. Trevino S, Gibbs M, Panchbhavi V. Evaluation of results of endoscopic gastrocnemius recession. Foot Ankle Int 26(5):35–364, 2005
21. Trevino S, Panchbhavi V. Technique of endoscopic gastrocnemius recession: cadaveric study. Foot Ankle Surg 8:45–47, 2002
22. Tashjian R, Appel A, Banerjee R, DiGiovanni C. Endoscopic gastrocnemius recession: evaluation in a cadaver model. Foot Ankle Int 24:607–613, 2003
23. Silverskiold N. Reduction of the uncrossed two-joints muscles of the leg to one-joint muscles in spastic conditions. Acta Chir Scand 56:315–30, 1924
24. DiGiovanni C, Kuo R, Tejwani N, Price R, Hansen T, Cziernecki J, Sangeorzan B. Isolated gastrocnemius tightness. J Bone Joint Surg 84A(6):962–970, 2002
25. Saxena A, Kim W. Ankle dorsiflexion in adolescent athletes. J Am Podiatr Assoc 93(4):312–314, 2003
26. Webb J, Moonjani N, Radford M. Anatomy of the sural nerve and its relation to the Achilles tendon. Foot Ankle Int 21(6):475–477, 2000
27. Barouk L, Barouk P. Techniques, results and comparison between the medial and lateral proximal gastrocnemius release. Presented at the International Spring Meeting, French Foot Society. Toulouse, France June 8–10, 2006

Percutaneous Reduction and Internal Fixation of the Lisfranc Fracture-Dislocation

3

Anish R. Kadakia and Mark S. Myerson

The success of minimally invasive percutaneous reduction and fixation of tarsometatarsal or Lisfranc injuries lies in understanding the appropriate injury pattern for this method of treatment. The eponym *Lisfranc dislocation* is derived from injuries sustained to cavalry troops in the Napoleonic era. These were associated with significant vascular and soft tissue injury, as they were treated with an amputation through the tarsometatarsal joints by Lisfranc, Napoleon's surgeon. Although the injuries secondary to equestrian activity have declined, the injury pattern is commonly associated with high-energy motor vehicle accidents, falls, and crushing injuries to the foot [1–4]. These mechanisms typically involve significant bony and soft tissue injury that rarely can be managed by closed methods (Fig. 3.1). Percutaneous fixation is most amenable in those patients with low-energy mechanisms, particularly in the athletic and elderly populations involving primarily a ligamentous injury (Fig. 3.2).

Mechanism of Injury

The indirect mechanism associated with the low-energy injury typically results from an axial longitudinal force with rotation on a plantar flexed foot [5, 6]. The plantar flexed position of the foot placed the weaker dorsal ligamentous restraints on tension, resulting in their failure allowing further displacement and rupture of the plantar ligamentous restraints or metatarsal base fracture [1, 6, 7]. This type of injury may not produce the obvious clinical picture associated with direct high-energy injuries of severe swelling, deformity, inability to bear weight, and neurovascular compromise [8]. Typical presentation includes swelling throughout the midfoot that improves after 1 week and therefore delayed presentations may not appear to have a significant injury upon visual examination [5]. Persistent pain and tenderness across the midfoot that is aggravated with stress testing of the tarsometatarsal joints is indicative of this injury pattern [9].

Radiographic Evaluation

The radiographic series for a suspected Lisfranc injury should include anteroposterior (AP), lateral, and 30° internal oblique views of both feet. Additionally, external oblique views in both 10° and 20° have demonstrated efficacy in delineating the amount of displacement in the transverse

A.R. Kadakia
Department of Orthopedic Surgery, University of Michigan, Ann Arbor, MI, USA

M.S. Myerson (✉)
Mercy Medical Center, Foot and Ankle Institute, Baltimore, MD, USA
e-mail: mark4feet@aol.com

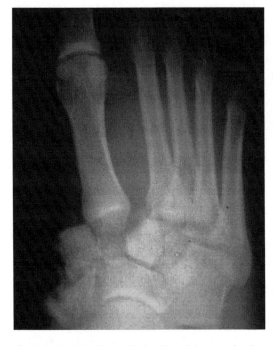

Fig. 3.1 An AP radiograph of a direct injury mechanism with significant displacement and bony comminution that is not amenable to percutaneous treatment

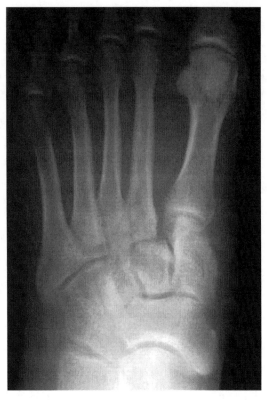

Fig. 3.2 An AP radiograph of a pure ligamentous injury that is ideally treated by percutaneous methods

plane [9]. In order to stress the midfoot and demonstrate the injury radiographically, the X-rays should be performed with as much weight-bearing as possible. Occasionally, weight bearing is too difficult for the patient, therefore, if the non-weight-bearing X-ray results are normal, repeat weight-bearing views should be performed at 10–14 days [6]. Stress radiographs can be performed to diagnosis the instability, however, they should be performed under anesthesia to prevent a false negative finding. The foot is stressed with pronation combined with abduction to detect subtle diastasis or angulation [5, 6, 10]. Coss et al. [11] have shown in a cadaveric model that disruption of the dorsal and Lisfranc ligamentous restraints resulted in a radiographic instability pattern consistently noted on abduction stress examination, verifying the utility of the clinical examination.

The anatomic relationships of the tarsometatarsal joints have consistent radiographic appearances, deviations from these patterns are consistent with injury [12]. The medial border of

the second metatarsal is in colinearity with the medial border of the middle cuneiform on the AP radiographic exam along with the first intermetatarsal space and the space between the medial and middle cuneiforms (Fig. 3.3a, b). The lateral border of the third metatarsal is colinear with the lateral border of the lateral cuneiform on the internal oblique radiograph. In addition, the medial border of the fourth metatarsal is colinear with the medial border of the cuboid. Subtle radiographic findings include minor angulation or displacement of the first metatarsal (Fig. 3.4). Myerson et al. [3] described the "fleck sign," a small avulsion fracture of either the medial cuneiform or the base of the second metatarsal, which is diagnostic of a Lisfranc disruption. Careful review of the radiographs should be performed so that Lisfranc variants with intercuneiform instability are not overlooked (Fig. 3.5).

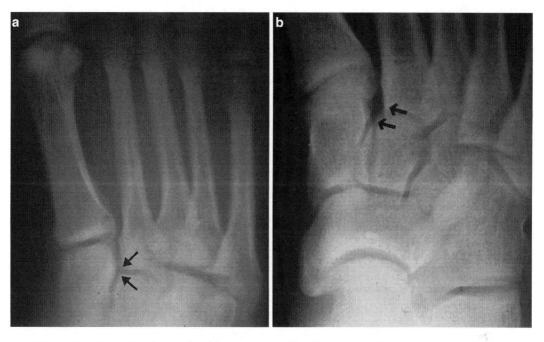

Fig. 3.3 (**a**) Note that the base of the second metatarsal is in continuity with the medial aspect of the middle cuneiform. (**b**) In a patient with a Lisfranc injury, note the lateral displacement of the second metatarsal in relation to the medial aspect of the middle cuneiform

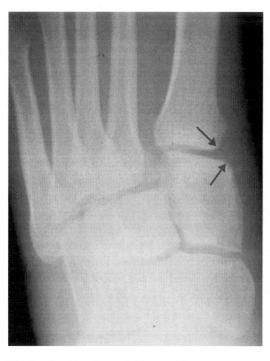

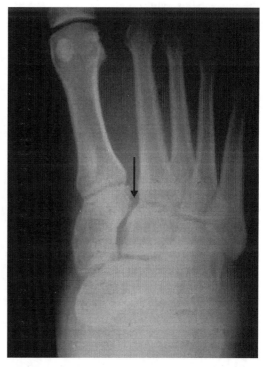

Fig. 3.4 An AP radiograph demonstrating lateral translation of the first metatarsal consistent with a Lisfranc injury

Fig. 3.5 Note that the diastasis exists between the medial and middle cuneiforms, consistent with a Lisfranc injury, despite the normal relationship between the second metatarsal and the middle cuneiform

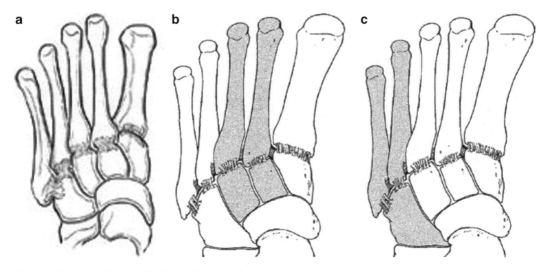

Fig. 3.6 The medial (**a**), middle (**b**), and lateral columns (**c**) are depicted

Classification

Multiple classification systems exist to describe the injury to this joint complex [2, 3, 13]. The use of the columnar classification developed by Myerson [6, 10, 14] divides the midfoot based on the respective motion segments. The medial column includes the first tarsometatarsal and the medial cuneiform-navicular joints (Fig. 3.6a). The middle column includes the second and third tarsometatarsal, intercuneiform, and the naviculocuneiform joints (between the middle and lateral cuneiforms) (Fig. 3.6b). The lateral column includes the articulations between the fourth and fifth metatarsals and the cuboid (Fig. 3.6c). This system of classification has prognostic implications based on the motion of the midfoot. The medial and middle columns have minimal motion (3.5 mm and 0.6 mm, respectively) and do not tolerate incongruity, suffering the highest incidence of posttraumatic arthritis [14, 15].

Nunley and Vertullo have proposed a classification system to define the midfoot sprain typically seen in athletes [16]. Stage 1 is consistent with pain at the Lisfranc joint without any evidence of diastasis on weight-bearing radiographs. Stage 2 involved 1–5 mm of diastasis between the first and second metatarsal on the AP radiograph, with evidence of lateral arch collapse. Stage 3 is greater than 5 mm of diastasis and loss of midfoot arch height. Patients with Stage 1 injuries were successfully treated with a nonoperative treatment protocol that included an initial 6 weeks of a non-weight-bearing fiberglass cast.

Treatment

Although recent literature may suggest that primary arthrodesis offers improved scores at a mean of 42.5 months of follow-up in ligamentous injuries over reduction and internal fixation, the longer-term complications of early arthrodesis may diminish these early results [17]. Therefore, treatment should consist of reduction and internal fixation of Lisfranc injuries and Stage 2 and 3 midfoot sprains via either percutaneous or open approaches. Non-operative treatment of these injuries is inappropriate as greater than 2 mm of displacement or 15° of angulation is associated with a poor outcome [3].

Surgical Technique

The use of a percutaneous technique requires a thorough understanding of the anatomy of the tarsometatarsal joints and their appearance under fluoroscopy. The undertaking of a percutaneous approach should not be performed unless the surgeon is capable of performing an open reduction,

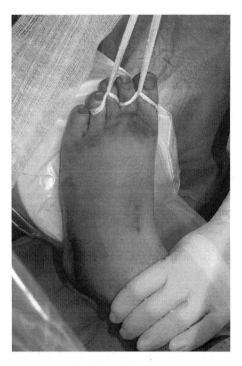

Fig. 3.7 Use of the gauze roll to create phalangeal slings to provide longitudinal traction and aid in closed reduction of the deformity

as, on occasion, soft tissue or bony fragment interposition may prevent an anatomic reduction using closed methods.

Initial attention must be performed to obtaining an anatomic reduction prior to any attempts at fixation. Longitudinal traction is required to reduce the tarsometatarsal joints and utilization of gauze rolls secured around the phalanges is a powerful aid in reduction (Fig. 3.7). Initial attention is paid to the medial column, which provides a stable post to which the middle column is reduced. The reduction maneuver involves grasping the hallux firmly and placing a medial- or lateral-directed force to the base of the metatarsal to reduce the deformity. Once an anatomic reduction is achieved, provisional fixation is achieved with a guidewire for a cannulated screw (Fig. 3.8a, b). A large bone clamp facilitates reduction of the second metatarsal into the mortise (Fig. 3.9a, b). If persistent diastasis remains despite adjustment of the clamp, then conversion to an open reduction should be performed. Typically, this realigns the third and fourth metatarsals into an anatomic position. A partially threaded screw is then placed obliquely from the medial cuneiform to the base of the second metatarsal. Stability of the lateral column is assessed fluoroscopically and, if persistent instability exists, stabilization is performed with either a 1.6-mm K-wire or screw

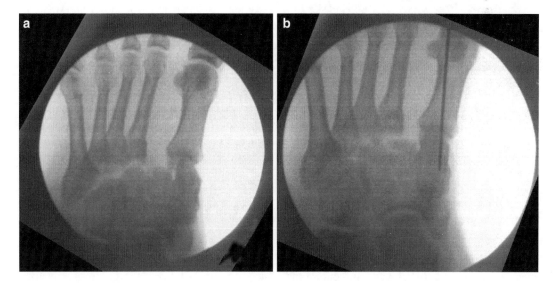

Fig. 3.8 Lisfranc injury with displacement (**a**) and after closed reduction with provisional fixation of the medial column (**b**)

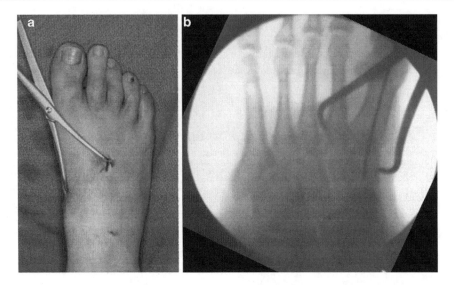

Fig. 3.9 Clinical (**a**) and fluoroscopic (**b**) depicting the use the bone clamp to reduce the base of the second metatarsal into the mortise

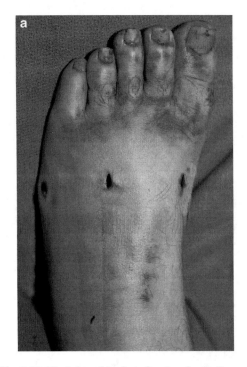

Fig. 3.10 Final view of the foot after closed reduction and fixation

fixation (Fig. 3.10a, b). If K-wire fixation is utilized for the lateral column, subcutaneous placement is important to prevent infection and premature removal.

Postoperative Rehabilitation

Initial immobilization is a below knee posterior plaster splint to decrease swelling and enhance wound healing. Early mobilization and range of motion is encouraged and rigid fixation with screws is important to prevent loss of reduction. Removal of the splint at 2 weeks is followed by placement into a removable boot, although non-weight bearing is continued for 8 weeks. Patients are allowed to begin range of motion and strengthening in a pool at 4 weeks and stationary biking is allowed at 6 weeks. Full weight bearing is allowed at 12 weeks, with conversion to an athletic shoe with an orthotic. Hardware removal is typically performed at 4 months, after which aggressive rehabilitation is performed under the direction of a therapist. Single plane running is initiated at 20 weeks and cutting sports are allowed at 24 weeks.

Summary

Disruptions of the tarsometatarsal joints can lead to significant disability if misdiagnosed and undertreated. Detailed review of weight-bearing radiographs of the affected extremity and a thorough understanding of the normal anatomic landmarks will consistently lead the clinician to diagnosis of even subtle injuries to the midfoot. Percutaneous treatment of these injuries is ideal as it avoids the risk of wound complications and morbidity associated with extensile incisions. However, if any question of malreduction exists, conversion to an open reduction must be performed.

References

 1. Myerson M. Tarsometatarsal arthrodesis: technique and results of treatment after injury. Foot Ankle Clin 1996;1:73–83.
 2. Hardcastle P, Reschauer R, Kutscha-Lissberg E, Schoffmann W. Injuries to the tarsometatarsal joint. Incidence, classification and treatment. J Bone Joint Surg Br 1982;64B(3):349–56.
 3. Myerson M, Fisher R, Burgess A, Kenzora J. Fracture dislocations of the tarsometatarsal joints: end results correlated with pathology and treatment. Foot Ankle 1986;6(5):225–42.
 4. Gossens M, De Stoop N. Lisfranc fracture dislocations: etiology, radiology, and results of treatment. A review of 20 cases. Clin Orthop Relat Res 1983;176:154–62.
 5. Curtis M, Myerson M, Szura B. Tarsometatarsal joint injuries in the athlete. Am J Sports Med 1993;21:497–502.
 6. Chiodo C, Myerson M. Developments and advances in the diagnosis and treatment of injuries to the tarsometatarsal joint. Orthop Clin North Am 2001;32(1):11–20.
 7. Buzzard B, Briggs P. Surgical management of acute tarsometatarsal fracture dislocation in the adult. Clin Orthop Relat Res 1998;353:125–33.
 8. Aronow M. Treatment of the missed Lisfranc injury. Foot Ankle Clin N Am 2006;11:127–42.
 9. Myerson M. The diagnosis and treatment of injuries to the Lisfranc joint complex. Orthop Clin North Am 1989;20:655–64.
10. Myerson M. The diagnosis and treatment of injury to the tarsometatarsal joint complex. J Bone Joint Surg (Br) 1999;81B:756–63.
11. Coss H, Manos R, Buoncristiani A, Mills W. Abduction stress AP weightbearing radiography of purely ligamentous injury in the tarsometatarsal joint. Foot Ankle Int 1998;19(8):537–41.
12. Stein R. Radiological aspects of the tarsometatarsal joints. Foot Ankle 1983;3:286–9.
13. Quenu E, Kuss G. Etude sur les luxations du metatarse. Reb Chir Paris 1909;39(281).
14. Komenda G, Myerson M, Biddinger K. Results of arthrodesis of the tarsometatarsal joints after traumatic injury. J Bone Joint Surg Am 1996;78:1665–76.
15. Ouzounian T, Shereff M. In vitro determination of midfoot motion. Foot Ankle 1989;10:140–6.
16. Nunley J, Vertullo C. Classification, investigation, and management of midfoot sprains. Lisfranc injuries in the athlete. Am J Sports Med 2002;30(6):871–8.
17. Ly T, Coetzee J. Treatment of the primarily ligamentous Lisfranc joint injuries: primary arthrodesis compared with open reduction and internal fixation. J Bone Joint Surg Am 2006;88A(3):514–20.

Arthroscopic Repair of Chronic Ankle Instability

4

Peter B. Maurus and Gregory C. Berlet

Lateral ankle ligament sprains are some of the most common injuries encountered in the orthopedic office, occurring in an estimated 1/10,000 persons per day [1]. These injuries can be seen in as many as 40% of all sports injuries [2]. While the majority of acute ankle sprains heal reliably with activity modification and physical therapy/ankle rehabilitation, approximately 29–42% of patients experience chronic functional ankle instability [3]. Functional lateral instability, as introduced by Freeman et al., describes a subjective complaint of giving way in the ankle joint [4]. Tropp's work further described this condition as motion beyond voluntary control, but not exceeding the physiologic range of motion [5]. Mechanical instability is motion beyond the normal physiologic limits of the ankle joint. This is manifested as excessive anterolateral ankle laxity.

The anterior talofibular ligament (ATFL) is the most commonly injured ligament during ankle sprains. Although described as mainly limiting anterior translation in relative plantarflexion, it serves as the primary restraint to inversion and translation at all angles of ankle flexion [6, 7]. During an inversion ankle sprain, the anterolateral capsule is typically injured first, followed by the ATFL, the calcaneofibular ligament (CFL),

and the posterior talofibular ligament (PTFL). Persistent failure (repeated giving way) of this lateral ligament complex is an indication for surgical stabilization of the ankle.

There are multiple surgical options for stabilization of the chronically unstable ankle, both anatomic and nonanatomic. Nonanatomic lateral ligament stabilizations are characterized by reconstruction with tendon grafts to recreate the lateral ligament complex. These techniques risk overconstraining the ankle joint and are not isometric in their kinematic effect on the ankle joint. Thus, they should be reserved for revisions or unique clinical situations.

Anatomic procedures maintain the natural ligament insertion points, but alter the tension on the native ligamentous structures. Isometry is not disturbed and overconstraint is rarely seen. Anatomic reconstructions include the modified Brostrom lateral ligament reconstruction and thermal capsular modification. Open techniques are not discussed in this chapter.

Whether an open or arthroscopic approach to treating instability is chosen, arthroscopy can and should be an important adjunct to the surgical treatment of ankle instability. Arthroscopy allows for a minimally invasive evaluation of the ankle joint and the ability to treat intraarticular pathology at the time of lateral ligament reconstruction. In the 1993 study by Taga et al. of 31 ankles, chondral lesions were found in 89% of the freshly injured ankles and 95% of the ankles with chronic injuries [8]. Hintermann et al. noted cartilage damage in 66% of ankles scoped prior to ligament reconstructions [9]. Komenda and Ferkel

P.B. Maurus
Steindler Orthopedic Clinic, Iowa City, IA, USA

G.C. Berlet (✉)
Ohio State University, Orthopaedic Foot and Ankle Center, Columbus, OH, USA
e-mail: gberlet@aol.com

G.R. Scuderi and A.J. Tria (eds.), *Minimally Invasive Surgery in Orthopedics: Foot and Ankle Handbook*,
DOI 10.1007/978-1-4614-0893-2_4, © Springer Science+Business Media, LLC 2012

found that 93% of 51 ankles had intraarticular abnormalities including loose bodies, synovitis, osteochondral lesions of the talus, ossicles, osteophytes, adhesions, and chondromalacia [10]. Takao et al. studied 72 patients with residual ankle disability lasting more than 2 months after injury and illustrated intraarticular pathology at the time of arthroscopy in 14 patients that was not identified on any clinical or radiologic testing [11].

Thermal-Assisted Capsular Modification

Thermal-assisted capsular modification for chronic lateral ankle instability was introduced recently [12, 13]. This technique has been successful in treating shoulder instability and early results in the ankle are encouraging. The concept is based on the fact that thermal energy between 65°C and 70°C shrinks collagen, which comprises more than 90% of joint capsules, ligaments, and tendons (TACS). Thermal energy may be applied using electrical energy (monopolar or bipolar) or laser energy.

Factors such as tissue properties themselves or variables related to the energy source (including the density, application time, and concentration area) determine the amount of energy delivered to the tissue [14]. *Pulsing* the energy can minimize tissue damage and control depth of penetration. In the authors' experience, electrical energy is more reliable and we have had success with the Mitek (Vapr TC; Mitek Products, Division of Ethicon, Somerville, NJ) or Arthrocare (CAPSure, ArthroCare Corporation, Austin, TX) devices.

Our decision to use thermal capsular modification for lateral ligament reconstruction is influenced by the patient's body habitus, activity pattern, and degree of ligament injury. Indications include patients with moderate build, intraligament stretching (not avulsed from bone), generalized ligamentous laxity with functional ankle instability, a commitment to adhere to the postoperative rehabilitation protocol, and no previous ankle ligament reconstructive surgery. Contraindications include muscle weakness, tendon tears and instability, subtalar instability, and tibiofibular joint instability.

Preoperatively, each patient undergoes a focused physical examination assessing ankle instability, muscle weakness, tendon tears and tendon instability, proprioceptive disorders, subtalar instability, and tibiofibular joint instability. Radiographs of the affected ankle are obtained and magnetic resonance imaging (MRI) should be performed if peroneal tears and chondral injuries of the talus are suspected.

Technique

After sterile preparation and draping of the ankle, a noninvasive ankle distractor strap is applied (Acufex, Smith & Nephew, Memphis, TN). Anteromedial and anterolateral portals are established. The surgeon should then perform a complete arthroscopic examination and treat any pathology encountered (e.g., synovitis, osteochondral defects) accordingly. Impingement lesions in the anterolateral gutter are encountered frequently and should be debrided aggressively with an arthroscopic trimmer to allow adequate exposure of the anterolateral gutter. The capsule should be preserved for use in the thermal procedure to follow.

Once visualization of the anterolateral capsule and distal fibula is confirmed, introduce a thermal control wand through the lateral portal and release the distraction device once the thermal wand is in position. The ATFL can be identified consistently [15]. With the maximum temperature set at 65°C (with the thermal feed backward or on level two with the Arthrocare system), the tissue of the anterolateral capsule (just distal and anterior to the distal fibula) and ATFL can be treated with the thermal wand by using a painting technique starting deep in the lateral gutter and working anteriorly, avoiding repetitive treatment of a specific location. Thermal treatment is below the equator of the lateral arthroscopy portal to avoid creating an iatrogenic impingement lesion. The treated capsule will show a blushing after treatment. Surgeons familiar with shoulder thermal modification will note that there is a visual contraction of the shoulder capsule that occurs while working in the inferior glenohumeral pouch. There is much less visual confirmation of contraction in the ankle. After adequate exposure to the thermal effects of the wand, the arthroscopic instrumentation can be removed. The ankle should be held in slight dorsiflexion and eversion as the portals are closed with suture and a well-padded posterior/gutter splint (with cooling pack) is applied to the operative extremity.

Results

Between February 1999 and December 2001, the authors performed 42 arthroscopic thermal-assisted capsular modifications of the anterolateral capsule and the ATFL [16]. The AOFAS hindfoot scores improved significantly: scores averaged 29.57 preoperatively (standard deviation [SD] 15.6) and improved to 55.36 (SD 13.56) at an average follow-up of 14.1 months ($p<0.001$).

One patient had skin breakdown over the calf where the ankle distracter strap had been, which resolved with conservative wound care. There were no infections.

Postoperatively, patients undergo physical examinations at 3-week intervals. Patients wear a non-weightbearing cast for the first 3 weeks, followed by a weightbearing cast for 3 weeks, and then a weightbearing boot walker for 3 weeks. Physical therapy ankle rehabilitation begins 9 weeks postoperatively.

Favorable outcomes using thermal stabilization have been reported, however, no prospective studies have been published reporting the use of thermal modification for ankle instability [12, 17–19].

The authors think that select patients with chronic lateral instability who have failed a course of conservative treatment are good candidates for arthroscopic thermal capsular and ATFL shrinkage. Longer follow-up will be necessary to determine whether the ankle will remain stable over time. Longer-term follow-up will determine how the outcomes compare with traditional surgical methods (i.e., modified Brostrom repair).

Thermal-assisted capsular modification has potential limitations. While the ATFL is easily visualized during arthroscopy, the CFL is not accessible. Therefore, the CFL cannot be addressed arthroscopically. Moreover, the extensor retinaculum, which is used in the open modified Brostrom procedure is not an intraarticular structure and cannot be incorporated into the repair. Both the CFL and the extensor retinaculum can be important restraints to medial talar tilt on varus stress. Perhaps a *hybrid* procedure that involves arthroscopic evaluation and treatment of the ATFL in conjunction with a mini-open approach to either the CFL or extensor retinaculum would be able to address the entire lateral ligament complex.

On the Horizon

As arthroscopists become more comfortable with arthroscopic knot tying techniques and new orthopedic implants are developed, we may see more novel ideas emerge. Early work is proceeding on a suture-based capsular ATFL imbrication technique. No published results are yet available.

References

1. Trevino SG, Davis P, Hecht PJ. Management of acute and chronic lateral ligament of the ankle. Orthop Clin North Am 1994;25:1–16
2. Holmer P, Sondergaard L, Konradsen L, Nielsen PT, Jorgensen LN. Epidemiology of sprains in the lateral ankle and foot. Foot Ankle Int 1994;15:72–74
3. Berlet GC, Anderson RB Davis WH. Chronic lateral ankle instability. Foot Ankle Clin 1999;4:(4):713–728
4. Freeman MAR. Instability of the foot after injuries to the lateral ligament of the ankle. J Bone Joint Surg 1965;47B:669–676
5. Tropp H, Ekstrand J, Gillquist J. Stabilometry in functional instability of the ankle and its value in predicting injury. Med Sci Sports Exerc. 1984;16:64–66
6. Colville MR, Marder RA, Boyle JJ, Zaring B. Strain measurement in lateral ankle ligaments. Am J Sports Med 1990;18:196–200
7. Johnson EE, Markolf KL. The contribution of the anterior talofibular ligament to ankle laxity. J Bone Joint Surg 1983;65:81–88
8. Taga I, Shino K, Inoue M, Nakata K, Maeda A. Articular cartilage lesions in ankles with lateral ligament injury. An arthroscopic study. Am J Sports Med 1993;21(1):120–126
9. Hintermann B, Boss A, Schafer D. Arthroscopic findings in patients with chronic ankle instability. Am J Sports Med 2002;30(3):402–409

10. Komenda GA, Ferkel RD. Arthroscopic findings associated with the unstable ankle. Foot Ankle Int 1999;20(11):708–713

11. Takao M, Uchio Y, Naito K, Fukazawa I, Ochi M. Arthroscopic assessment for intra-articular disorders in residual ankle disability after sprain. Am J Sports Med 2005;33(5):686–692 (Epub 2005 Feb 16)

12. Ryan AH, Lee TH, Berlet GC. Arthroscopic thermal assisted capsular shrinkage in anterolateral ankle instability: a retrospective review of 13 patients. AOFAS Annual Summer Meeting, Vail, CO, July 2000

13. Myers JB, Lephart SM, Bradley JP, et al. Proprioception following thermal capsulorrhaphy. AAOS Annual Meeting, San Francisco, CA, 2001

14. Arnoczky SP, Aksan A. Thermal modification of connective tissues: basic science considerations and clinical implications. J Am Acad Orthop Surg 2000; 8:305–13

15. Leyes M, Hersch J, Sferra J. Arthroscopic identification of the anterior talofibular ligament. AOSSM, Orlando, FL, July 2002

16. Berlet GC, Saar WE, Ryan A, et al. Thermal-assisted capsular modification for functional ankle instability. Foot Ankle Clin 2002;7:567–76

17. Orecchio A. "Running Start," Study reports heat shrinkage technique for ankle instability. Biomechanics April 2000, 14–15

18. Berlet GC, Raissi A, Lee TH. Thermal capsular modification for chronic lateral ankle instability, AOFAS Annual Summer Meeting, Traverse City, MI, July 2002

19. Fanton GS. Thermal ankle stabilization – clinical Update 2002. AOSSM Annual Meeting, Orlando, FL, July 2002

Arthroscopic Subtalar Arthrodesis: Indications and Technique

Dominic S. Carreira and Pierce Scranton

The subtalar joint is an important joint, playing a major role in eversion and inversion of the foot as it transmits and dissipates forces applied to the calcaneus proximally. Arthrosis of the subtalar joint may be a significant source of pain and dysfunction. It may have a rheumatoid, inflammatory, posttraumatic, or degenerative etiology. In patients with painful subtalar arthrosis with or without progressive deformity, arthrodesis is an accepted form of salvage [1]. If the arthritic subtalar joint is well aligned, a simple subtalar arthrodesis without the use of bone graft has been shown to be effective. Mann and Baumgarten reported a high rate of success by denuding the posterior facet articular surface, *feathering* the bony surface, and using internal fixation [2]. This and other open techniques for subtalar arthrodesis may be significantly painful and may require hospitalization for pain control.

In an effort to decrease potential morbidity and reduce costs, alternative techniques have been introduced. Arthroscopic procedures have demonstrated decreased morbidity in a variety of joints. The theoretic advantages include smaller incisions, less blood loss, less pain, and a shorter rehabilitation time.

The indications for arthroscopy of the subtalar joint are similar to those for open procedures, including removal of loose bodies, evaluation of chondral and osteochondral fractures, excision of intraarticular adhesions, and arthrodesis. If one chooses to perform an arthroscopic-assisted arthrodesis, relative contraindications include significant deformity, bone loss, severe edema, and poor vascularity. An absolute contraindication is infection.

A retrospective comparison study has been reported between arthroscopic and open procedures. This nonrandomized study of in situ, isolated subtalar arthrodesis compared open treatment with autogenous bone graft versus arthroscopic treatment using injectable morphogenic protein-enhanced grafts [3]. Eight patients were treated by open arthrodesis and five patients were treated arthroscopically. During follow-up, in each group, one AO screw required removal. There was one diabetic patient who was treated open and who was the sole patient requiring an additional procedure (revision bone grafting) to achieve fusion. Tourniquet time averaged 5 min longer in the arthroscopic group (63 vs. 58 min). Average savings in the arthroscopy group was related to the length of stay (approximately $600/day at the time of that report).

In a study of arthroscopic fusions, Tasto et al. reported on 24 patients with an average follow-up of 31 months [4]. All 24 patients had a successful fusion with an average time to union of 8.9 weeks. Tasto et al. cited additional advantages

D.S. Carreira
Broward Health Orthopedics,
Fort Lauderdale, FL, USA

P. Scranton (✉)
Department of Orthopedics, University of Washington,
Seattle, WA, USA
e-mail: piercescranton@hotmail.com

of preservation of the blood supply to the hindfoot joints and a low complication rate.

In a report of open isolated subtalar arthrodesis, Easley and Myerson reported on 148 patients [5]. The union rate was 84%. Complications reported included prominent hardware (20%), sural nerve injury (9%), infection (3%), lateral impingement (10%), and malalignment of the hindfoot (6%). Of the 30 nonunions, all had 2 mm or more of avascular bone noted at the time of the procedure.

The routine use of supplementary bone graft is not always necessary for isolated subtalar fusions as reported by Mann and Baumgarten [2] and Mangone et al. [6]. Its use is dependent on the amount of deformity and bone stock, and may be indicated in cases of poliomyelitis, spastic cerebral palsy, or posttraumatic calcaneal fracture care [6–8]. Further, Thordarson and Kuehn were not able to demonstrate a superior union rate with the use of Grafton putty or Orthoblast compared with historical controls or between one another [9].

The use of pulsed electromagnetic fields at the time of hindfoot arthrodesis was studied in 64 consecutive patients [10]. All patients who underwent open elective triple/subtalar arthrodesis were randomized into control and pulsed electromagnetic field study (PES) groups. Subjects in the PES group were treated and an electromagnetic field was applied for 12 h per day with its application over the cast. All joint fusions, as evaluated by radiographic union, occurred over less time in the study group. For subtalar arthrodesis, the average time was 14.5 weeks in 33 primary subtalar arthrodeses with 4 nonunions. In the study group, the average time was 12.9 weeks to fusion, with no nonunions. Of note, the average cost was $3,000 and most insurance companies did not cover the cost in a primary arthrodeses.

Anatomy

The subtalar joint is divided by the sinus tarsi and tarsal canal into an anterior and posterior part. The tarsal canal is formed by a sulcus on the undersurface of the talus and the superior surface of the calcaneus, and laterally this opening is termed the sinus tarsi. The borders of the tarsal canal include the anterior portion of the posterior subtalar joint capsule, which forms the posterior border of the canal. The anterior boundary is the posterior portion of the talocalcaneal navicular joint capsule. The contents of the tarsal canal include the cervical ligament, the interosseous talocalcaneal ligament, the medial part of the inferior extensor retinaculum, vessels, and fatty tissue.

The anterior part of the subtalar joint is formed by the anterior and medial joint facet, the talonavicular joint, and the spring ligament. There is usually no communication between the anterior and posterior parts of the subtalar joint because of the thick interosseous ligament, which fills the tarsal canal.

The posterior portion of the subtalar joint is very close to the posterior ankle joint. As the talus tapers posteriorly, the posterior talofibular ligament is just proximal to the posterior subtalar joint line. The axis of the posterior joint facet is directed 40° laterally in relation to the longitudinal axis of the foot. The calcaneal surface is shaped in a convex fashion, whereas the talar joint surface is concave. The lateral joint capsule is reinforced by the calcaneofibular and the talocalcaneal ligaments. The capsule contains a posterior pouch and a small lateral recess.

The ligamentous support of the subtalar joint has been divided into three layers [11]. The superficial layer consists of the lateral root of the inferior extensor retinaculum, the lateral talocalcaneal ligament, the calcaneofibular ligament, the posterior talocalcaneal ligament, and the medial talocalcaneal ligament. The intermediate layer consists of the intermediate root of the inferior extensor retinaculum and the cervical ligament. The deep layer consists of the medial root of the inferior extensor retinaculum and the interosseous talocalcaneal ligament.

Portal Anatomy

Parisien described an anterior and posterior portal. Frey and coworkers described the middle portal. Mekhail described the medial portal, and

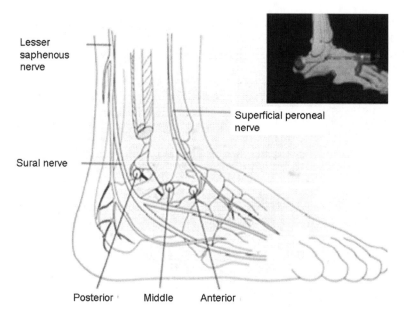

Fig. 5.1 Subtalar arthroscopy portal placement and relationship to verves (From Frey CC, DiGiovanni C. Gross and arthroscopic anatomy of the foot. In: Guhl JF, Parisien MD, Boyton JS (eds.) Foot and Ankle Arthroscopy, 2004, with kind permission of Springer Science + Business Media.)

Ferkel described the accessory anterolateral and posterolateral portals. One must maintain enough separation between portals to prevent instrument crowding.

The posterior portal (named the posterolateral portal by Ferkel) is approached from the lateral side. It has the greatest risk of causing sural nerve injury. The lesser saphenous vein, peroneal tendons, and Achilles tendon can also be injured with posterior portal placement. The sural nerve is typically located 2 cm posterior and 2 cm inferior to the lateral malleolus. After making a superficial small skin incision, a hemostat should be used to spread through the subcutaneous tissue down to the level of the capsule. The trocar is angled upward and in a slightly anterior direction (Fig. 5.1).

In a study by Frey [12] describing portal anatomy and safety, the portal is located, on average, 25 mm (range, 20–28 mm) posterior and 6 mm (range, 0–10 mm) proximal to the tip of the fibula, behind the saphenous vein and nerve and anterior to the Achilles tendon. In seven of ten dissection cases, the posterior portal was located posterior to the sural nerve, and in two cases it was anterior. One sural nerve was transected, and in another case, a small transection of the lesser saphenous vein was made. The peroneal tendon sheath was located on average 11 mm anterior to the portal and the Achilles tendon an average of 15 mm posterior to the portal.

For the anterior portal (named the anterolateral portal by Ferkel), the point of entry is 2 cm anterior and 1 cm distal to the tip of the lateral malleolus. The trocar is angled slightly upward and approximately 40° posterior [13]. In the study by Frey et al. [14] this portal was located an average of 28 mm (range, 23–35 mm) anterior to the tip of the fibula. Structures at risk with placement of this portal include the dorsal intermediate cutaneous branch of the superficial peroneal nerve, the dorsolateral cutaneous branch of the sural nerve, the peroneus tertius tendon, and a small branch of the lesser saphenous vein. The dorsal intermediate cutaneous branch of the superficial peroneal nerve is located an average of 17 mm (range, 0–28 mm) anterior to the portal (Fig. 5.1).

The accessory anterolateral portal is usually slightly anterior and superior to the anterior portal.

This portal is best made under direct visualization from either the posterior or anterior portal. The accessory posterolateral portal is made lateral to the posterior portal, using caution to avoid the abovementioned structures and under direct visualization.

The middle portal is approximately 1 cm anterior to the tip of the fibula, directly over the sinus tarsi [14]. It places no structures at risk and is therefore relatively safe.

Mekhail et al. [15] described the establishment of a medial portal. A blunt-ended trocar is placed into the sinus tarsi and is pushed through the tarsal canal in a posteromedial and slightly cephalad direction. While the ankle is in equinus and the foot is inverted in order to relax the posteromedial neurovascular bundle and slightly displace it posteriorly, the trocar is advanced to exit the skin medially and is angled approximately 45° to the lateral border of the foot. The portal entry lies along a line between the medial malleolus and the medial calcaneal tubercle, at the point where the anterosuperior ¾ meets the posteroinferior ¼. Improved visualization was described of the posteromedial and anterolateral aspects of the posterior subtalar joint. The authors also warned that in feet with significant adipose tissue or edema, the portal would be situated more posteriorly and therefore in closer approximation to the neurovascular bundle. The indications for use of this portal are rare.

The best combination for portal access to the cartilage of the posterior facet involves placement of the arthroscope through the anterior portal and instrumentation through the posterior portal [16]. This allows for direct visualization and instrumentation of nearly the entire posterior facet, the posterior aspect of the interosseous ligament, the lateral capsule and its small recess, and the posterior pouch.

Instrumentation through the anterior portal allows for improved visualization of the lateral aspect of the posterior facet. Access to the anterior and lateral compartments of the posterior facet, as well as structures of the extraarticular sinus tarsi, is best obtained by placing the arthroscope in the anterior portal and the instrumentation through the middle portal.

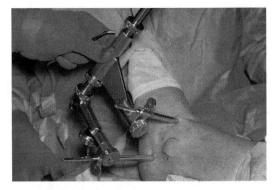

Fig. 5.2 Setup of AO distractor for subtalar arthrodesis

Arthroscopic Technique

For patient positioning, the preferred technique is to place the patient supine with a bolster under the ipsilateral buttock. Other options for positioning include the lateral decubitus or 90° flexion at the knee. The procedure can be performed with the patient under general or regional anesthesia. A sciatic nerve block can provide additional prolonged postoperative anesthesia. Relaxation is critical and therefore local anesthesia is not recommended. A tourniquet is applied and used as necessary. Distraction is applied with invasive or noninvasive instrumentation. Tasto has reported the use of a lamina spreader in sinus tarsi to allow for easier introduction of instrumentation [17]. We prefer the use of AO distraction pins, which are inserted manually and confirmed fluoroscopically. The calcaneal pin is inserted from the lateral side, just posterior to the vascular triangle. The threaded tip engages the opposite medial cortex without penetrating it. The talar pin is inserted across the neck of the talus just anterior to the anterior talofibular ligament insertion. The AO distractor then is attached and gradual distraction applied (Fig. 5.2).

The superficial anatomy is outlined: the fibula, sinus tarsi, and anterior, middle, and posterior portals. An 18-gauge needle may be used to distend the joint and check for backflow. Care should be taken to ensure the ankle joint has not been entered by checking for distension about the ankle joint. A number 11 blade is used to initiate the portals. As the distraction progresses, the borders of the cervical and interosseous ligaments increase in tension and are sequentially cut using the number 11 blade. A 30°, 2.7-mm or 4.0-mm arthroscope (depending on patient size) is then introduced through the anterior portal. A 70° scope also may be quite useful to look around corners for further visualization. Gravity is usually sufficient to fill the joint with fluid and an arthroscopic pump usually is not usually necessary. A shaver is introduced through the middle portal and obscuring synovial debris is removed. A number of sizes of shaver-type blades may be used, including 1.9 mm, 2.0 mm, 2.9 mm, and 4.0 mm.

The primary fusion is performed at the posterior facet, which makes up most of the area of the subtalar joint. The middle facet is also debrided and fused after resecting the contents of the sinus tarsi. Fusion of the anterior facet requires extensive ligamentous resection and is generally avoided. A 4-mm burr is used to abrade the bone to ensure a good bleeding base of bone.

A cannulated pin is driven from the anteromedial shoulder of the talar neck until the pin protrudes from the superior talar surface of the posterior facet (Fig. 5.3). Keep the pin away from the anterior ankle joint so that the screw does not impinge and interfere with ankle dorsiflexion. Once the position is confirmed, the guide pin is backed away from the joint surface and the 4-mm burr is reintroduced. A bone slurry is then generated by burring both sides of the joint, keeping the suction turned off (Fig. 5.4). If bone graft is used, the arthroscope only is then removed and 5 mL of osteoinductive gel is injected through the arthroscopic sheath. The obturator is used as a plunger to push the gel into place.

The distractor is removed and the joint is held reduced (0–5° valgus, neutral in the sagittal and axial planes) by compressing the talar and calcaneal pins. The cannulated talar pin is driven across the subtalar joint and into the calcaneus. The cannulated screw is then driven across and confirmed fluoroscopically (Fig. 5.5). An alternative method is to drive one or more screws up from the calcaneus into the talus. Closure is

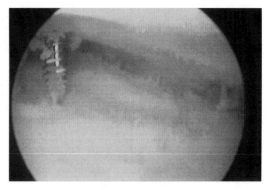

Fig. 5.3 Intraarticular view of posterior facet demonstrating adequate pin placement

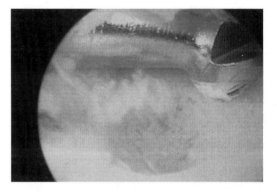

Fig. 5.4 A 4-mm burr at the posterior facet demonstrating creation of bone slurry

performed with 4–0 nylon sutures. Compression dressings are applied along with a posterior splint.

Postoperative Rehabilitation

Patients are seen in follow-up at 7–14 days for a wound check, and then placed either in a cast or boot walker. They are placed on crutches nonweightbearing for 6 weeks and then are placed in a boot walker for 6 weeks. If there is radiographic evidence of union, a good intermediate transition shoe is an aerobics shoe that has good arch support and a slight rocker-bottomed sole. If there is doubt regarding the completeness of the arthrodesis, the patient may be recasted for another 4–6 weeks.

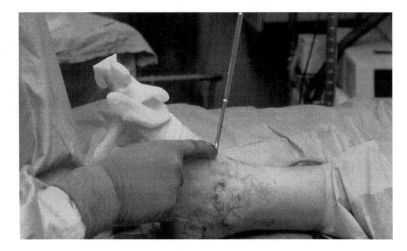

Fig. 5.5 Insertion of cannulated screw

References

1. Scranton PE. Results of arthrodesis of the tarsus: talo-calcaneal, midtarsal, and subtalar joints. Foot Ankle Int 12:156–164, 1991
2. Mann RA, Baumgarten M. Subtalar fusion for isolated subtalar disorders. Clin Orthop Relat Res 226:260–265, 1988
3. Scranton PE. Comparison of open isolated subtalar arthrodesis with autogenous bone graft versus outpatient arthroscopic subtalar arthrodesis using injectable bone morphogenic protein-enhanced graft. Foot Ankle Int 20(3):162–165, 1999
4. Tasto JP, Frey C, Laimans P, et al. Arthroscopic ankle arthrodesis. Instr Course Lect 49:259–280, 2000
5. Easley ME, Trnka H-J, Schon LC, et al. Isolated subtalar arthrodesis. J Bone Joint Surg 82A:613–624, 2000
6. Mangone PG, Fleming LL, Fleming SS, Hedrick MR, Seiler JG III, Bailey E. Treatment of acquired adult planovalgus deformities with subtalar fusion. Clin Orthop Relat Res, 341:106–112, 1997
7. Grice DS. An extra-articular arthrodesis of the subastragalar joint for correction of paralytic feet in children. J Bone Joint Surg 34A:927–930, 1952
8. Scranton PE, McMaster JH, Kelly E. Dynamic fibular function: a new concept. Clin Orthop Relat Res 118:76–82, 1976
9. Thordarson DB, Kuehn S. Use of demineralized bone matrix in ankle/hindfoot fusion. Foot Ankle Int 24(7):557–60, 2003
10. Dhawan SK, Conti SF, Towers J, Abidi NA, Vogt M. The effect of pulsed electromagnetic fields on hindfoot arthrodesis: a prospective study. J Foot Ankle Surg 43(2):93–96, 2004
11. Harper MC. The lateral ligamentous supports of the subtalar joint. Foot Ankle Int 12:354, 1991
12. Frey C, Gasser S, Feder K. Arthroscopy of the subtalar joint. Foot Ankle Int 15:424–428, 1994
13. Parisien JS (ed.). Arthroscopic Surgery. New York, McGraw-Hill, 1988
14. Frey C, Gasser S, Feder K. Arthroscopy of the subtalar joint. Foot Ankle Int 15:424–428, 1994
15. Mekhail AO, Heck BE, Ebraheim NA, et al. Arthroscopy of the subtalar joint: establishing a medial portal. Foot Ankle Int 16:427–431, 1995
16. Frey C. Subtalar arthroscopy. In: Myerson MS (ed.) Foot and Ankle Disorders. Philadelphia, PA, Saunders, 1999, pp. 1494–1501
17. Tasto JP. Subtalar arthrodesis. Presented at the Arthroscopy Association of North America, Orlando, FL. February, 1995

Minimally Invasive Ankle Arthrodesis

6

Jamal Ahmad and Steven M. Raikin

The ankle joint is a constrained mortise and tenon-type joint consisting of the distal tibial plafond and fibula articulating with the dome of the talus. Arthritis of the ankle can result in pain, joint incongruence, decreased motion, and functional disability. The most common etiology of ankle arthritis is posttraumatic, which includes cartilaginous injury and ligamentous insufficiency [1]. Other less common causes of arthritis include the inflammatory arthritides, osteonecrosis, infection, and Charcot neuroarthropathy [2].

To date, the ankle remains one of the few major extremity joints in which arthrodesis is the gold standard surgical treatment for advanced arthritis that has failed nonoperative management. Open ankle arthrodesis was first described by Albert in 1879 [3]. Fusion through an open arthrotomy has received numerous modifications since that time, but remains a widely used technique for surgical exposure. Currently, the most common surgical exposure for open ankle arthrodesis is the lateral transfibular approach. Upon osteotomy, the distal fibula can be used either as bone graft or as a lateral strut to increase the stability of the arthrodesis construct. Preparations of the distal tibia and talar dome through these open techniques include either "dome" cuts or flat cuts. Dome cuts allow for minimal loss of height, but do not offer much

in terms of angular correction. Straight, flat cuts allow for correction of significant deformity, but can result in loss of joint height.

However, ankle arthrodesis through an open arthrotomy is not without its shortcomings. Skin slough, wound dehiscence, and wound infection may occur with a sizable wound at the ankle. As the distal fibula and syndesmotic ligaments are removed during the open fusion, the ankle's mortise and lateral stability are lost. This is undesirable should the arthrodesis be taken down and later converted to an ankle arthroplasty. Greisberg et al. recently showed that patients who received a distal fibula resection with their fusion had a more complicated postoperative course in terms of pain and loosening following conversion to arthroplasty than patients in whom the fibula was spared for their fusion [4]. Distal fibular osteotomy also often sacrifices the peroneal artery, which may affect healing of the ankle fusion and wound. At the ankle, the peroneal artery gives rise to the artery of the tarsal sinus to supply the lateral one eighth to one fourth of the talus. The artery of the tarsal sinus then links to the artery of the tarsal canal at the tarsal canal to form the artery of the tarsal sling. This artery enters the talar neck inferiorly to supply it and the remainder of the bone in a distal-to-proximal direction. Without the peroneal artery, the blood supply to the ankle fusion may not be optimal. Additionally, open ankle fusion techniques typically involve a high degree of soft tissue stripping, which can damage the extraosseous blood supply of the fusion site. When the blood supply is compromised in some

J. Ahmad • S.M. Raikin (✉)
Department of Orthopaedic Surgery,
Rothman Institute and Thomas Jefferson
University Hospital, Philadelphia, PA, USA
e-mail: steven.raikin@rothmaninstitute.com

manner, the quality and time to union may be deleteriously affected. Finally, there is concern that, after resection of the distal fibula during the approach to the ankle joint, the peroneal tendons will lose their biomechanical fulcrum around which they act during eversion of the hindfoot.

To avoid these shortcomings of open ankle arthrodesis, the technique of arthroscopic fusion was proposed [5–7]. For this procedure, a standard two or three portal ankle arthroscopy is performed. With the joint distracted, the articular cartilage and subchondral bone is removed with curettes and mechanical burrs. Two or three percutaneous cannulated cancellous screws are then placed across the ankle under fluoroscopic guidance to achieve fusion. Since first being described in 1983, several authors have reported their experience [5]. Ogilvie-Harris et al. presented an 89% union rate among 19 arthroscopic fusions with a mean time to union of 10.5 weeks [8]. Zvijac et al. reported a 95% union rate among 21 arthroscopic fusions with an average time to fusion of 8.9 weeks [9]. Myerson and Quill retrospectively compared arthroscopic with open arthrodesis in 33 patients [10]. The arthroscopic group showed 100% union at a mean of 8.7 weeks while the open population displayed a 94% union rate at a prolonged mean of 14.5 weeks after surgery. However, patients who had more deformity or osteonecrosis were selectively placed in the open population due to the study's inherent retrospective nature. In one of the largest studies to date, Winson et al. described a 7.6% nonunion rate in 105 arthroscopic ankle arthrodeses, with 20% of patients describing their results as fair or poor [11]. In the literature to date, arthroscopic ankle arthrodesis has been mainly reserved for patients with minimal deformity.

However, this technique of arthroscopic ankle arthrodesis is not without its own shortcomings. The technique itself is technically demanding and has a steep learning curve [1]. Because a burr is used to prepare the distal tibia and talar dome surfaces, there is a genuine concern of thermal injury to the bony surfaces, which can increase the risk of nonunion [12].

To combine the advantages of the open and arthroscopic ankle fusion methods while limiting their respective disadvantages, a minimally invasive or "mini-open" technique was detailed in 1996 [1, 12]. The advantages of this newer procedure are as follows: (1) decreased incision sizes to minimize morbidity, which include the risks of skin slough, wound dehiscence, and postoperative infection; (2) distal fibula preservation, which is preferred should the fusion later be converted to an arthroplasty; (3) preservation of the peroneal artery; (4) elimination of burrs to prepare bony surfaces, which could otherwise cause thermal necrosis; and (5) decreased time to union.

Indications

The primary indication for minimally invasive ankle arthrodesis is pain and dysfunction from severe ankle arthritis that has failed conservative treatment. Such nonoperative modalities may include nonsteroidal anti-inflammatory medications (NSAIDs), soft-laced ankle gauntlets, and motion-limiting braces. However, this specific technique of ankle arthrodesis is best reserved for patients with minimal or absent deformity of the ankle [1, 12]. An additional theoretical advantage is the younger patient who is not a candidate for ankle arthroplasty on the basis of their age, but who wishes to potentially pursue this option in the future.

Contraindications

The following factors are relative contraindications for performing minimally invasive ankle arthrodesis: (1) significant ankle deformity or subluxation; (2) bone loss at the ankle; and (3) osteonecrosis involving a significant portion of the talus or distal tibia. This is because it is difficult to address the above conditions through a minimally invasive technique. Correcting a significant ankle deformity usually necessitates correction via bony cuts at the tibial plafond and the talar dome, combined with more extensive soft tissue release and rebalancing that is not possible with small incisions. Ankles that display significant bone loss, osteonecrosis, and collapse often require thorough debridement of pathologic bone and supplementation with structural bone graft. Such situations are best suited for an open ankle arthrodesis via a transfibular approach.

Preoperative Planning

Weightbearing radiographs of the ankle in the anteroposterior (AP), lateral, and mortise plane are critical to planning a minimally invasive ankle arthrodesis (Fig. 6.1). Weightbearing films allow for more accurate evaluation of malalignment and loss of joint space. As stated earlier, ankles that exhibit minimal radiographic deformity on weightbearing remain best suited for minimally invasive fusion techniques. Characteristic radiographic findings of ankle arthritis are decreased joint space, subchondral sclerosis, subchondral cysts, osteophytes, loose bodies, and malalignment [13].

A complete and informed discussion with the patient should be undertaken to prepare the patient for realistic postoperative expectations. Patients

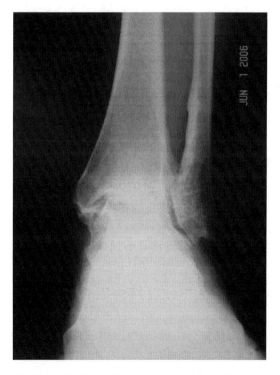

Fig. 6.1 AP radiograph of a severely arthritic ankle without significant varus or valgus deformity

should be informed that the risks of minimally invasive ankle fusion include but are not limited to bleeding, infection, nerve injury, and nonunion. Patients should also be advised about the potentials to require prolonged weightbearing restrictions and accommodative footwear postoperatively.

Operative Procedure

The patient is administered a general or spinal anesthetic for the operation supplemented with a regional nerve block for postoperative pain control. The patient is positioned supine with a bump underneath the ipsilateral hip rotating the pelvis to bring the foot into a straight upright position, aligning the tibial tubercle with the web space between the first and second toes. A radiolucent table is used to facilitate fluoroscopy assistance throughout surgery. A "mini image" dose radiation fluoroscopy device is usually adequate for visualization in this procedure. A pneumatic tourniquet is applied to the proximal calf and inflated to 250 mmHg after exsanguination during the procedure. Surgical drapes are applied to leave the foot, ankle, and leg distal to the tourniquet exposed in the surgical field. Preoperative prophylactic antibiotics are routinely indicated for this procedure, prior to tourniquet inflation.

Technique

Two 2-cm vertical incisions are utilized for this technique. These incisions are centered over the standard portal sites for ankle arthroscopy. An 18-gauge needle should be inserted into the joint at each proposed incision site to confirm the appropriate level of the incision and that adequate access to the ankle can be achieved. The anteromedial incision is made immediately medial to the tibialis anterior tendon, between the tendon and the notch of the medial malleolus. Care must be taken with this incision to avoid injury to a branch of the saphenous nerve, which could result in painful neuroma formation. The anterolateral incision is made in the space between the lateral border of the peroneus tertius tendon and the

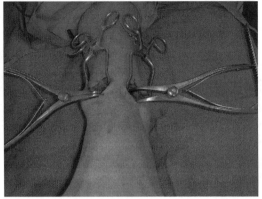

Fig. 6.3 Incisions are extended through the retinaculum to expose the ankle joint

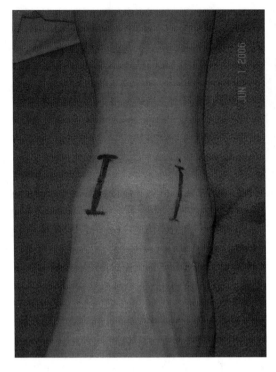

Fig. 6.2 Incision sites marked out for the minimally invasive ankle arthrodesis

anterior border of the fibular. Special care should be taken not to injure the lateral cutaneous branch of the superficial peroneal nerve, which should be identified and retracted medially with the peroneus tertius tendon (Fig. 6.2). Through both incisions, blunt dissection is continued down to the ankle joint capsule, which is incised longitudinally to expose the joint. Subperiosteal dissection around the anterior aspect of the ankle is performed with an elevator to optimize joint exposure. Anterior ankle osteophytes are removed with a sharp chisel to enhance visualization of the joint. The joint is then denuded of articular cartilage through one of the incisions while distraction is maintained via the other incision. Upon proper exposure of the ankle joint, a laminar spreader is placed in one of the incisions to distract the joint (Fig. 6.3). Proper insertion of the laminar spreader within the joint is crucial so as not to excessively plantarflex the ankle. With the joint distracted, a sharp chisel and/or angled curette is placed in the other incision and used to remove cartilage through the other incision

(Fig. 6.4a, b). Enough cartilage is removed from the distal tibia and talar dome to penetrate through the subchondral plate and observe bleeding cancellous bone from each surface. This layer of resection is typically 1–2 mm. Once one side (medial or lateral) of the ankle joint is devoid of cartilage, the laminar spreader is switched to the other incision. The chisel and curettes are placed in their corresponding alternate incision to remove cartilage from the other side of the ankle. Great care must be utilized to ensure that the medial and lateral gutters are adequately debrided to allow the ankle joint to be appropriately aligned for the arthrodesis (Fig. 6.5). It is our recommendation that no power saws or burrs be utilized to limit potential thermal necrosis of the bone, which may lead to nonunion of the arthrodesis. All of the resected bone and cartilage is removed utilizing a rongeur. Once all of the cartilage has been removed from the ankle, the joint is copiously irrigated with saline to remove loose bodies and bone shavings.

To date, there is a general lack of consensus regarding the use of bone autograft or allograft during minimally invasive ankle arthrodesis. The senior author routinely enhances this arthrodesis with autogenous cancellous bone graft [1]. This is harvested from the lateral aspect of the calcaneal body [14].

The ankle is then held in an appropriate position for fusion, which is checked fluoroscopically. The ankle is fused in 5° of valgus, 0° of

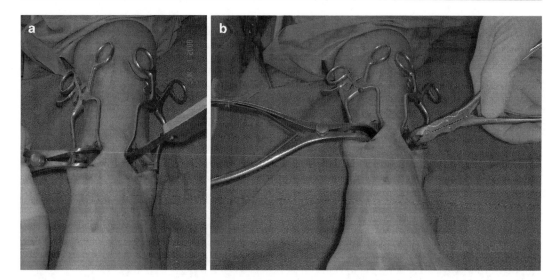

Fig. 6.4 (**a, b**) One side of the ankle joint is distracted with a laminar spreader while the other side is debrided with a rongeur and/or chisel

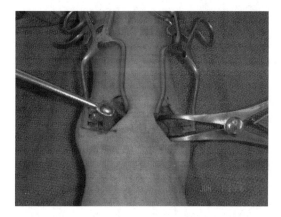

Fig. 6.5 With one side of the ankle joint distracted, the gutter of the opposite side is debrided

dorsiflexion, and 10° of external rotation [15]. This position is optimal as it results in a plantigrade foot and maximal functional results [16]. Note that it may be tempting for the surgeon to fuse a female's ankle in slight plantarflexion such that she may wear shoes with raised heels. However, this should be avoided for two reasons. The first is that fusing the ankle in equinus increases the stress and risk of developing secondary arthritis at the transverse tarsal joints. In addition, this ankle position causes genu recurvatum while walking without a raised heeled shoe [17, 18]. Provided that there is no hindfoot or

midfoot arthritis, compensatory motion after ankle arthrodesis often allows for walking in as much as a 2-in. heel.

Once an optimal alignment is obtained, guide pins for screw fixation are inserted under fluoroscopic guidance. The ankle arthrodesis is held with three 7.3-mm (or 6.5-mm) short-threaded cannulated cancellous screws. Using three screws to achieve an ankle arthrodesis has been shown biomechanically to impart the greatest amount of rigidity to the fusion [19–21]. A method of using three screws involves the following technique of two crossing screws and a third posterior to anterior (PA) "home run" screw [1, 22]. The first guidewire is placed percutaneously from the medial distal tibia to the lateral talar body. The second guidewire is placed percutaneously from the anterolateral distal tibia to the medial talar body. Both wires are placed crossing each other. This configuration of the two screws has shown increased rigidity in laboratory tests [12, 23]. The positions of these wires are checked under fluoroscopy to confirm they have sufficient purchase of distal tibia and talus and that they do not penetrate the subtalar joint (Fig. 6.6). Once wire positioning is deemed acceptable, the length of both is measured. The two guidewires are overdrilled and a 7.3-mm (or 6.5-mm) short-threaded

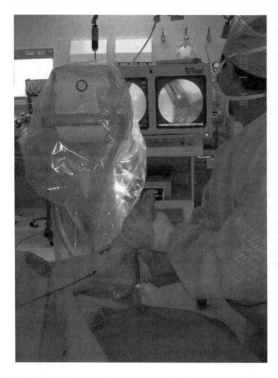

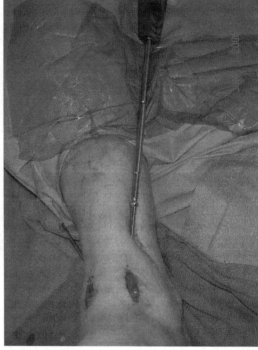

Fig. 6.6 Correct position of the arthrodesis is confirmed under fluoroscopy

Fig. 6.7 Screws to achieve fusion are placed percutaneously

cannulated cancellous screw for each are inserted over them (Fig. 6.7). Typically, screws selected for use are 5–10 mm shorter than the measured length of their respective guidewires. This allows for compression of the ankle fusion during screw fixation without the screws themselves violating the subtalar joint. After placement of these two screws, the guidewires are removed. While screw length is determined by the size of the individual patient's bone size, these two screws are usually approximately 50 mm in length.

A third guidewire is then placed from the posterior distal tibia, just lateral to the Achilles tendon, into the neck and head of the talus. The position of this wire is assessed under fluoroscopy to confirm that it has adequate purchase of distal tibia and talar neck and that it does not penetrate the talonavicular joint. Once wire positioning is deemed acceptable, its length is measured. The guidewire is overdrilled and a 7.3-mm short-threaded cannulated cancellous screw is inserted over it. Akin to the first two screws, the third

screw selected for use is 5 mm shorter than the measured length of the guidewire. This allows for compression of the ankle fusion during screw fixation without the screw violating the talonavicular joint. Again, while variable, dependent on individual bone size, this screw is usually approximately 65 mm in length. After screw placement, the guidewire is removed. For any of the three screws, adding a washer may improve compression in osteopenic bone. Final fluoroscopy is performed to confirm proper alignment of the ankle fusion and screw placement. When performing this procedure we routinely leave preexisting hardware in place unless it blocks the reduction of the joint or the placement of one of the arthrodesis screws.

All wounds are closed in a routine fashion. The ankle retinaculum is closed with interrupted 0 Vicryl suture. The subcutaneous tissue of all three wounds is closed with interrupted 2.0 Vicryl suture. The skin of all of the wounds is closed with a skin stapler.

The wounds are then dressed in sterile fashion. Sterile Xeroform, gauze, and Webril are applied to the wounds in a layered fashion. At this point, the tourniquet is deflated and the sterile drapes are removed. Immediately after surgery and application of the dressing, the patient is placed in a nonweightbearing posterior and "U" coaptation plaster splint.

Postoperative Care

The initial postoperative splint remains intact for 2 weeks. At 2 weeks postoperatively, the splint is removed and the patient is placed in a nonweight-bearing short leg cast for 4 weeks.

Typically, at 6 weeks postoperatively, radiographs start to show bony union across the fusion. So long as this is the case, the cast is removed and the patient is placed into a fracture boot to allow for progressive weightbearing. Currently, there is no uniform postoperative weightbearing regimen for patients following a minimally invasive ankle fusion. The senior author instructs patients to begin 25–50% weightbearing in the boot at 6 weeks postoperatively so long as there is radiographic evidence of bony consolidation. The patient may then apply an additional 25% of weight in the boot every 2 weeks as comfort allows. Thus, patients should be fully weight-bearing on the ankle arthrodesis in the boot by 12 weeks postoperatively. Once the patient is fully weightbearing in the boot without discomfort, and radiographs show adequate fusion of the arthrodesis (Fig. 6.8), the patient may gradually wean out of the fracture boot and return to their previous level of activity. Footwear modifications such as a rocker-bottom sole with a solid ankle cushioned heel (SACH) may help patients to resume a more normal gait.

After minimally invasive ankle arthrodesis, patients should be provided with conservative guidelines regarding postoperative activity level. Bicycle riding, swimming, and other low-impact activities are encouraged for aerobic exercise. Patients may return to playing golf at 9–12 months postoperatively. Jogging and running are discouraged after ankle arthrodesis. The repetitive

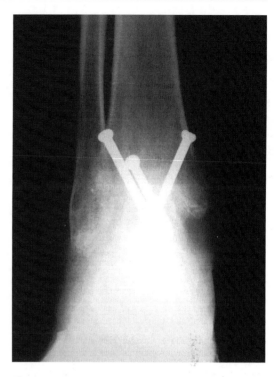

Fig. 6.8 Radiograph of a patient with a completely healed ankle arthrodesis done through a minimally invasive technique

high-impact loading of the ankle fusion can irritate and place additional load upon the knee, hindfoot, and midfoot.

Published Results

To date, very little published data exists for the mini-open ankle arthrodesis. Myerson et al. described the procedure and published their results in two separate studies [12]. In the same paper where the technique was first described and the compromise of vascularity with the fibular resection was studied, Miller et al. reported on 32 ankles undergoing the mini-arthrotomy technique [24]. They described a 96.8% union rate in 32 ankles, with two delayed unions. Their average time to union was 8 weeks, with a range of 6–22 weeks. Paremain et al. separately reported a union rate of 100% at a mean time of 6 weeks (range, 3–15 weeks) in 15 ankles undergoing this minimally invasive technique of arthrodesis [12].

No specific studies have been published on takedown of the mini-open ankle arthrodesis for conversion to total ankle arthroplasty. However, Greisberg et al. did report on conversion of 23 open ankle arthrodeses to arthroplasty [4]. They reported 3 of 19 patients who were available for follow-up finally choosing to undergo below-knee amputation for recalcitrant pain, but the remaining 16 patients improved their AOFAS ankle hindfoot score from an average of 42 points to an average of 68 points out of 100. They did comment that all patients who had undergone a distal fibular resection as part of their initial arthrodesis had complicated courses after arthroplasty. This supports the theory that the mini-open fibular preserving technique may result in superior arthroplasty conversion results in the future.

Senior Author's Experience

The senior author (SMR) has performed 16 minimally invasive ankle arthrodeses in 16 ankles, with longer than 12 months follow-up. Patients' ages ranged from 28 to 52 years (average 24.1 years), with ten male patients six female patients. The right and left ankle were equally involved, with eight cases each. The most common underlying diagnosis was posttraumatic arthritis, which was present in 14 (87%) patients, with one patient having a history of juvenile rheumatoid arthritis (JRA) and one patient with talar osteonecrosis secondary to steroid use for asthma. All patients had minimal or no deformity at the ankle joint without significant bone loss or collapse. Postoperative follow-up averaged 37.5 months, with the range being from 15 to 68 months. The rate of union in this population was 100%. Mean time to union was 11.4 weeks after surgery, with the range being from 10 to 16 weeks. When asked if they were satisfied with their postoperative outcome, all of the patients (100%) stated they would have their respective procedure done identically unless an arthroplasty could be done as an alternative. There were no observed postoperative complications such as wound infections, nerve injuries, or delayed healing. Of incidental note, none of these

patients were involved in the workers compensation system, litigation, or secondary gain related to their injuries. To date, none of these fusions have been attempted to be taken down and converted to an ankle arthroplasty.

References

1. Raikin S. Arthrodesis of the ankle: arthroscopic, mini-open, and open techniques. Foot Ankle Clin North Am 8:347–359, 2003
2. Coughlin M. Arthritides. In: Coughlin M (ed.) Surgery of the foot and ankle. St. Louis: Mosby; pp. 560–650, 1999
3. Albert E. Beitrage zur operativen chiurgie. Zur resection des kniegelenkes. Wien Med Press 20:705–708, 1879
4. Greisberg J, Assal M, Flueckiger G, Hansen, ST. Takedown of ankle fusion and conversion to total ankle replacement. Clin Orthop Relat Res 424:80–88, 2004
5. Schneider D. Arthroscopic ankle fusion. Arth Video J 3, 1983
6. Morgan C. Arthroscopic tibio-talar arthrodesis. Jefferson Orthop J 16:50–52, 1987
7. Myerson M, Allon S. Arthroscopic ankle arthrodesis. Contemp Orthop 19:21–27, 1989
8. Ogilvie-Harris D, Lieberman I, Fitsialos D. Arthroscopically assisted arthrodesis for osteoarthrotic ankles. J Bone Joint Surg 75A:1167–1173, 1993
9. Zvijac J, Lemak L, Schurhoff M, Hechtman K, Uribe J. Analysis of arthroscopically assisted ankle arthrodesis. Arthroscopy 18(1):70–75, 2002
10. Myerson M, Quill G. Ankle arthrodesis: a comparison of an arthroscopic and an open method of treatment. Clin Orthop Relat Res 268:84–95, 1991
11. Winson IG, Robinson DE, Allen PE. Arthroscopic ankle arthrodesis. J Bone Joint Surg Br 87(3):343–347, 2005
12. Paremain G, Miller S, Myerson M. Ankle arthrodesis: results after the miniarthrotomy technique. Foot Ankle Int 17(5):247–252, 1996
13. Demetriades L, Strauss E, Gallina J. Osteoarthritis of the ankle. Clin Orthop Relat Res 349:48–57, 1998
14. Raikin SM, Brislin K. Local bone graft harvested from the distal tibia or calcaneus for surgery of the foot and ankle. Foot Ankle Int 26(6):449–453, 2005
15. Buck P, Morrey BF, Chao EY. The optimum position of arthrodesis of the ankle. A gait study of the knee and ankle. J Bone Joint Surg 69A:1052–1062, 1987
16. Mann R, Van Manen J, Wapner K, et al. Ankle fusion. Clin Orthop Relat Res 268:49–55, 1991
17. King H, Watkins T Jr, Samuelson K. Analysis of foot position in ankle arthrodesis and its influence on gait. Foot Ankle 1:44–49, 1980

18. Wu W, Su F, Cheng Y, et al. Gait analysis after ankle arthrodesis. Gait Posture 11:54–61, 2000
19. Dohm M, Benjamin J, Harrison J, et al. A biomechanical evaluation of three forms of internal fixation used in ankle arthrodesis. Foot Ankle Int 15:297–300, 1994
20. Ogilvie-Harris D, Fitsialos D, Hedman T. Arthrodesis of the ankle. A comparison of two versus three screw fixation in a crossed configuration. Clin Orthop Relat Res 304:195–199, 1994
21. Verkelst M, Mulier J, Hoogmartens M, et al. Arthrodesis of the ankle joint with complete removal of the distal part of the fibula: experience with the transfibular approach and three different types of fixation. Clin Orthop Relat Res 118:93–99, 1976
22. Holt E, Hansen S, Mayo K, et al. Ankle arthrodesis using internal screw fixation. Clin Orthop Relat Res 268:21–28, 1991
23. Nasson S, Shuff C, Palmer D, et al. Biomechanical comparison of ankle arthrodesis techniques: crossed screws vs. blade plate. Foot Ankle Int 22:575–580, 2001
24. Miller SD, Paremain GP, Myerson MS. The miniarthrotomy technique of ankle arthrodesis: a cadaver study of operative vascular compromise and early clinical results. Orthopedics 19(5):425–430, 1996

Arthroscopic Ankle Arthrodesis

C. Christopher Stroud

The benefits of minimally invasive surgery have received significant attention in the lay press as well as in scientific meetings. Often patients will ask whether such a "minimalistic" approach is available for treatment of their specific problem. While ankle fusion has long been treated via an open approach with generally excellent results [1, 2], there has been a push to perform this procedure through smaller incisions. While the extended lateral approach to the ankle has been the norm in the past, we have seen the evolution of the "mini-open" procedure as a technique used in a significant proportion of these procedures today [3]. Following this line of thinking, the arthroscopic approach has been used in performing arthrodesis procedures of the ankle and foot. However, with the use of these novel techniques, it is incumbent on us, as the treating physicians, to ensure surgical results that equate or surpass these historical results.

The benefits of a standard arthroscopic procedure are clear and well documented in the literature. Less perioperative pain experienced by the patient, smaller and more cosmetically appealing incisions, less surgical dissection, and a procedure that can be performed as an outpatient are clear advantages. What remains to be seen are the definite indications for the procedure, including the extent of deformity and bone loss that can be

handled with the arthroscopic approach. It also should be noted that this "lesser" approach does not reduce the time to healing or to fusion. This chapter focuses on the surgical technique for those appropriately selected patients who will undergo an arthroscopic ankle arthrodesis.

Indications

Arthrosis of the ankle is generally uncommon, despite the ankle being a major weight-bearing joint [4]. Posttraumatic causes are the most common etiology, followed by primary osteoarthrosis, osteonecrosis, inflammatory arthropathy, and neuropathic causes. Patients typically present with complaints of pain globally about the ankle, usually of insidious onset. Potential causes for ankle pain should be investigated and include a history of trauma, instability, or systemic illnesses such as diabetes or other inflammatory or autoimmune diseases. The pain is usually described as a dull ache while sedentary and at times a sharp pain with weightbearing and pivoting. Patients may note a "grind" or a "click" with activity or movement. On examination, swelling is often present and tenderness is noted about a portion of, or the entire ankle joint itself. The presence of a deformity should be noted. Examination of limb alignment is particularly important, paying close attention the knee and hindfoot. Any deformity about the knee should be investigated with mechanical axis, weightbearing radiographs, and symptoms associated

C.C. Stroud (✉)
Department of Surgery, William Beaumont
Hospital-Troy, Troy, MI, USA
e-mail: stroudmdrn@aol.com

G.R. Scuderi and A.J. Tria (eds.), *Minimally Invasive Surgery in Orthopedics: Foot and Ankle Handbook*, 45
DOI 10.1007/978-1-4614-0893-2_7, © Springer Science+Business Media, LLC 2012

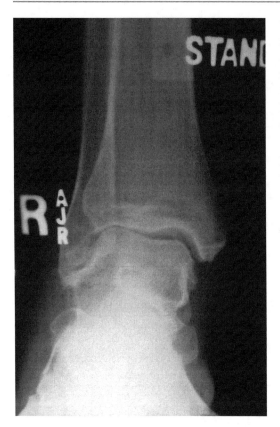

Fig. 7.1 AP radiograph of a patient with symptomatic right ankle arthrosis noting joint space narrowing and a slight valgus deformity. This minimal deformity is amenable to an arthroscopic arthrodesis

with the knee sought. Range of motion of the ankle, hindfoot, and midfoot should be recorded, noting any restriction of movement. The patient's neurovascular status is also assessed.

Radiographs consisting of weightbearing anteroposterior (AP), lateral, and mortise views of the ankle and foot are required (Fig. 7.1). These X-rays should be examined for the degree of arthrosis and the presence of osteophytes, cystic changes, and deformity. An anterior tibiotalar osteophyte of significant size will make the initial arthroscopic approach more difficult. If a bone defect is noted, the judgment will have to be made whether this defect is contributing to any ankle deformity and whether a grafting procedure will need to be performed. While smaller cystic defects are common and can be dealt with arthroscopically, larger defects that need to be filled with autograft or those that occur on the

tibial side probably are best dealt with in an open fashion. There are no clear guidelines as to when an arthroscopic procedure should be abandoned in favor of the open approach but roughly a defect 30% or larger of the talar or tibial surface is best handle with direct visualization, i.e., a traditional open approach [5]. Additionally radiographs should be examined for any deformity that is present. If the deformity if extraarticular, consideration should be given to a supramalleolar or calcaneal osteotomy. If the deformity occurs at the ankle joint, then the decision becomes one of judgment. If the patient has a correctable ankle, that is, it can be placed in a plantigrade position passively, then one can proceed with an arthroscopic approach. If the deformity is rigid and exceeds 10–15°, the arthroscopic procedure should be abandoned in favor of the open approach [5]. This is especially true if there is a bony defect preset.

A patient who presents with ongoing complaints of ankle pain as a result of arthrosis should initially be treated with conservative measures. These include the use of oral analgesics or anti-inflammatories and limitations or modulations in their activities. It is difficult to totally restrict normal activities, but patients will often find it helpful to note that fewer weight-bearing activities can reduce their symptoms. Use of a pool or a stationary bike can often help the active patient stay healthy yet reduce the load on their symptomatic ankle. Proper footwear is important as well. This would include a soft-soled tennis type shoe and perhaps an accommodative orthotic that would lessen pain about the ankle. There are a multitude of braces available ranging from a lace-up ankle brace to an ankle foot orthosis or a custom semi-rigid ankle gauntlet type brace, all in order to diminish the pressure and load that the ankle bears. Judicious use a steroid injection can, at times, offer some temporary relief to the symptomatic ankle.

The patient that has failed these conservative measures and that has radiographic evidence of advanced arthrosis is a candidate for an arthrodesis procedure. The benefits of such a procedure include the elimination or significant reduction in pain, and the ability to increase their normal activities of daily living. Potential disadvantages of an

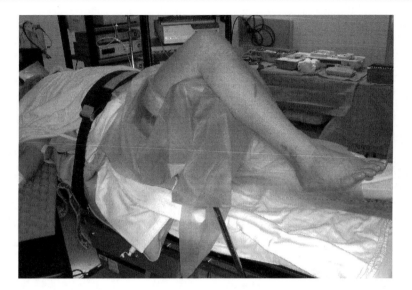

Fig. 7.2 A well-padded leg holder is placed under the thigh to suspend the ankle with room for instrumentation from the posterolateral portal

arthrodesis procedure include loss of motion of one segment of the ankle/foot complex. This may, with time, transfer stress to other areas of the foot and ankle, namely the subtalar joint complex, which may in turn become symptomatic at a future date. Other disadvantages include limb shortening, chronic swelling, and a limp. Overall, however, the results have been extremely satisfactory to patients in long-term follow-up studies to date.

The arthroscopic ankle fusion can offer the advantages noted above, but with less perioperative pain, less surgical dissection, and can be done as an outpatient procedure. The downside of this approach includes the demanding surgical technique and its relatively steep learning curve. One must be very patient and extremely facile with arthroscopic instrumentation in order to take on this procedure.

Contraindications

Arthroscopic arthrodesis is contraindicated in the presence of infection, or in the neuropathic joint. Relative contraindications include severe bony deformity in which tibiotalar alignment exceeds 15° or there is greater than 1 cm of translation in the sagittal plane. Bony defects or significant osteonecrosis greater than 30% of the

Table 7.1 Instruments required for arthroscopic ankle arthrodesis

Thigh holder
Ankle distractor
30/70°, 2.7-mm, short arthroscope
Short, straight, and angled curettes
Short, straight, and angled open curettes
Arthroscopic elevator
Motorized shaver/burr

talar or tibial area are also difficult to treat arthroscopically.

Technique

The patient is brought to the operative suite and placed supine on the table. Preoperative prophylactic antibiotics are administered within 1 h of incision time. A general anesthetic coupled with a paralyzing agent is useful for complete muscle relaxation. Otherwise a spinal, or regional, anesthetic is used. A thigh tourniquet is placed. The patients' leg is placed in an angled thigh holder, which elevates the leg and ankle off the table (Fig. 7.2). One should ensure that there is adequate clearance under the foot and ankle for maneuvering instrumentation during the case (Table 7.1). The limb is then prepped and draped. At this point, a commercially available ankle

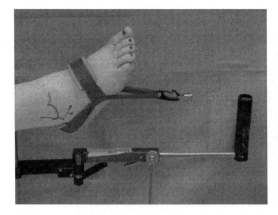

Fig. 7.3 A commercially available ankle distractor is available for autodistraction purposes

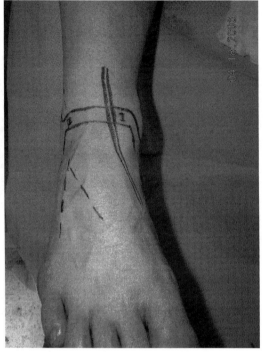

Fig. 7.4 The landmarks are noted on the anterior aspect of the ankle. Note the anteromedial portal just medial to the tibialis anterior tendon. The anterolateral portal lies just lateral to the peroneus tertius tendon and usually lies adjacent to the superficial branch of the peroneal nerve, visible just under the skin in most patients

distractor can be used (Fig. 7.3). The ankle strap is attached to a sterile side post attached directly to the table. This can obviate the use of an assistant for distraction purposes. The limb is exsanguinated and the thigh tourniquet inflated.

A standard anteromedial portal is made with a #15-blade scalpel. This portal lies immediately medial to the tibialis anterior tendon (Fig. 7.4). The skin is incised and the soft tissues are spread down to the capsule with a mosquito clamp. The blunt obturator is angled approximately 30° laterally and the ankle joint is entered. Inflow can be accomplished through the scope or through a separate posterolateral portal. Gravity inflow can be used or alternatively the pump is usually set at 40 mmHg. At this point, often there is significant scarring and adhesions present precluding adequate visualization. The anterolateral portal is then established using a 23-gauge needle placed just lateral to the peroneus tertius muscle. Care is taken to avoid the branch of the superficial peroneal nerve, which often can be visualized just under the skin (Fig. 7.5). Proper placement of this portal is crucial. The needle should be visualized from inside the ankle and moved around, simulating instrument placement. The skin about the anterolateral ankle is then incised and the soft tissues are again spread down to the capsule. A larger blunt obturator will dilate the portal for future instrument passage (Fig. 7.6).

At this point, the anterior tibial osteophyte should be taken down with a motorized shaver or

a burr. Care should be taken to point the instruments toward the ankle joint itself and not anteriorly, because significant bleeding can occur with disruption of the anterior neurovascular structure, obscuring visualization. An arthroscopic elevator, often found in the shoulder arthroscopic instruments, can be useful to elevate a capsule that is scarred down to the anterior aspect of the joint. An aggressive removal of anterior osteophytes, from the tibiofibular joint to the notch of Hardy is often required as one often underappreciates the extent of these spurs noted on preoperative radiographs. Extreme care and patience are required at this point of the procedure, because careful debridement at this point can make the remainder of the case significantly less difficult.

Next, the lateral gutter is debrided (Fig. 7.7). Curettes are used progressing from posterior to anterior, alternating with the shaver to remove

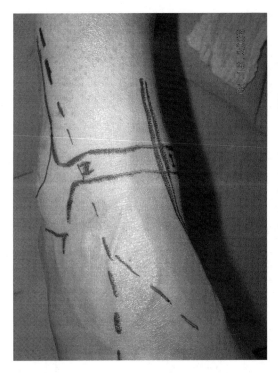

Fig. 7.5 A close up of the anterolateral portal lies adjacent to the superficial peroneal nerve branch

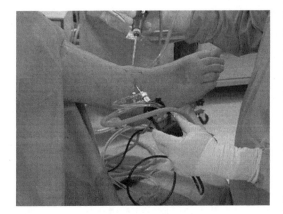

Fig. 7.6 The ankle joint is suspended allowing enough clearance for instrumentation

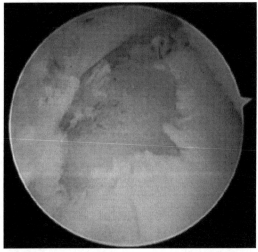

Fig. 7.7 The lateral ankle gutter often has significant scarring and cartilaginous debris, which needs to be cleared during the procedure

extraneous debris and osteophytes. One should then be able to visualize the inferior fibula and anterior talofibular ligament. The portals are switched and a debridement of the medial ankle gutter is accomplished in a similar fashion. Again it can be helpful to use a posterolateral portal for inflow purposes in order to avoid *clogging* of the

arthroscope or shaver with suction/irrigation. Once the debridement has been performed, which again often takes a significant amount of time, the remaining articular cartilage about the tibiotalar joint is removed. Open, curved curettes are useful for this step. Progressing posterior to anterior and from lateral to medial, on both sides of the joint, in a step-wise fashion is helpful. The portals are again switched and the cartilage removed from medial to lateral. The curettes are placed through the posterolateral portal and the posterior cartilage is removed. Any cystic defects are thoroughly debrided with a curette and shaver to remove fibrous tissue. The decision is then made as to whether a bone grafting procedure will need to be performed concurrently.

Once the damaged cartilage has been removed and the ankle joint lavaged, a motorized egg-shaped burr is used to remove 1–2 mm of sclerotic bone to a bleeding surface. This is done in the stepwise fashion noted above. The inflow can be turned off at this point to ensure an adequate amount of resection. If necessary, a 1.6-mmK wire can be used to create small perforations in the tibia and talus bone to act as channels for future vascular ingress and aid in healing. Use of the MICRO VECTOR drill guide (Smith & Nephew, Andover, MA) can aid in placement of this wire if done via a transtibial approach.

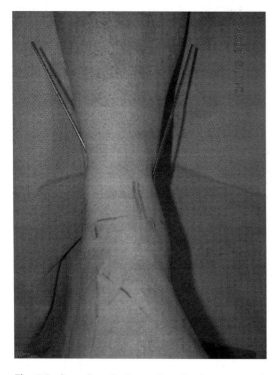

Fig. 7.8 Once the articular cartilage has been removed, two guidewires are placed percutaneously, with the ankle in the proper position

Once the joint has been debrided, guide wires from a large fragment cannulated screw set are placed. Through a 1-cm incision placed approximately 3–4 cm proximal to the joint line, one wire is placed medially and advanced just to the articular surface. This wire should be aimed centrally or slightly posteriorly. A second wire is placed either through the fibula to the joint surface, or from the lateral tibia, aiming slightly anteriorly (Fig. 7.8). There is debate about the number of screws required and their placement. Most authors recommend at least a minimum of two screws with satisfactory purchase and placement. A third wire is preferred and is placed through an incision posteriorly, just lateral to the Achilles tendon, approximately 4 cm proximal to the joint line. This guidewire is advanced just to the articular surface aiming down the neck of the talus, slightly medially. The instruments are removed and the joint reduced. Reduction should be confirmed clinically in the appropriate position. That is, neutral in the sagittal plane, and neutral to 5° valgus in the coronal plane, with

external rotation equivalent to the contralateral side (roughly 10°). At this point, inspection of the position of the hindfoot and limb alignment should be performed. The tibial crest should be in line with the second metatarsal and the hindfoot should be in slight valgus. One should not attempt to correct an extraarticular malalignment with compensation through the ankle joint. Rather, a calcaneal or supramalleolar osteotomy should be performed at this time.

Mini C-arm fluoroscopic views in the AP, oblique, and lateral planes are obtained. If any incongruency exists at this point, the instruments are reinserted and the surfaces smoothed. If at this point, alignment cannot be obtained, then the incisions should be extended and a formal "mini-open" procedure performed.

If the alignment is satisfactory, the joint is held reduced by an assistant and the pins are advanced. Again, proper length of the pins and alignment is confirmed fluoroscopically, taking care to avoid violation of the subtalar joint complex. Once confirmed, the 6.5- or 7.3-mm cannulated screws are placed. Excellent fixation should be accomplished. Final radiographs are then obtained again.

The portals are reapproximated with nylon sutures and a padded dressing with posterior and U-shaped splints are applied. A popliteal nerve block applied at this time (or preoperatively) is helpful in postoperative analgesia.

The patient is instructed to elevate and ice the limb and remain nonweightbearing until the first postoperative visit at 10 days. At that time, the limb can be placed in a cast or a removable boot brace. The patient remains nonweightbearing for 6–8 weeks time and can begin weight bearing when swelling has resided and there are signs of radiographic consolidation (Fig. 7.9a, b).

Literature Review

Since the year 2000, the number of published reports noting the results of arthroscopic ankle arthrodesis has doubled. This highlights the push toward minimally invasive surgery advocated both by physicians experienced in this arena as well as the lay public. But are the results comparable to

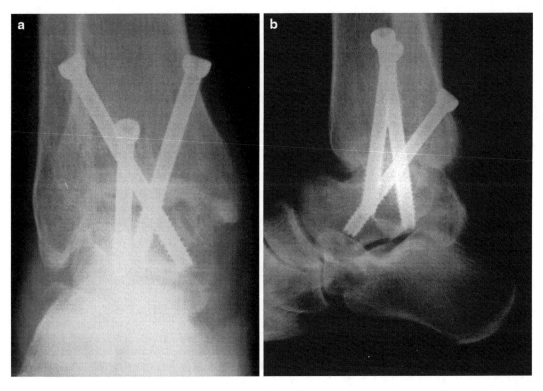

Fig. 7.9 (**a**) Final AP radiograph showing consolidation of the tibiotalar fusion site at 8 weeks. (**b**) Final lateral radiograph showing proper position of the screws placed during the arthroscopic procedure

the traditional open experience, which as noted, has a long and reasonably satisfactory track record? While the nonunion rate of the traditional open procedure has been reported to occur in up to 41% of patients, recent reports note the nonunion rate to be in the 1–5% range [1]. Other disadvantages of the open approach include the significant soft tissue stripping required for the procedure as well as the discomfort associated with such an approach.

Myerson and Quill [6] retrospectively compared open versus arthroscopic arthrodesis in 33 patients. They noted a shortened time to fusion in the arthroscopic group (8.7 weeks) versus the open procedure (14.5 weeks). Additionally the fusion rate as well as the complication rate was similar in the two groups. O'Brien et al. [7] also retrospectively reviewed a group of patients who underwent an arthroscopic fusion procedure, noting similar fusion rates between the two groups. Both studies noted a shortened hospital stay in the arthroscopic group, but limitations included being retrospective in nature with a bias toward

more difficult cases, i.e., those with more deformity, undergoing the open procedure.

Ferkel and Hewitt [8] reported on 35 patients who underwent the procedure at their institution, with a follow-up averaging 72 months. They noted the average time to fusion of 11.8 weeks and three delayed unions, with one requiring revision surgery. The most common complication was prominent hardware with 11 patients requiring screw removal. They noted 83% excellent or good results using a consistent (Mazur) scoring system. Glick et al., [5] in a retrospective multicentered study, noted a 97% fusion rate at an 8-year follow-up study on 35 arthroscopic arthrodeses. Eighty-six percent of their patients were rated as good or excellent. Deformity greater than 15° and/or 1 cm of translation presented significant difficulties in achieving a good result.

While older literature reports noted prolonged union rates with a significant nonunion percentage in groups of patients treated with an arthroscopic approach to ankle fusion [9–11], most recent reports have noted fusion rates of 90–95% with healing times between 8 and 12 weeks [12–20]. Complication rates appear to be similar to the open procedure, with nonunion, infection, prominent hardware, and thromboembolic event, among the most events noted [10]. The rate of radiographic hindfoot arthrosis has been reported to be high in the follow-up of patients with an ankle arthrodesis [2]. However, Winson et al. [16] have shown that this condition is probably present preoperatively in a significant number of patients, but that most do not need specific treatment for this condition at the index procedure.

Conclusion

As has been shown, the arthroscopic technique can be utilized in the arthrodesis of the ankle [21–26], albeit with a reasonably steep learning curve. The results appear to be at least equivalent to the standard open procedure with the benefits of less perioperative pain and shorter hospitalization times. This procedure, similar to arthroscopic shoulder techniques, should increase in popularity in the future.

References

1. Munroe MT, Beals TC, Manoli A. Clinical outcome of arthrodesis of the ankle using rigid internal fixation with cancellous screws. Foot Ankle Int 20:227–231, 1999
2. Coester LM, Saltzman CL, Leupold J, Pontarelli W. Long-term results following ankle arthrodesis for post-traumatic arthritis. J Bone Joint Surg 83-A: 219–228, 2001
3. Paremain GD, Miller SD, Myerson MS. Ankle arthrodesis: results after the miniarthrotomy technique. Foot Ankle Int 17:247–252, 1996
4. Schon LC, Ouzounian TJ. The ankle. In: Jahss MH (ed.). Disorders of the Foot and Ankle, Vol. 2, Edition 2. Philadelphia, WB Saunders, pp. 1417–1460, 1991
5. Glick JM, Morgan CD, Myerson MS, Sampson TG, Mann JA. Ankle arthrodesis using an arthroscopic method: long-term follow-up of 34 cases. Arthroscopy 12(4):428–434, 1996
6. Myerson MS, Quill G. Ankle arthrodesis. A comparison of an arthroscopic and an open method of treatment. Clin Orthop Relat Res 268:84–95, 1991
7. O'Brien TS, Hart TS, Shereff MJ, Stone J, Johnson J. Open versus arthroscopic ankle arthrodesis: a comparative study. Foot Ankle Int 20(6):368–374, 1999
8. Ferkel RD, Hewitt M. Long-term results of arthroscopic ankle arthrodesis. Foot Ankle Int 26(4):275–280, 2005
9. Dent CM, Patil M, Fairclough JA. Arthroscopic ankle arthrodesis. J Bone Joint Surg 75-B(5):830–832, 1993
10. Crosby LA, Yee TC, Formanek TS, Fitzgibbons TC. Complications following arthroscopic ankle arthrodesis. Foot Ankle Int 17(6):340–342, 1996
11. DeVriese L, Dereymaeker G, Fabry G. Arthroscopic ankle arthrodesis preliminary report. Acta Arthop Belg 60(4):389–392, 1994
12. Ogilvie-Harris DJ, Lieberman I, Fitsialos D. Arthroscopically assisted arthrodesis for osteoarthrotic ankles. J Bone Joint Surg 75-A(8):1167–1174, 1993
13. Kats J, van Kampen A, de Waal-Malefijt MC. Improvement in technique for arthroscopic ankle fusion: results in 15 patients. Knee Surg Sports Traumatol Arthrosc 11:46–49, 2003
14. Turan I, Wredmark T, Felländer-Tsai L. Arthroscopic ankle arthrodesis in rheumatoid arthritis. Clin Orthop Relat Res 320:110–114, 1995
15. Zvijac JE, Lemak L, Schurhoff MR, Hechtman K, Uribe J. Analysis of arthroscopically ankle arthrodesis. Arthroscopy 18(1):70–75, 2002
16. Winson IG, Robinson DE, Allen PE. Arthroscopic ankle arthrodesis. J Bone Joint Surg 87-B(3):343–347, 2005
17. Cameron SE, Ullrich P. Arthroscopic arthrodesis of the ankle joint. Arthroscopy 16(1):21–26, 2000
18. Fisher RL, Ryan WR, Dugdale TW, Zimmermann GA. Arthroscopic ankle fusion. Conn Med 61(10):643–646, 1997
19. Corso SJ, Zimmer TJ. Technique and clinical evaluation of arthroscopic ankle arthrodesis. Arthroscopy 11(5):585–590, 1995
20. Fleiss DJ. Arthroscopic arthrodesis of the ankle joint. Arthroscopy 16(7):788, 2000
21. Wasserman LR, Saltzman CL, Amendola A. Minimally invasive ankle reconstruction: current scope and indications. Orthop Clin North Am 35:247–253, 2004
22. Raikin SM. Arthrodesis of the ankle: arthroscopic, mini-open, and open techniques. Foot Ankle Clin 8(2):347–359, 2003
23. Stroud CC. Arthroscopic arthrodesis of the ankle, subtalar, and first metatarsophalangeal joint. Foot Ankle Clin 7(1):135–146, 2002
24. Tasto JP, Frey C, Laimans P, Morgan CD, Mason RJ, Stone JW. Arthroscopic ankle arthrodesis. Instr Course Lect 49:259–280, 2000
25. Fitzgibbons TC. Arthroscopic ankle debridement and fusion: indications, techniques, and results. Instr Course Lect 48:243–248, 1999
26. Stone JW. Arthroscopic ankle arthrodesis. Foot Ankle Clin 11(2):361–368, 2006

Endoscopic Calcaneoplasty

8

P.A.J. de Leeuw and C.N. van Dijk

The first case of a patient with posterior heel pain, caused by hypertrophy of the posterosuperior part of the calcaneus in combination with wearing rigid low-back shoes, was described by Haglund in 1928 [1]. Nowadays in Haglund's disease, we describe a clinical situation of tenderness and pain of the posterolateral aspect of the calcaneus. On physical examination, a bony prominence can be palpated at this location. This entity is described by a variety of different names such as "pump-bump," [2] cucumber heel [3], winter heel [4], etc. In Haglund's syndrome, the retrocalcaneal bursa is inflamed and therefore swelled, sometimes in combination with insertional tendinopathy of the Achilles tendon. The syndrome is caused by repetitive impingement between the anterior aspect of the Achilles tendon and the enlarged posterosuperior aspect of the calcaneus. The patient typically describes the onset of pain when starting walking after a period of rest. Operative treatment consists of removal of the inflamed retrocalcaneal bursa and resection of the bony calcaneal prominence.

A distinction between Haglund's disease and other pathologic conditions of the posterior aspect of the heel, most importantly Achilles tendinitis, must be made. Achilles tendon pathology can be divided in insertional and noninsertional problems [5, 6]. Noninsertional pathology can be divided into tendinopathy, paratendinopathy, or a combination of both. Symptoms typically occur 4–6 cm proximal of the insertion to the calcaneus. Insertional tendinopathy is defined as a tendinopathy of the tendon at its insertion. The pain is most frequently located in the midline at the insertion into the calcaneus. Coexistence with retrocalcaneal bursitis is known. In retrocalcaneal bursitis, as part of Haglund's syndrome, pain can be reproduced by palpating laterally and medially of the Achilles tendon at the level of the posterosuperior calcaneal prominence. With dorsiflexion of the ankle, the anterior part of the tendon impinges against the posterosuperior rim of the calcaneus, leading to retrocalcaneal bursitis. In the cavus foot, the calcaneus is not only varus, but is also more vertical, which results in a more prominent projection posteriorly [7].

Multiple treatments have been described to treat chronic retrocalcaneal bursitis. Conservative treatment of retrocalcaneal bursitis includes avoidance of tight shoe heel counters, nonsteroidal anti-inflammatory drugs, activity modification, the use of padding, physiotherapy, and a single injection with corticosteroids into the retrocalcaneal space. If the conservative treatment fails, there are basically two distinct operative methods and one endoscopic surgical treatment. The open operative alternatives include resection of the posterosuperior part of the calcaneus or a calcaneal wedge osteotomy. Complications include skin breakdown, tenderness around the operative scar, ugly operative scars, and altered sensation around the heel [8–12]. Complications

P.A.J. de Leeuw • C.N. van Dijk (✉)
Department of Orthopaedic Surgery,
Academic Medical Centre, University of Amsterdam,
Amsterdam, the Netherlands
e-mail: m.lammerts@amc.uva.nl

G.R. Scuderi and A.J. Tria (eds.), *Minimally Invasive Surgery in Orthopedics: Foot and Ankle Handbook*,
DOI 10.1007/978-1-4614-0893-2_8, © Springer Science+Business Media, LLC 2012

that are more serious include Achilles tendon avulsions and calcaneal (stress) fractures [10, 12, 13]. Also recurrent persistent pain secondary to an inadequate amount of bone resected and stiffness of the Achilles tendon resulting in decreased dorsiflexion have been reported [14]. Wound-healing problems have been described in 30% of the patients treated with open procedures [15].

Endoscopic treatment offers the advantages that are related to any minimal invasive surgical procedure, such as a low morbidity, excellent scar healing, functional aftertreatment, short recovery time, and quick sports consumption as compared with open surgical approaches. In this article we describe the technique of endoscopic calcaneoplasty and will compare the results of this minimal invasive technique [16] with those reported for the open surgical techniques.

Indication Endoscopic Calcaneoplasty

Patient complaints include pain at rest, when standing, (uphill) walking, running, and walking on hard surfaces. X-ray shows hypertrophy of the posterosuperior aspect of the calcaneus (Fig. 8.1). If conservative treatment fails, endoscopic surgery is indicated.

Surgical Technique

The operation is performed with the patient in the prone position under general or regional anaesthesia. The involved leg is marked by the patient with an arrow to avoid wrong-side surgery. The feet are positioned just at the edge of the operation table. The involved leg is slightly elevated by placing a small support under the lower leg (Fig. 8.2). The position of the foot is in plantarflexion through gravity. Dorsiflexion of the foot can be controlled by leaning into the plantarflexed foot with the surgeon's body, thereby still having both hands free to manipulate the arthroscope and instruments. Prior to the surgery, important anatomical structures are marked. These include the medial and lateral border of the

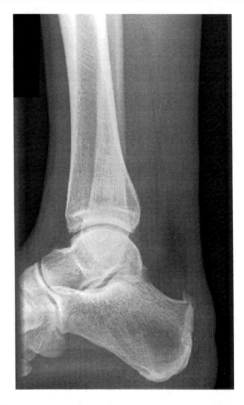

Fig. 8.1 Lateral X-ray of a right ankle in a patient with persistent posterior heel pain showing a hypertrophic posterosuperior calcaneal aspect (Haglund's syndrome)

Achilles tendon and the calcaneus. The lateral portal is situated just lateral of the Achilles tendon at the level of the superior aspect of the calcaneus. This portal is created first as a small vertical incision through the skin only. The retrocalcaneal space is penetrated by a blunt trocar. A 4.5-mm arthroscopic shaft with an inclination angle of 30° is introduced (Fig. 8.3a, b). Irrigation is performed by gravity flow or pressured flow at 100 mmHg. A 70° arthroscope can also be useful but is seldom necessary. Under direct vision, a spinal needle is introduced just medial to the Achilles tendon, again at the level of the superior aspect of the calcaneus, to locate the medial portal (Fig. 8.4a, b). After having made the medial portal by a vertical stab incision, a 5.5-mm bonecutter shaver (Dyonics Bonecutter, Smith & Nephew, Andover, MA, USA) is introduced and visualized by the arthroscope. The inflamed retrocalcaneal bursa is removed first (Fig. 8.5a, b). Next, the superior surface of the calcaneus is

Fig. 8.2 For an endo-scopic calcaneoplasty, the patient is placed in the prone position with a support in the hip (1), a tourniquet around the upper leg (2), and a small support is placed under the lower leg (3), making it possible to move the ankle freely

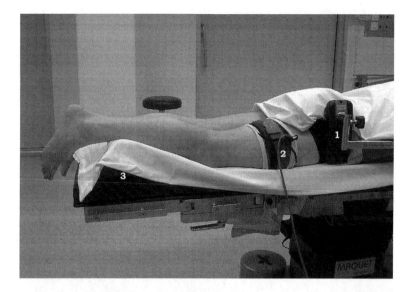

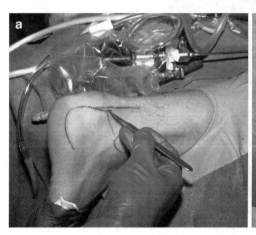
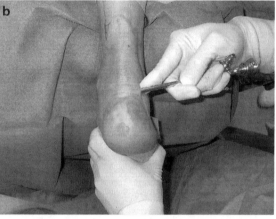

Fig. 8.3 (a) The lateral portal is situated just lateral of the Achilles tendon at the level of the superior border of the calcaneus. The important landmarks are indicated. (b) The portal is made by a vertical skin incision followed by introduction of a 4.5-mm arthroscopic shaft with an inclination angle of 30°

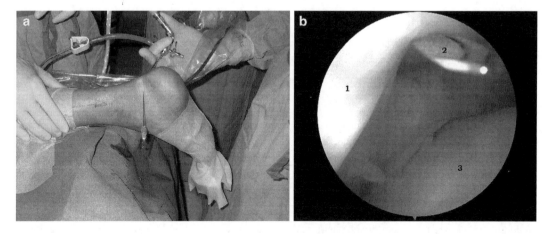

Fig. 8.4 (a) The exact position of medial portal is deter-mined with a spinal needle that approximately needs to be introduced just medial of the Achilles tendon at the superior level of the calcaneus. (b) Under direct endoscopic view, the location of the spinal needle (at the location of medial portal) is checked. *1* Achilles tendon; *2* spinal needle; *3* calcaneus

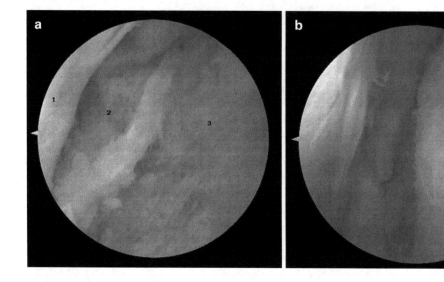

Fig. 8.5 (a) Endoscopic picture of the right ankle with the arthroscope in the posterolateral portal showing the inflamed retrocalcaneal bursa (*1* Achilles tendon; *2* inflamed retrocalcaneal bursa; *3* superior border calcaneus after partial resection). (**b**) Endoscopic picture after complete removal of the inflamed retrocalcaneal bursa with the full radius resector

visualized and its fibrous layer and periosteum are stripped off. During the resection of the bursa and the fibrous layer and periosteum of the superior aspect of the calcaneus, the full radius resector is facing the bone to avoid damage to the Achilles tendon. When the foot is brought into full dorsiflexion, impingement between the posterosuperior calcaneal edge and the Achilles tendon can be detected. The foot is subsequently brought into plantarflexion and now the posterosuperior calcaneal rim is removed. This bone is quite soft and can be removed by the aggressive synovial full radius resector or bonecutter. A burr is not needed at this point. The portals are used interchangeably for both the arthroscope and the resector, in order to remove the entire bony prominence. It is important to remove enough bone at the posteromedial and lateral corner (Fig. 8.6a, b). These edges have to be rounded off by moving the synovial resector beyond the posterior edge onto the lateral respectively medial wall of the calcaneus. The Achilles tendon is protected throughout the entire procedure by keeping the closed end of the resector against the tendon. With the foot in the fully plantarflexed position, the insertion of the Achilles tendon can be visualized.

The bonecutter is placed on the insertion against the calcaneus to smoothen this part of the calcaneus. Finally, the resector is introduced to clean up loose debris and to smooth possible rough edges (Fig. 8.6c). To prevent sinus formation, at the end of the procedure, the skin incisions are sutured with 3.0 Ethilon. The incisions and surrounding skin are injected with 10 ml of a 0.5% bupivacaine/morphine solution. A sterile compressive dressing is applied (Klinigrip, Medeco BV, Oud Bijerland, The Netherlands). Postoperatively, the patient is allowed weight bearing as tolerated and is instructed to elevate the foot when not walking. The dressing is removed 3 days postoperatively and the patient is allowed to shower. The patient is encouraged to perform active range of motion exercises for at least three times a day for 10 min each. The patient is allowed to return to regular footwear as soon as this is tolerated. Two weeks postoperatively, the stitches are removed. An X-ray is made to ensure that sufficient bone has been excised (Fig. 8.6d). With satisfaction of the surgeon and patient, no further outpatient department contact is necessary. Patients with limited range of motion are directed to a physiotherapist.

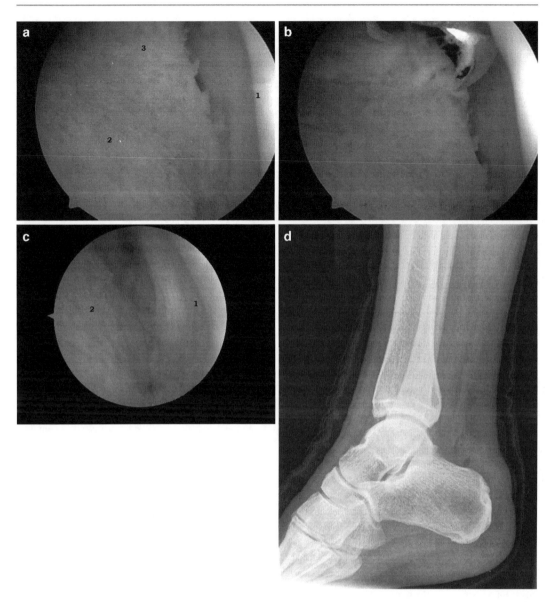

Fig. 8.6 (**a**) Endoscopic picture of the right ankle with the arthroscope in the posteromedial portal. Via the posteromedial portal, part of the bony prominence has been removed by means of a full radius resector (2). After switching portals, the bony prominence is now visualized (3) (1 Achilles tendon). (**b**) Shaver on top of the remaining bony prominence. The closed end of the resector is facing the Achilles tendon. (**c**) Situation after total resection of the bony prominence. (**d**) Postoperative lateral X-ray showing the result of the endoscopic calcaneoplasty operation of the patient presented in Fig. 8.1

Patient Outcomes

Between 1995 and 2000 in the Academic Medical Centre in Amsterdam, we performed 39 procedures in 36 patients. The average age was 35.0 years (range 16–50 years). Patients had a painful swelling of the soft tissue of the posterior heel, medial and lateral of the Achilles tendon on physical examination, without pain on palpation of the tendon itself. Conservative treatment for at least 6 months did not relieve the symptoms. The X-rays showed a superior calcaneal angle of more than 75°. The mean follow-up was 4.5 years (range 2–7.5 years). There were no surgical complications except from one patient who experienced an area of hypoaesthesia over the heel pad. Postoperatively, there were no infections, no sore or ugly scars, and all patients were happy with their small incisions. Except for two patients, all patients were improved. The Ogilvie-Harris score [17] for fair results was rated by 4 patients, 6 rated good, and 24 had an excellent result. Work and sports resumption took place at an average of 5 weeks (range 10 days–6 months) and 11 weeks (range 6 weeks to 6 months), respectively.

Discussion

Conservative therapy for retrocalcaneal bursitis includes a single cortisone injection in the retrocalcaneal bursa [14, 18, 19]. Repeated injections are not advised because these can weaken the tendon with the potential danger of a rupture. The aim of operative treatment for retrocalcaneal bursitis, after failure of the conservative treatment, is preventing impingement between the Achilles tendon and os calcis. This can be accomplished by means of removal of the inflamed retrocalcaneal bursa followed by either resection of the posterosuperior calcaneal rim or by means of a closing wedge osteotomy. Posterosuperior calcaneal resection can be performed via a posterolateral or posteromedial incision or via a combination of both [8, 11, 20].

Endoscopic calcaneoplasty offers a good, minimal invasive, alternative to open surgery. Surgeons familiar with the endoscopic approach tend to favour this procedure, because it has better visualization as compared with the open procedure. Due to an inappropriate visualization of the Achilles tendon during the open procedure, weakening or even rupture of the tendon have been reported [10, 13]. Full recovery time after the open resection can take as long as 2 years [21]. Our patient series shows a high percentage of good to excellent results based on the Ogilvie-Harris score. These results are comparable with the reports of Morag et al. [22] and Jerosch and Nasef [23]. Morag et al. treated four patients with

endoscopic calcaneoplasty and after an average follow-up of 2 years (range 1–3.5 years) no complications, pain, decrease in range of motion, or disability were reported [22]. In the report of Jerosch and Nasef in 2003, ten patients were treated with the endoscopic calcaneoplasty approach and after a mean follow-up of 5.2 months (range 2–12 months); three patients rated good results and seven excellent, based on the Ogilvie-Harris score. There were no intraoperative or postoperative complications. Full recovery lasted 2–5 weeks, except for two patients who did not follow the study protocol advising no weight bearing immediately after the surgery [23].

The advantage of the endoscopic procedure over the open procedure are the small incisions, avoiding the complications such a wound dehiscence, painful and/or ugly scars, and nerve entrapment within the scar, as was described for the open procedure by Huber et al. [9] He found a considerable amount of residual complaints in 32 clinically and radiologically examined patients treated by resection of the posterosuperior calcaneal prominence for Haglund's exostoses at a mean follow-up of 18.6 years (range 2–41 years). Fourteen of the 32 patients had soft tissue problems including excessive scar formation and persistent swelling. In eight patients, not enough bone was excised and two had new bone formation, both resulting in persistent painful swelling. The function of the Achilles tendon was disturbed in eight patients [9].

There is no consensus regarding the ideal surgical approach, medial, lateral, or both [8, 11, 24]. Jones and James performed ten partial calcaneal ostectomies for retrocalcaneal bursitis followed by a short walking cast and rehabilitation period for aftertreatment. All patients were back to their desired level of activity within 6 months [24]. Angermann operated on 40 heels for the same indication using the posterolateral approach in 32 patients. Postoperatively, 29 patients were allowed immediate weight bearing. Complications consisted of one superficial heel infection, one haematoma, and two patients with delayed skin healing. At an average follow-up of 6 years (range 1–12 years) 50% of the patients were cured, 20% improved, 20 remained unchanged, and in 10%

the preoperative symptoms worsened [8]. The rate of poor results in this study corresponds to the results of Taylor, who reported 36% poor results after the same type of surgery [25]. Pauker et al. operated 28 heels in 22 patients with Haglund's disease. All patients received a walking cast for 4 weeks followed by mobilization exercises for aftertreatment. At a mean follow-up of 13 years in 19 patients (range 3–20 years), 15 had a good result, 2 fair, and 2 poor. The authors advocate using one incision, because many patients have complaints of tenderness over the operative scar up to 1 year postoperatively, which might be exaggerated by a more extensive approach [11]. In a study of Schepsis et al., 24 patients with retrocalcaneal bursitis 6 (25%) had a fair result requiring reoperation [26]. In the study of Schneider, 49 heels were operated from a consecutive group of 36 patients with a mean follow-up of 4.7 years (range 1–11 years). Early complications were reported in four cases (haematomas and a superficial infection) and late complications resulting in revision surgery in three cases. Seven patients noted some improvement, one patient described no change, and seven patients reported worsening of their symptoms after surgery [27]. Brunner et al. operated on 39 heels from 36 patients and reported at an average follow-up of 51 months, with an average improvement of the AOFAS score of 32 points as compared with the mean preoperative score. Recovery time took up from 6 months to 2 years. Six of the 36 patients reported persistent posterior heel pain after surgery [21].

Because no consensus exists whether Haglund's deformity needs to be treated by endoscopy or by an open procedure, comparative studies were done. Leitze et al. compared the endoscopic approach ($n=30$; 22 months follow-up) with the open surgical technique ($n=17$; 42 months follow-up). The endoscopic approach revealed 19 excellent, 5 good, 3 fair, and 3 poor results, which was numerically but not significantly better than the open surgical procedure. The recovery time was identical, nevertheless the operation time and the amounts of complications and scar tissue favorite the endoscopic approach [28]. In the recent study of Lohrer et al. a comparison was made between the endoscopic and open resection for Haglund's disease. In this anatomic study, nine cadaver feet were operated on by means of open surgery and six were operated on with endoscopic calcaneoplasty. After the procedure, the feet were dissected to determine the amount of damage after surgery. Comparable amounts of damage were found for the sural nerve, the plantaris tendon, and the medial column of the Achilles tendon [29]. Since this is an anatomic study, no data could be gathered regarding recovery time and scar healing, which seems to be the advantage points of the endoscopic procedure. In addition, the cadaver feet could have been stiffer as compared with patients, which makes the endoscopic approach more difficult to perform.

In summary, whether the operation is performed by endoscopic or open surgery, enough bone has to be removed to prevent impingement between the calcaneus and Achilles tendon. The endoscopic calcaneoplasty has demonstrated to show several advantages including low morbidity, functional aftertreatment, outpatient treatment, excellent scar healing, a short recovery time, and quick sports resumption as compared with the results for the open technique.

References

1. Haglund P. Beitrag zur Klinik der Achillessehne. Zeitschr Orthop Chir 1928;49:49–58
2. Dickinson PH, Coutts MB, Woodward EP, Handler D. Tendo Achillis bursitis. Report of twenty-one cases. J Bone Joint Surg Am 1966;48(1):77–81
3. Fowler A., Philip JF. Abnormalities of the calcaneus as a cause of painful heel: Its diagnosis and operative treatment. Br J Surg 1945;32:494–498
4. NISBET NW. Tendo Achillis bursitis (winter heel). Br Med J 1954;2(4901):1394–1395
5. Clain MR, Baxter DE. Achilles tendinitis. Foot Ankle 1992;13(8):482–487
6. Saltzman CL, Tearse DS. Achilles tendon injuries. J Am Acad Orthop Surg 1998;6(5):316–325
7. Fuglsang F, Torup D. Bursitis retrocalcanearis. Acta Orthop Scand 1961;30:315–323
8. Angermann P. Chronic retrocalcaneal bursitis treated by resection of the calcaneus. Foot Ankle 1990;10(5):285–287
9. Huber HM, Waldis M. [The Haglund exostosis - a surgical indication and a minor intervention?]. Z Orthop Ihre Grenzgeb 1989;127(3):286–290

10. Miller AE, Vogel TA. Haglund's deformity and the Keck and Kelly osteotomy: a retrospective analysis. J Foot Surg 1989;28(1):23–29

11. Pauker M, Katz K, Yosipovitch Z. Calcaneal ostectomy for Haglund disease. J Foot Surg 1992;31(6): 588–589

12. Leach RE, DiIorio E, Harney RA. Pathologic hindfoot conditions in the athlete. Clin Orthop Relat Res 1983; (177):116–121

13. Le TA, Joseph PM. Common exostectomies of the rearfoot. Clin Podiatr Med Surg 1991;8(3):601–623

14. Nesse E, Finsen V. Poor results after resection for Haglund's heel. Analysis of 35 heels in 23 patients after 3 years. Acta Orthop Scand 1994;65(1):107–109

15. Segesser B, Goesele A, Renggli P. [The Achilles tendon in sports]. Orthopade 1995;24(3):252–267

16. van Dijk CN, van Dyk GE, Scholten PE, Kort NP. Endoscopic calcaneoplasty. Am J Sports Med 2001; 29(2):185–189

17. Ogilvie-Harris DJ, Mahomed N, Demaziere A. Anterior impingement of the ankle treated by arthroscopic removal of bony spurs. J Bone Joint Surg Br 1993;75(3):437–440

18. Myerson MS, McGarvey W. Disorders of the Achilles tendon insertion and Achilles tendinitis. Instr Course Lect 1999;48:211–218

19. Subotnick SI, Block AJ. Retrocalcaneal problems. Clin Podiatr Med Surg 1990;7(2):323–332

20. Kolodziej P, Glisson RR, Nunley JA. Risk of avulsion of the Achilles tendon after partial excision for treatment of insertional tendonitis and Haglund's

21. Brunner J, Anderson J, O'Malley M, Bohne W, Deland J, Kennedy J. Physician and patient based outcomes following surgical resection of Haglund's deformity. Acta Orthop Belg 2005;71(6):718–723

22. Morag G, Maman E, Arbel R. Endoscopic treatment of hindfoot pathology. Arthroscopy 2003;19(2):E13

23. Jerosch J, Nasef NM. Endoscopic calcaneoplasty – rationale, surgical technique, and early results: a preliminary report. Knee Surg Sports Traumatol Arthrosc 2003;11(3):190–195

24. Jones DC, James SL. Partial calcaneal ostectomy for retrocalcaneal bursitis. Am J Sports Med 1984; 12(1):72–73

25. Taylor GJ. Prominence of the calcaneus: is operation justified? J Bone Joint Surg Br 1986;68(3):467–470

26. Schepsis AA, Wagner C, Leach RE. Surgical management of Achilles tendon overuse injuries. A long-term follow-up study. Am J Sports Med 1994;22(5):611–619

27. Schneider W, Niehus W, Knahr K. Haglund's syndrome: disappointing results following surgery – a clinical and radiographic analysis. Foot Ankle Int 2000;21(1):26–30

28. Leitze Z, Sella EJ, Aversa JM. Endoscopic decompression of the retrocalcaneal space. J Bone Joint Surg Am 2003;85-A(8):1488–1496

29. Lohrer H, Nauck T, Dorn NV, Konerding MA. Comparison of endoscopic and open resection for haglund tuberosity in a cadaver study. Foot Ankle Int 2006;27(6):445–450

deformity: a biomechanical study. Foot Ankle Int 1999;20(7):433–437

Arthroscopy of the First Metatarsophalangeal Joint

9

Nicholas Savva and Terry Saxby

Attempts to arthroscope small joints in the 1930s failed due to the disparity in size between the arthroscope and joint. In 1968, a new light-emitting material known as Selfoc was developed jointly by the Nippon Sheet Glass Company, Osaka and the Nippon Electrical Company, Tokyo. In 1970, the Selfoc arthroscope was developed for arthroscopy of small joints by Watanabe using a Selfoc glass rod. The gauge of the scope was 1.7 mm and the outer diameter of the sheath was 2 mm. The first report of arthroscopy of the first metatarsophalangeal (MTP) joint was by Watanabe reporting on five cases in his book titled *Atlas of Arthroscopy* published in 1972 [1].

Anatomy

The first MTP joint is a ball and socket joint, which gains little support from its shallow articulation. The major stabilising elements are the capsule and the medial and lateral collateral ligaments. Abductor and adductor hallucis and the short flexor and extensor tendons contribute to stability. Most of the stabilizing structures are on the plantar aspect making the dorsum the obvious choice for portal placement. The dominant landmark on the dorsum is the extensor hallucis longus (EHL) (Fig. 9.1).

The metatarsal head has the central crista on its plantar surface. Both tendons of flexor hallucis

brevis contain a sesamoid bone, which sit either side of the crista. The tendons then go on to insert into the base of the proximal phalanx as well as sending fibres to the thick plantar plate. The flexor hallucis longus is both superficial to the plantar plate and between the two heads of the flexor hallucis brevis as it passes distally to insert into the distal phalanx.

Structures most at risk during arthroscopy are cutaneous nerves, principally the dorsomedial branch of superficial peroneal, which provides much of sensation of hallux. It passes 6–18 mm medial to the EHL at the level of the joint [2]. The plantar aspect is supplied by the digital nerves, which are branches of the medial plantar nerve. These lie just plantar to the collateral ligaments and superficial to the transverse metatarsal ligament on the lateral side.

Arthroscopic Anatomy

Ferkel has described a systematic sequential examination of the MTP joint starting laterally and progressing medially [3]. He developed a 13-point examination through the dorsolateral portal. The structures of the plantar surface, including the sesamoids as well as the centre of the metatarsal head may be better visualised through the dorsomedial or direct medial portal.

1. Lateral gutter
2. Lateral corner of metatarsal head
3. Central portion of metatarsal head
4. Medial corner of metatarsal head

N. Savva • T. Saxby (✉)
Brisbane Private Hospital, Brisbane, Australia

G.R. Scuderi and A.J. Tria (eds.), *Minimally Invasive Surgery in Orthopedics: Foot and Ankle Handbook*,
DOI 10.1007/978-1-4614-0893-2_9, © Springer Science+Business Media, LLC 2012

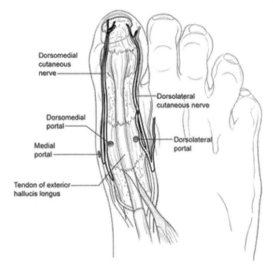

Fig. 9.1 Dorsal view of portals. Note the relative position of portals to the extensor hallucis longus tendon and the neurovascular structures

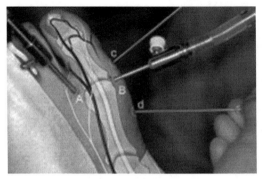

Fig. 9.2 The 1.9-mm 30° arthroscope and finger trap

assisted arthrodesis has also been described, although it was noted to be time consuming and technically difficult [5, 6]. Arthroscopic excision of the medial and lateral sesamoids has also been described but may require extra portals or a small arthrotomy [7–9].

5. Medial gutter
6. Medial capsular reflection
7. Central bare area
8. Lateral capsular reflection
9. Medial portion of proximal phalanx
10. Central portion of proximal phalanx
11. Lateral portion of proximal phalanx
12. Medial sesamoids
13. Lateral sesamoid

Equipment

Because of the small size of the joint, a small arthroscope is required (Fig. 9.2). Ideally, a short 1.9-mm arthroscope with a 30° oblique viewing lens is used. Great care should be taken because this is a very fragile instrument. If this is not available, a 2.7-mm scope is acceptable but much more difficult to manoeuvre.

Shoulder traction system
Thigh tourniquet
Sterile finger trap
1.9-mm 30° arthroscope
Small joint shaver system
2-mm probe
2-mm curette
Small joint grasper
Two 23-gauge needles
10-cc syringe

Indications

Plain radiographs, bone scans, and computed tomography (CT) scans are all useful investigations in the diagnosis of first MTP joint pathology. Magnetic resonance imaging (MRI) of the first MTP joint has improved considerably in the last 10 years, rendering diagnostic arthroscopy almost obsolete. However, a diagnostic arthroscopy may be performed if persistent pain, swelling, stiffness, and locking or grinding symptoms continue despite conservative treatment. Therapeutic indications include treatment of chondromalacia, synovitis, osteochondral lesions, osteophytes, loose bodies, and arthrofibrosis. More recently, cheilectomy has been described for hallux rigidus [4]. The technique of arthroscopically

Portals

Three portals are commonly used to visualise the joint (Fig. 9.1). The dorsomedial portal is placed just medial to the tendon of EHL at the level of the joint. This is placed close to the tendon to

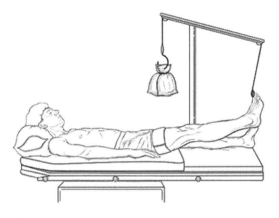

Fig. 9.3 Patient on an operating table with a tourniquet in place and great toe suspended from finger trap. A suspension gantry is fixed to the opposite side of the operating table

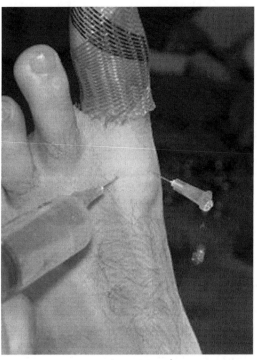

Fig. 9.4 Two 23-gauge needles, correctly placed intraarticularly, demonstrated by the free flow of normal saline

avoid injury to the dorsomedial branch of the superficial peroneal nerve. The dorsolateral portal is placed just lateral to the tendon of EHL and the medial portal, midway between the dorsal and plantar aspects of the joint. This can be done under direct vision if necessary.

Technique

Arthroscopy of the first MTP joint can be carried out under general, spinal, epidural, or local anaesthesia. The patient is placed supine on the operating table and with skin preparation applied to the level of the knee with standard draping. Distraction is helpful to allow full visualisation, although manual traction has been reported as being adequate to visualise the whole joint. A sterile finger trap is applied to the great toe and a pulley system rigged over the shoulder traction system. Two to three kilograms of traction is usually ample to allow full visualisation of the joint (Fig. 9.3). A 23-gauge needle is inserted into the joint just medial to the tendon of EHL at the level of the joint. The joint is then distended with normal saline. A second needle is then placed into the joint just lateral to the tendon of EHL at the level of the joint. When free flow has been established (Fig. 9.4), longitudinal incisions are made through the skin only using a #15 blade. Small artery forceps are then used to spread soft tissues

and identify the capsule. This minimises risk of injury to neurovascular structures, in particular, the dorsomedial cutaneous nerve close to the dorsomedial portal. The capsule is penetrated through either portal using a 2-mm cannula with a blunt-tipped obturator and the arthroscope is introduced. A 2-mm probe is inserted through the other dorsal portal. The medial portal can be made under direct vision to ensure correct placement, which is helpful to view the plantar structures and also to avoid injury to the digital nerve. Arthroscope and instruments are swapped around the portals during the procedure to aid visualisation and allow access to pathology (Fig. 9.5).

After the procedure is completed, the joint is washed out, instilled with local anaesthetic, and the wounds closed with 4–0 nylon sutures. A bulky dressing is applied. Postoperatively, the patient is encouraged to elevate the limb to reduce swelling and the risk of infection. Patients are allowed to mobilise in a stiff-soled shoe until approximately 10 days, when the wound is reviewed and sutures removed. Mobilisation then depends upon the

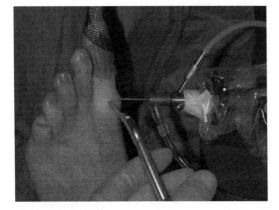

Fig. 9.5 Arthroscope and instrument successfully placed into the joint

pathology treated. If a fusion has been undertaken, then the patient is mobilised in the shoe for a further 4–5 weeks, otherwise range of motion and strengthening exercises are started as comfort allows.

Results

The first report of arthroscopy of the first MTP joint was by Watanabe reporting on five cases in his book titled *Atlas of Arthroscopy* published in 1972 [1]. The results of the first series of 22 arthroscopies of the first MTP joint were reported by Watanabe in his book *Equipment and Procedures of Small Joint Arthroscopy* published in 1986 [10]. In the same year, Yovich and McIlwraith reported arthroscopic debridement of osteochondral defects in the MTP joint of the horse [11]. In 1988, Bartlett described debridement of an osteochondral lesion of the first MTP joint in an adolescent that allowed return to sport and complete resolution of symptoms at 1 year [12]. Since these first reports, there have been four case series reported and numerous case reports.

In his book titled *Arthroscopic Surgery: The Foot and Ankle* published in 1996, Ferkel described the technique and indications of first MTP joint arthroscopy [3]. He also reported on 22 patients who underwent the procedure with

follow-up at a mean of 54 months. The following pathologies were identified.

Degenerative joint disease	5
Arthrofibrosis	4
Synovitis	3
Osteophytes	3
Osteochondral lesions of the metatarsal	3
Loose bodies	2
Chondromalacia	2

Good results were found in 73% of patients, with the remainder going on to arthrodesis. For most patients who had a limited movement preoperatively, the range of motion was improved by surgery. There were no specific complications.

In 1987, Iqbal and Chana reported on 15 patients, with a mean follow-up of 9.4 months, who underwent arthroscopic cheilectomy for hallux rigidus [4]. All patients were at least satisfied with the outcome with complete resolution of pain in two thirds of the patients. Return to nonathletic activity at an average of 3.7 weeks shows an advantage over the open technique, but a mean postoperative range of movement of 47.6° is less than might be expected after an open procedure. In some cases, an inferomedial portal was required to fully access the osteophyte. It was also noted that distraction was not beneficial because this tightened the dorsal capsule over the osteophyte, making its excision more difficult. There were no complications in this series.

In 1998, van Dijk et al. published their review of 25 first MTP joint arthroscopies at a mean of 2 years [9]. Twelve procedures were performed for dorsal impingement with removal of the dorsal osteophyte arthroscopically, of which eight had a good or excellent result. Three of four patients treated for osteochondritis dissecans by debridement of the lesion and removal of loose bodies had good or excellent results. Treatment of hallux rigidus by debridement of osteophytes was less successful. Five patients had sesamoid pathology warranting excision, of which, three gained good or excellent results. Two extra portals were necessary, one proximal and in the

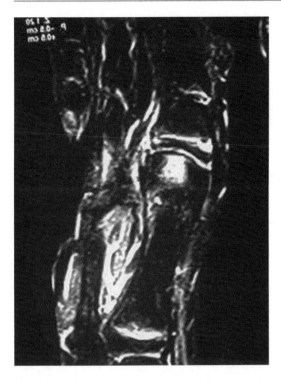

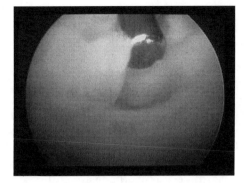

Fig. 9.7 Intraoperative photograph of an osteochondral lesion of the metatarsal head (From Davies and Saxby [13], by permission of J Bone Joint Surg (Br))

Fig. 9.6 MRI scan of an osteochondral lesion of the metatarsal head

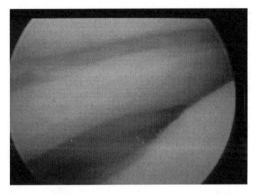

Fig. 9.8 Meniscoid lesion (From Davies and Saxby [13], by permission of J Bone Joint Surg (Br))

medial midline and one in the first dorsal web space. Two patients had the lateral sesamoid removed arthroscopically but a small separate incision was required to remove the medial sesamoids in three patients. Overall in this series, one patient suffered transient loss of sensation on the medial aspect of the hallux and one other patient on the lateral side, which continued to follow-up.

In the author's series of 12 arthroscopies in 11 patients, 6 patients had suffered an injury [13]. In six patients, there was no radiological abnormality detected on plain radiography but isotope, CT, and MRI bone scans were helpful in some cases. The true diagnosis was only established at arthroscopy in some cases. At arthroscopy, seven joints were noted to have synovitis, including one case of pigmented villonodular synovitis (PVNS). A chondral lesion was noted in four cases and an osteochondral lesion of the metatarsal head was found in four joints (Figs. 9.6 and 9.7). There was one dorsal osteophyte, one proximal phalangeal cyst, one loose body, and one meniscoid lesion

(Fig. 9.8). The latter lesion was thought to be a condensation of fibrous tissue akin to the soft tissue lesion in the ankle described by Wolin et al. [14]. All pathologies were dealt with arthroscopically at the time. In three cases, a small arthrotomy was required to complete the surgical procedure. In one case, early on in the series, an arthrotomy was performed to exclude other pathology, none was found. On another occasion, an arthrotomy was performed due to equipment failure and on another to complete an extensive synovectomy. Apart from a minor wound infection, there were no complications relating to surgery. At a mean of 19.3 months, all patients had minimal or no pain with an increased range of movement. The one patient who had residual stiffness was known to have degenerative joint disease and had fractured a dorsal osteophyte.

Arthroscopy of the first MTP joint has a small but well-defined role in the armamentarium of the foot surgeon. It is indicated in patients with persistent pain, swelling, stiffness, and locking or grinding symptoms despite conservative measures and in whom the diagnosis is not clear. It can be used to treat multiple pathologies including chondromalacia, synovitis, osteochondral lesions, osteophytes, loose bodies, and arthrofibrosis, particularly in those whose symptoms do not warrant arthrodesis or arthroplasty. Arthroscopic arthrodesis and cheilectomy for hallux rigidus have been demonstrated to be effective but technically demanding procedures, but have yet to demonstrate any significant advantage over the open procedure. Dealing with sesamoid pathology is also technically demanding and may require extra portals.

References

1. Watanabe M, Takeda S, Ikeuchi H. Atlas of Arthroscopy, 2nd edition. Igakui-Shoin, Tokyo, 1969
2. Solan MC, Lemon M, Bendall PS. The surgical anatomy of the dorsomedial cutaneous nerve of the hallus. J Bone Joint Surg Br 2001;83B:250–252
3. Ferkel RD. Arthroscopic Surgery. The Foot and Ankle. Lippincott-Raven, Philadelphia. 1996
4. Iqbal MJ, Chana GS. Arthroscopic cheilectomy for hallux rigidus. J Arthrosc Relat Surg 1998;14:307–310
5. Perez-Carro L, Busta-Vallina B. Arthroscopic-assisted first metatarsophalangeal joint arthrodesis. J Arthrosc Relat Surg 1999;15:215–217
6. Stroud CC. Arthroscopic arthrodesis of the ankle, subtalar, and first metatarsophalangeal joint. Foot Ankle Clin N Am 2002;7:135–146
7. Chan PK, Lui TH. Arthroscopic fibular sesamoidectomy in the management of the sesamoid osteomyelitis. Knee Surg Sports Traumatol Arthrosc 2005;14:1–4
8. Perez Carro L, Escevarria Llata JI, Martinez Agueros JA. Arthroscopic medial bipartite sesamoidectomy of the great toe. J Arthrosc Relat Surg 1999;15:321–323
9. van Dijk CN, Veenstra KM, Nuesch BC. Arthroscopic surgery of the metatarsophalangeal first joint. J Arthrosc Relat Surg 1998;14:851–855
10. Watanabe M, Ito K, Fuji S. Equipment and procedures of small joint arthroscopy. In: Watanabe M (ed.) Arthroscopy of Small Joints. Igakui-Shoin, Tokyo. 1986
11. Yovich JV, McIlwraith CW. Arthroscopic surgery for osteochondral fractures of the proximal phalanx o the metacarpophalangeal and metatarsophalangeal fetlock) joints in horses. J Am Vet Med Assoc 1986; 188:273–279
12. Bartlett DH. Arthroscopic management of osteochondritis of the first metatarsal head. Arthroscopy 1988;4:51–54
13. Davies MS, Saxby TS. Arthrosopy of the first metatarsophalangeal joint. J Bone Joint Surg Br 1999; 81B:203–206
14. Wolin J, Glassman F, Sideman S. Internal derangement of the talofibular component of the ankle. Surg Gynaecol Obstet 1950;91:193–200

Arthroscopic Management of Disorders of the First Metatarsal–Phalangeal Joint

10

A.C. Stroïnk and C.N. van Dijk

Arthroscopic surgery is one of the basic types of procedures in orthopaedic surgery. In the 1980s, there was a drift toward performing arthroscopic procedures on smaller joints [1–4]. Although nowadays arthroscopic surgery of the knee, shoulder, elbow, ankle, and wrist have become routine procedures, arthroscopy of the first metatarsophalangeal (MTP-I) joint has received scant attention [5] and has scarcely been reported in articles. Watanabe [1] was the first to describe an arthroscopic procedure of the big toe in 1986. In 1999, Frey et al. [6] reported that arthroscopic surgery of the MTP-I was still a developing procedure with a grey area for application. We published our first 27 MTP-I joint arthroscopic procedures in 1998, and, in a further publication, we reported the most important indications: osteochondral defect, dorsal impingement, and infectious arthritis [7]. Currently, we lack evidence based on long-term follow-up studies on arthroscopic surgery of the MTP-I joint. After all these years, the procedure is still considered investigational. Although the arthroscopic procedure of the MTP-I joint is technically feasible and amenable for arthroscopy, the procedure is dependent on the skills of the surgeon. In this chapter, we describe the basic anatomy of the joint, the indication, the arthroscopic procedure, and the outcome.

Anatomy

Marked variations occur in the skin and the subcutaneous tissue of the foot. The skin on the dorsal side is less sensitive and much thinner in comparison with the plantar side. The majority of the stability of the MTP-I joint is obtained by the soft tissues surrounding the joint, such as the capsule, the ligaments, and the musculotendinous structures. A minor stability contribution is obtained from the shallow ball of the distal metatarsal head and the socket form of the proximal phalanx [6]. From the dorsal view of the joint, the extensor hallucis longus tendon divides the joint into a medial and a lateral part. The medial part of the joint is innervated by branches of the superficial peroneal nerve and the lateral part of the joint by the deep peroneal nerve. The medial side of the great toe is innervated by the terminal branches of the saphenous nerve. The plantar blood supply is from the medial and lateral plantar artery, which are branches of the posterior tibial artery. They form anastomoses with the vessels from the dorsal side, which have their origin from the dorsalis pedis artery.

The MTP-I joint has two sesamoid bones at the plantar side, which are situated on the medial and lateral side of the flexor hallucis brevis

A.C. Stroïnk • C.N. van Dijk (✉)
Department of Orthopaedic Surgery,
Academic Medical Center, University of Amsterdam,
Amsterdam, The Netherlands
e-mail: m.lammerts@amc.uva.nl

G.R. Scuderi and A.J. Tria (eds.), *Minimally Invasive Surgery in Orthopedics: Foot and Ankle Handbook*,
DOI 10.1007/978-1-4614-0893-2_10, © Springer Science+Business Media, LLC 2012

Table 10.1 Indications for arthroscopy of the MTP-I joint

Dorsal osteophytes
Hallux limitus
Hallux rigidus
Osteochondritis dissecans/chondromalacia
Corpora libera
Impingement syndrome
Pathology of the sesamoid bone
Inflammation/infection
Arthritis
Synovitis
Diagnostic procedure

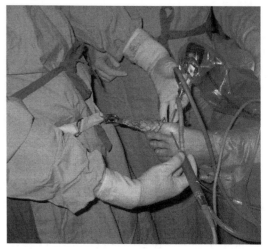

Fig. 10.1 Position during surgery

tendon. The fibres of this tendon are subsequently attached to the plantar plate and the proximal part of the proximal phalanx. The superficial tendon of the hallucis longus tendon is situated between the two tendons of the flexor hallucis brevis.

Indications

Along with the development of the arthroscopic technique and the instrumentation of the arthroscopic equipment, it is important to understand the relative advantage of the arthroscopic surgery of the MTP-I joint; meanwhile, it should be kept in mind that arthroscopic surgery is a patient-centred procedure.

Open surgery of the first metatarsophalangeal joint can result in restriction of range of motion, prolonged swelling, poor wound healing, and difficulties finding footwear [6]. The arthroscopic approach results in a good intraarticular visualization, minimal surgical joint trauma, and minimal soft tissue dissection, with excellent cosmetic and functional results [7, 8]. Another advantage of the arthroscopic procedure is a faster rehabilitation to sports and work. The indications of the arthroscopic procedure of the MTP-I joint are listed in Table 10.1. For pathology of the medial sesamoid bone, the arthroscopic procedure of the MTP-I joint does not have any great advantages compared with the more conservative techniques.

Operative Technique

The arthroscopic procedure can be performed under spinal, general, or regional anaesthesia, using a tourniquet at the homolateral thigh. The patient is placed in the operating room in the supine position with the heel resting on the edge of the operation table [7]. To improve the joint space and to give the best direction of traction, a sterile finger trap is placed on the first toe and connected to the belt of the surgeon (Fig. 10.1).

For the majority of procedures, enough working space is created with two main portals; a dorsolateral portal and a dorsomedial portal, these accessory portals are placed at the level of the joint line on either side of the extensor hallucis longus tendon [7].

A complete overview of the first metatarsophalangeal joint is attained by the insertion of two extra portals, the true medial portal and the proximal plantar portal, which are placed at the joint line midway between the dorsal and plantar side of the foot. The proximal plantar portal is placed 4 cm proximal to the joint line in between the flexor hallucis brevis and the flexor hallucis longus (Fig. 10.2).

The operation starts by placing the dorsomedial portal, just medial from the extensor hallucis longus tendon. Before placing the portals, a 4-mm

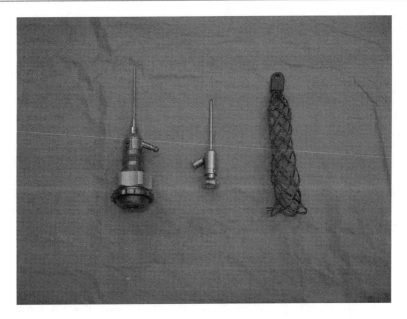

Fig. 10.2 Insertion of the two main portals (**a, b**) and the two extra portals (**c, d**). (**a**) dorsomedial portal; (**b**) dorsolateral portal; (**c**) true medial portal; (**d**) proximal plantar

longitudinal, through the skin only, stab incision is made. To prevent neurovascular injury, especially of the medial dorsal cutaneous branch of the superficial peroneal nerve, the subcutaneous layer is divided by a haemostat until the capsule is identified.

The 2.7-mm shaft with blunt trocar is introduced into the joint, followed by the 2.7-mm arthroscope with a 30° inclination angle. The joint is distended with saline. The clarity can be enhanced by a high-flow system of normal saline. After achieving visualisation of the joint, the remaining portals can be introduced by using a spinal needle under direct vision.

The working instruments are situated in the dorsomedial portal and the arthroscopic examination is performed through the dorsolateral portal. The nine major areas that should be inspected are the lateral and medial gutter; the lateral and medial corner and the central portion of the metatarsal head; the medial, central, and lateral portion of the proximal phalanx; and the medial sesamoid bone. For inspection of the lateral sesamoid bone, the two additional portals are necessary. A basic list of required instruments is listed in Table 10.2.

Table 10.2 List of required equipment for arthroscopy of the first metatarsophalangeal joint

2.7-mm arthroscope (30°)
Blunt trocar
Blade (No. 11)
Haemostat
Mosquito clamp
Shaver system
Acromionizer
Spinal needle
Thigh/ankle tourniquet
Sterile finger trap
Belt
Saline

A dorsal osteophyte of the metatarsal head is best visualized by bringing the MTP-I joint into dorsal flexion. Subsequently, they can be removed, working from distal to proximal and from medial to lateral, by the abrader, shaver, or a small acromionizer. To improve the range of motion, up to one third of the articular surface can be eliminated [6]. Before removing the osteophyte, the finger trap should be unstressed to prevent the capsule from pulling against the osteophyte [6]. In case of a large osteophyte, it is

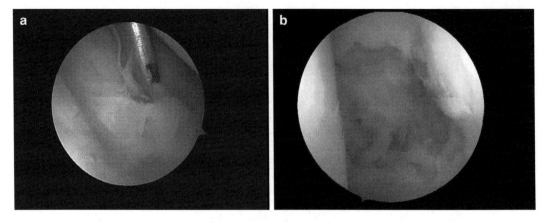

Fig. 10.3 Osteochondritis dissecans of the basis from the proximal phalanx of the first digit. Before (**a**) and after (**b**) debridement

recommended to convert the operation to an open cheilectomy.

The arthroscopic cheilectomy can be performed through the two main portals. In the presentation of osteochondritis dissecans or a corpora libra, the defect is curetted and debrided until a bleeding surface is exposed; subsequently, the loose fragments are removed (Fig. 10.3). When the lateral sesamoid bone needs to be resected, the two additional portals, as described above, are mandatory.

In case of an infection of the MTP-I joint, the arthroscopic procedure allows differentiation between arthritis, synovitis, and osteitis; material for culture should be collected. The infected synovia will be treated by a shaver or a whisker. When arthritis is present, drainage through the system should be performed, whereupon the joint should be rinsed with saline.

A diagnostic arthroscopic procedure of the MTP-I joint is indicated in the following situations: presentation of recurrent inflammatory symptoms, with locking complaints, which have failed to respond to any conservative treatment; [6] or appearance of swelling, persistent pain, and a reduced range of motion without any improvement after conservative treatment in patients who are classified as "too good" for arthrodesis or arthroplasty [5].

After the procedure, the small portal wounds are closed with 4/0 nylon sutures, which can be removed 10–14 days after the operation. To prevent formation of fistula, a bulky dressing is placed for 4–7 days and the patient is given two elbow crutches. Normal shoe wearing is resumed as comfort and swelling allows [5]. After removing a dorsal osteophyte, the patient starts flexion–extension exercises immediately after the operation, and weight bearing is permitted 5 days after surgery [6]. After debridement of the joint, the range of motion exercises are started 5 days after the operation and the patient is allowed full weight bearing 14 days after the intervention.

Complications

Similar to other arthroscopic operations, the arthroscopic procedure of the MTP-I joint can be complicated by an infection or a fistula formation. However, the most specific complication is a (transient) loss of sensation on the medial or lateral side of the first toe, induced by neurapraxia or compression of the peroneus profundus nerve [5].

Results

We performed 27 arthroscopic procedures [7, 9], concluding that the main diagnosis for this procedure are: osteochondritis dissecans, infectious arthritis, dorsal impingement syndrome, and removal of pathologic sesamoid bone. For patients with a dorsal impingement syndrome, the arthroscopic procedure gives good relief of symptoms and increased range of motion.

In 1998, Iqbal et al. [10] compared 15 patients with an arthroscopic cheilectomy with previous results from the open procedure. Their main outcomes were the recurrence rate of exostosis, which was 10% in the open procedure, compared with none in their arthroscopic cheilectomy series.

Compared with the arthrotomy, an arthroscopic approach provides a better assessment of the intraarticular conditions of the MTP-I joint [8]. However, the open procedure causes more extensive soft tissue dissection and disruption of ligamentous and tendinous structures around the sesamoid bones, which may result in hallux varus and cock-up deformity [8].

Other chief advantages of the arthroscopic procedure is the shorter revalidation period with a faster resumption of sports and work; [9, 10] excision methods appear to allow a shorter hospitalisation, less postoperative pain and stiffness, and a better cosmetic result [7].

Discussion

Arthroscopy of the MTP-I gives an excellent view of the joint. The main indications are treatment of osteochondritis dissecans, removal of loose bodies, and removal of dorsal osteophytes in cases of dorsal impingement syndrome. Intraarticular evaluation in patients with persistent pain and swelling despite conservative therapy is another indication for performing a diagnostic procedure (recurrent inflammatory symptoms and locking complaints, failure of conservative treatment; persistent swelling and reduced range of motion) [5].

MTP-I arthroscopy has not yet had the attention it deserves; when performed for the correct indication, it is just as rewarding as for the ankle, knee, and shoulder joints. Technically, the procedure is limited only by the skills of the surgeon, the pathology, and the available instrumentation. As a result of the smaller operation incisions with a smaller chance of scar fibrosis, the range of motion in the MTP-I joint is less affected by the procedure. Thus the MTP-I arthroscopy has an added value, especially for athletes and dancers whose performances are dependent on their range of motion from their great toe [9].

References

1. Watanabe M, Ito K, Fuji. Equipment and procedures of small join arthroscopy. In: Watanbe M, editor. Arthroscopy of small joints. NewYork: Igaku-Shoin, 1986
2. Lundeen R. Arthroscopic approaches to the joints of the foot. J Am Podiatr Med Assoc 1987;77:41–55
3. Richard O, Lundeen D. Review of diagnostic arthroscopy of the foot and ankle. J Foot Surg 1987;26:33–36
4. Bartlett M. Arthroscopic management of osteochondritis dissecans of the first metatarsal head. Arthroscopy 1988;4:51–54
5. Davies M, Saxby T. Arthroscopy of the first metatarsophalangeal joint. J Bone Joint Surg 1999; 81-B:203–06
6. Frey C, Van Dijk C. Arthroscopy of the great toe. AAOS Instr Course Lect 1999;48:343–346
7. Van Dijk C. Arthroscopy of the first metatarsophalangeal joint. In: James F, Serge Parisien J, Melbourne D, eds. Foot and ankle arthroscopy. New York: Springer, 2004:207–14
8. Chan K, Lui T. Arthroscopic fibular sesamoidectomy in the management of the sesamoid osteomyelitis. Knee Surg Sports Traumatol Arthrosc 2006; 14:664–67
9. Van Dijk C, Kirsten M, Veenstra M. Arthroscopic surgery of the metatarsophalangeal first joint. Arthroscopy 1998;14:851–55
10. Iqbal M, Gursharan S, Chana F. Arthroscopic cheilectomy for hallux rigidus. Arthroscopy 1998; 14:307–10

Steven L. Shapiro

Plantar fasciitis is the most common cause of heel pain in adults. The predominant symptom is pain in the plantar region of the foot when initiating walking. The etiology is a degenerative tear of part of the fascial origin from the calcaneus, followed by a tendinosis-type reaction.

Anatomy

The plantar fascia is a ligament with longitudinal fibers attaching to the calcaneal tuberosity. The normal medial band is the thickest, measuring up to 3 mm. The central and lateral bands measure 1–2 mm in thickness [1]. Distally, the plantar fascia divides into five slips, one for each toe. The plantar fascia provides support to the arch. As the toes extend during the stance phase of gait, the plantar fascia is tightened by a windlass mechanism, resulting in elevation of the longitudinal arch, inversion of the hindfoot, and external rotation of the leg. Endoscopically, the pertinent anatomy is the abductor hallucis muscle medially, then the plantar fascia. After fasciotomy, the flexor digitorum brevis comes into view as well as the medial intermuscular septum.

Pathogenesis

Specimens of plantar fascia obtained during surgery reveal a spectrum of changes including degeneration of fibrous tissue to fibroblastic proliferation. The fascia is usually markedly thickened and gritty. These pathologic changes are more consistent with fasciosis than fasciitis, but fasciitis remains the accepted description in literature.

Natural History

The typical patient is an adult who complains of plantar heel pain aggravated by activity and relieved by rest. Start-up pain when initiating walking is common. Strain of the plantar fascia can result from prolonged standing, running, or jumping. Excessive pronation is a common mechanical cause. The rigid cavus foot type can also predispose to plantar fasciitis. Obesity is present in up to 70% of patients. Plantar fasciitis is common among runners and ballet dancers. About 15% of cases are bilateral. Women are affected more than men.

Physical Findings

Localized tenderness over the calcaneal tuberosity is the most common physical finding. Pain is usually medial, but occasionally lateral. Rarely, pain may be located distally and this condition is called

S.L. Shapiro (✉)
Savannah Orthopaedic Foot and Ankle Center,
Savannah, GA, USA
e-mail: savannahfoot@bellsouth.net

G.R. Scuderi and A.J. Tria (eds.), *Minimally Invasive Surgery in Orthopedics: Foot and Ankle Handbook*,
DOI 10.1007/978-1-4614-0893-2_11, © Springer Science+Business Media, LLC 2012

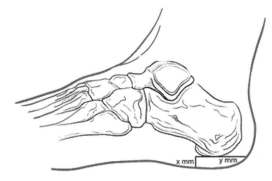

Fig. 11.1 Diagram of preoperative nonweightbearing lateral X-ray demonstrating the appropriate measurements to identify the location of the medial portal incision

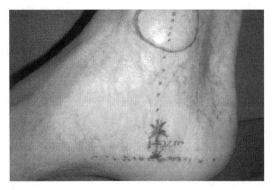

Fig. 11.2 Photograph of a second method to determine the placement of the medial incision. The incision is made along a line that bisects the medial malleolus 1–2 cm superior to the junction of keratinized and nonkeratinized skin

distal plantar fasciitis. Frequently, there may be soft tissue swelling of the plantar medial heel. Careful comparison with the contralateral heel is essential to observe this finding (Fig. 11.1).

Imaging

X-rays are ordered routinely in patients with plantar heel pain. Plantar calcaneal spurs occur in up to 50% of patients but are not thought to cause heel pain. Stress fractures, unicameral bone cysts, and giant cell tumors can usually be seen on plain films. Bone scans are rarely necessary but are positive in up to 95% of cases of plantar fasciitis. Magnetic resonance imaging (MRI) can be used in questionable cases and elegantly demonstrates thickening of the plantar fascia, and rules out soft tissue and bone tumors, subtalar arthritis, and stress fractures. Ultrasound is cost-effective and easily measures the thickness of the plantar fascia, documenting plantar fasciitis when thickness exceeds 3 mm (Fig. 11.2).

Differential Diagnosis

Plantar fascia rupture generally occurs acutely following vigorous physical activity. There may be visible ecchymosis in the arch. MRI or ultrasound confirms the diagnosis.

Tarsal tunnel syndrome occurs with compression of the T posterior tibial nerve, which can cause numbness, and pain in the heel, sole, or toes. A positive percussion test is elicited and electromyogram (EMG) and nerve conduction study results are positive in 50% of cases.

Stress fractures may sometimes be diagnosed on plain film, but can always be diagnosed on MRI.

Neoplasms can be visualized on plain film at times. MRI is diagnostic. Pain is typically constant and nocturnal.

In *infection*, pain is often constant. There may be swelling, redness, or fluctuance. Plain films, MRI, and/or Ceretec Scan can be diagnostic. Laboratory results may show increased erythrocyte sedimentation rate (ESR), C-reactive protein (CRP), or white blood cell count (WBC).

Painful heel pad syndrome occurs most often in runners, and is thought to result from disruption of fibrous septae of the heel pad.

Heel pad atrophy occurs in the elderly, and is usually not characterized by morning pain.

Inflammatory arthritis is usually bilateral and diffuse in nature. It may be associated with positive results for rheumatoid arthritis (RA), HLA, B27, and increased ESR.

Nonsurgical Management

Conservative management includes rest, ice, nonsteroidal anti-inflammatory drugs (NSAIDs), plantar fascia and Achilles tendon stretching, silicone heel pads, prefabricated and custom orthoses, night splints, CAM walkers, casts, physical therapy, athletic shoes, judicious use of steroid injections, and shockwave therapy. Ninety-five percent of patients will respond to conservative management. Surgery is indicated after 6–12 months of no improvement with conservative treatment.

Surgical Management

Plantar fasciotomy is indicated in the small percentage of patients who fail to respond to conservative treatment. Although open techniques have yielded good results, endoscopic plantar fasciotomy (EPF) offers several important advantages: (1) minimal soft tissue dissection; (2) excellent visualization of the plantar fascia; (3) precision in transecting only the medial one third to one half of the plantar fascia; (4) minimal postoperative pain with early return to full weightbearing status; and (5) earlier return to activities and work.

Preoperative Planning

Nonweightbearing lateral X-rays of the affected foot are performed. A point just anterior and inferior to the calcaneal tubercle is marked and measurements are made to the inferior and posterior skin lines [2]. These measurements are used to help select the incision site.

Positioning and Anesthesia

The patient is positioned supine with a bump under the buttock of the affected side to provide external rotation of the limb. The operative foot is then elevated on a foot prop, with a tourniquet in place at the distal calf. The limb is prepped and draped in this position. One gram of Ancef is administered. Anesthesia may be regional or general. Ankle block or popliteal nerve block is used with general anesthesia or intravenous sedation. The procedure is performed on an outpatient basis.

Equipment

The equipment required includes the Instratek Endotrac System (Houston, TX), consisting of a plantar fascia elevator, cannula and obturator, probe, nondisposable knife handles, and disposable hook and triangle knives. A 4-mm 30° short arthroscope is used. Finally, several Q-tips lightly fluffed with a Bovie scratch pad will be needed (Fig. 11.3).

Surgical Technique

The foot is prepped and draped on the foot prop and then exsanguinated with an Esmarch bandage. The tourniquet is inflated at the distal calf to 250 mmHg. An 8-mm vertical incision is made just anterior and plantar to the medial tubercle of the calcaneus. The measurements from the nonweightbearing lateral X-ray are used as a guide. Another good landmark is the medial malleolus. The incision can be placed on a line dropped from the midpoint of the medial malleolus or the junction of the middle and posterior third of the medial malleolus. Portal placement is critical to the success of the procedure.

The incision is deepened with blunt tenotomy scissors. Next, the plantar fascia elevator is placed through the incision and swept from medial to lateral just plantar to the plantar fascia. The obturator and cannula are then passed through this pathway and brought out through a lateral incision overlying the tip of the obturator. The obturator is then removed from the cannula and the cannula is cleared of fat with Q-tips. The cannula should be perpendicular to the long axis of the foot (Fig. 11.4).

The 4-mm 30° scope is then brought into the medial portal. The abductor hallucis muscle is visualized medially and then the plantar fascia is visualized. The probe is passed from the lateral portal and advanced medially to palpate the medial band of the plantar fascia. The probe is removed and the triangle knife is then advanced to the medial band. The foot is dorsiflexed to place tension on the plantar fascia. With a controlled

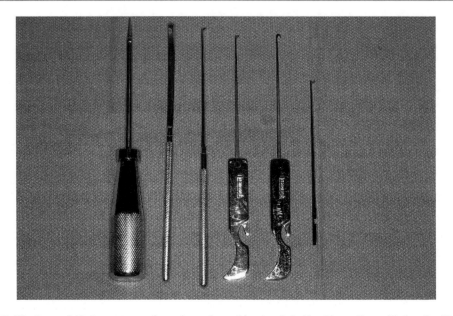

Fig. 11.3 The Instratek Endotrac system for endoscopic plantar fasciotomy. From left to right: (1) obturator with cannula, (2) plantar fascia elevator, (3) probe, (4) dispos- able triangle knife with nondisposable handle, (5) dispos- able hook knife with nondisposable handle, (6) disposable triangle knife without handle

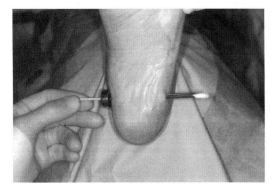

Fig. 11.4 Clearing fat from the cannula with a fluffed Q-tip to allow good visualization of the plantar fascia

motion, the triangle knife is pulled across the medial band of the plantar fascia. Several passes are often necessary to completely divide this band. The flexor digitorum brevis muscle belly should be visible after the medial band is divided. The fasciotomy is complete when the medial intermuscular septum is visualized. The amount of fascia divided is usually 14 mm, which can be measured off markings on the probe. The hook knife can be used to cut the fascia, but the triangle knife can be more easily manipulated with less likelihood of cutting into the muscle. After

performing a partial fasciotomy, the scope is moved into the lateral portal to check to see if any bands of fascia remain uncut. The triangle knife can be passed through the medial portal to cut these bands. The two-portal system allows this versatil- ity, which is lacking in the single-portal system.

The wound is irrigated through the cannula. The trochar is reinserted and the trochar and can- nula are removed together. The incisions are closed with 4–0 nylon suture. A light dressing and posterior splint are applied. Prints and/or CD of before and after fasciotomy are made (Fig. 11.5).

Postoperative Care

Ice and elevation are recommended for 48–72 h postoperatively. Minimal postoperative pain medication is required. Sutures are removed at 1 week postoperatively and a CAM walker, weight bearing as tolerated, is applied and used for 3 weeks to minimize the risk of lateral column pain. Most patients can resume normal activities at 6 weeks and vigorous athletic activities at 12 weeks postoperatively.

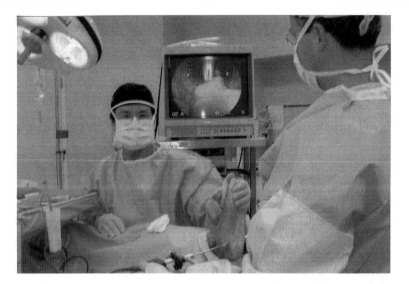

Fig. 11.5 Intraoperative set-up with foot draped on the foot prop, and the monitor on the same side as the foot, the scope placed in the cannula through the medial portal, and the probe through lateral portal. The plantar fascia is visualized on the monitor with the probe palpating the fascia

Outcomes

All published literature on EPF reports greater than 90% success with shorter recovery times than traditional open surgery [1–7]. My experience mirrors the literature with no infections or nerve damage and only four cases of lateral column pain in more than 400 procedures in the last 11 years. The success rate of EPF is significantly higher than extracorporeal shockwave treatment. In addition, EPF is reimbursed by all insurance companies, whereas shockwave procedures still have erratic insurance reimbursement.

EPF is minimally invasive with a simple, easy-to-learn surgical technique. The equipment is minimal and cost-effective. The incision is 8 mm compared with open procedures, where the incision is at least 4 cm and, with some more extensile approaches, as long as 10 cm.

Surgeons with prior arthroscopic experience should find EPF to be a straightforward procedure to master. DVDs and technique guides are readily available through Instratek. Training courses with cadavers are also given through the Orthopaedic Learning Center or Instratek. After ten cases, the surgeon should feel confident with this procedure. With experience, the average surgery time should be 10–15 min.

Complications

Lateral column pain and arch pain have been the most common complications reported in up to 3–5% of cases. Immobilization in a CAM walker for 4 weeks and limiting the division of the plantar fascia to the medial and central bands should reduce this complication even further. The Instratek System has single and double lines etched into the cannula to guide the surgeon to limit the plantar fasciotomy to 14 mm. The probe also has 1-cm markings. The disposable knives can also be marked with a marking pen to 14 mm. Finally, using the intermuscular septum as a guide for where to stop the fasciotomy is probably the best anatomic reference to indicate where the central band ends and the lateral band begins.

Infection rates are extremely low with EPF. I have had just one superficial wound infection (in a diabetic patient) in more than 400 cases. Injury to the medial and lateral plantar nerves is discussed extensively, but rarely reported. Cadaver studies reveal a reasonable safe zone as long as the incision is appropriate. One case of pseudoaneurysm of the lateral plantar artery and one case of a cuneiform stress fracture have been reported. With appropriate technique and postoperative immobilization, these complications should be rare.

Perils and Pitfalls

Performing the procedure on a prep stand or prop and ensuring that the foot and ankle are stable is vital to the smooth operation of this procedure. U-shaped padded foot-prepping devices that attach to the side of the operating room table are ideal. We also use the Lift-A-Limb foot prop, which cradles the limb and is an excellent device.

The placement of the incision is critical. The ideal placement is 1.5–2.0 cm superior to the junction of keratinized and nonkeratinized skin on a plumb line from the midpoint of the medial malleolus. Fluffed Q-tips and a defogging liquid to apply to the tip of the scope allow good visualization (Fig. 11.6).

Maintaining tension on the plantar fascia while cutting is key. The triangle knife is usually more predictable than the hook knife. Staying in the center of cannula and not skiving are important elements of technique. Although it is possible for the surgeon to hold the scope in one hand and the knife in the other hand, it is usually easier to have the assistant hold the scope and dorsiflex the foot, while the surgeon makes precise and controlled cuts with both hands on the knife, if necessary (Fig. 11.7).

In some cases, the central band is incredibly thick and gritty. Several passes of the triangle knife may be needed. Using the hook knife as well in such cases may be helpful. Remember also to clearly see the complete separation of the plantar fascia with the flexor digitorum brevis muscle plainly visible. Failure of EPF is usually due to incomplete or inadequate division of the plantar fascia (Fig. 11.8).

Other causes of failure include portal placement that is too proximal. It is difficult to release the fascia so proximally, directly off the calcaneus. Finally, misdiagnosis may lead to a poor result. Careful evaluation of the patient to rule out other etiologies in the differential diagnosis (described in detail previously) should be performed preoperatively.

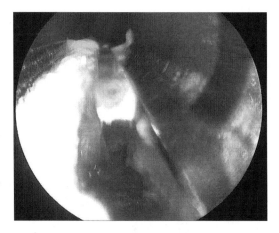

Fig. 11.7 Endoscopic plantar fasciotomy performed with a triangle knife as seen through a cannula

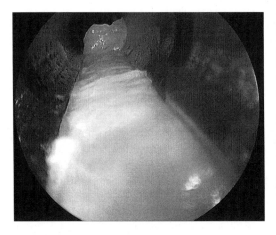

Fig. 11.6 Plantar fascia prior to fasciotomy as seen through a cannula

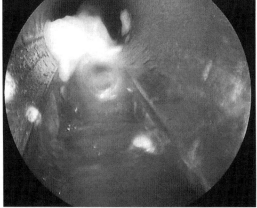

Fig. 11.8 Flexor digitorum brevis muscle seen after endoscopic plantar fasciotomy. Note that the central and lateral bands remain intact

References

1. Barrett SL, Day SV. Endoscopic plantar fasciotomy: preliminary studies with cadaveric specimen. J Foot Surg. 1991 30:170–172.
2. Barrett SL, Day SV. Endoscopic plantar fasciotomy two portal endoscopic surgical techniques – clinical results of 65 procedures. J Foot Surg. 2004 32:248–256.
3. Buchbinder R. Clinical practice. Plantar fasciitis. N Engl J Med. 2004 350(21):2159–2166.
4. Hofmeister EP, Elliott MJ, Juliano PJ. Endoscopic plantar fascia release: an anatomic study. Foot Ankle Int. 1995 16(H):719–723.
5. Hogan KA, Weber D, Shereff M. Endoscopic plantar fascia release. Foot Ankle Int. 2004 25(12):875–881.
6. Sabir N, Debirlenk S, Yagzi B, Karabulut N, Cubukus S. Clinical utility of sonography in diagnosing plantar fasciitis. J Ultrasound Med. 2005 24(8);1041–1048.
7. Saxena A. Uniportal endoscopic plantar fasciotomy: a prospective study on athletic patients. Foot Ankle Int. 2004 25(12):882–889.

Uniportal Endoscopic Decompression of the Interdigital Nerve for Morton's Neuroma

12

Steven L. Shapiro

Morton's neuroma represents a nerve entrapment syndrome in which the intermetatarsal nerve in the second and/or third webspace becomes compressed by the intermetatarsal ligament, enlarges, and undergoes perineural fibrosis [1–4].

Endoscopic Anatomy

The most important soft tissue structure is the transverse intermetatarsal ligament (TIML). The TIML is a continuation of the plantar plates. This structure becomes taut during the late midstance and push-off phases of gait. The TIML should be well visualized. It measures 10–15 mm in length and 2–3 mm in thickness [1].

The lumbrical tendon will be located on the plantar lateral aspect of the TIML. It is the most likely structure to be severed during endoscopic decompression of the intermetatarsal nerve, but with proper identification it can be spared. Inadvertent severing of the lumbrical tendon, however, has not resulted in any adverse sequelae. The plantar interossei muscles are superior to the TIML in the second, third, and fourth intermetatarsal spaces.

The intermetatarsal nerve is plantar to the TIML and should not be visualized during endo-

scopic division of the TIML; the nerve, however, may be seen by rotating the cannula 180° to the 6 o'clock position. This will be discussed in the Surgical Technique section.

Pathogenesis

The clinical symptoms of this condition were first described by Durlacher in 1845 and later by Morton in 1876. It is Morton's name that has remained linked to this condition. The most recent literature attributes Morton's neuroma to nerve entrapment, which has been confirmed by electron microscopy. Perineural fibrosis is seen at the level of nerve compression.

Natural History

The symptoms of Morton's neuroma are dull, aching pain in the ball of the foot, often radiating into the second, third, and/or fourth toes. This may be associated with tingling, burning, or numbness. This may occur gradually over several months or progress more acutely. Overuse activities, and compression by narrow-toed shoes and high heels have been implicated. Seventy-five percent of patients are women. The average age of onset is 54 years [5]. Occasionally, trauma can result in formation of an interdigital neuroma. Pain is sometimes relieved by removing the shoe.

S.L. Shapiro (✉)
Savannah Orthopaedic Foot and Ankle Center,
Savannah, GA, USA
e-mail: savannahfoot@bellsouth.net

Physical Findings

Classic findings include localized tenderness in the second and/or third webspace. Subtle swelling may be present in the affected webspaces. The two adjacent toes may be slightly separated. Mulder's click (a palpable snap) may be elicited in the affected webspace. Finally, the metatarsal compression test may be positive. This is performed by grasping and squeezing the patient's forefoot with the examiner's hand. The results of this maneuver are positive if it reproduces the patient's symptoms.

Imaging

Plain films should routinely be performed to rule out other pathologies. If the diagnosis or correct webspace is in doubt, sonographic imaging can be performed with a high degree of accuracy in experienced hands. MRI is not operator dependent, but yields a large percentage of false negatives and positives and is also much more costly. On ultrasound, a neuroma appears as a hypoechoic oval mass in the interspace at the level of the metatarsal heads. The size of the neuroma can be measured [5].

Differential Diagnosis

Differential diagnosis should include metatarsal stress fracture, Frieberg's disease (avascular necrosis [AVN] of the metatarsal head), synovitis, intermetatarsal bursitis, metatarsophalangeal (MTP) synovitis, peripheral neuropathy, lumbar radiculopathy, tarsal tunnel syndrome, vascular claudication, and spinal stenosis.

Nonsurgical Management

Conservative treatment may include metatarsal pads, orthotics, shoes with a wide toebox, steroid injections, and, more recently, alcohol injections. In my experience, conservative treatment has been successful in approximately 70% of patients.

Surgical Management

Preoperative Planning

Surgery is indicated when conservative treatment has failed to relieve pain after 6 months. All patients should have plain films preoperatively. Preoperative ultrasound is valuable if available. Otherwise, the surgeon should determine which webspace is most tender. Diagnostic lidocaine injection may also pinpoint the appropriate webspace. If both the second and third webspaces are symptomatic, consider endoscopy on both spaces.

Positioning and Anesthesia

The patient should be positioned supine. A bump under the buttock and thigh is used when the leg is externally rotated. The toes should extend just beyond the end of the operating room (OR) table with the heel firmly resting on the table. Anesthesia may be general or regional (popliteal or ankle block). Local anesthesia should be avoided because it may distort the endoscopic anatomy.

Prophylaxis and Equipment

Prophylactic intravenous antibiotics are given when the patient comes to the OR. An ankle tourniquet inflated to 250 mmHg is routinely used. Equipment required includes the AM Surgical set and a 30° 4-mm scope. The AM Surgical system includes an elevator, slotted cannula and obturator, locking device, and disposable knife blade.

Surgical Technique

The advantage of division of the TIML without excision of the interdigital neuroma is that there is no loss of sensation or possible formation of a stump neuroma, which is a very difficult problem to treat. Barrett and Pignetti introduced endoscopic decompression of the intermetatarsal nerve, which offers several advantages including

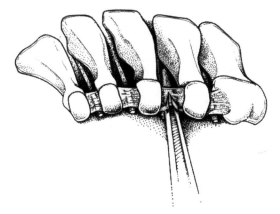

Fig. 12.1 Illustration of surgical technique for UDIN. The cannula is in the interspace just plantar to the TIML and dorsal to the intermetatarsal (interdigital) nerve. The TIML is being transected from distal to proximal (Courtesy of A.M. Surgical, Inc., Smithtown, NY.)

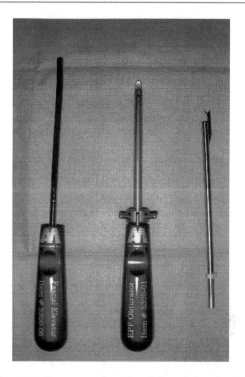

Fig. 12.2 Instrumentation. From left to right: elevator, cannula and obturator, and disposable knife

a smaller incision, faster postoperative recovery, and reduced incidence of hematoma and infection [1]. Although Barrett reported good and excellent results in 88% of patients, the original technique was difficult with a steep learning curve. He has since modified his technique, changing from two portals to a single portal.

Presented here is a single-portal technique using the AM Surgical system originally designed by Dr. Ather Mirza for endoscopic carpal tunnel release. I have adapted the instrumentation for uniportal endoscopic decompression of the intermetatarsal nerve (UDIN) (Fig. 12.1). The following is a step-by-step guide to the procedure (Fig. 12.2) [6].

1. Make a 1-cm vertical incision in the appropriate webspace.
2. Spread the subcutaneous tissue gently with blunt Steven's scissor.
3. Use the AM Surgical elevator to palpate and separate the TIML from the surrounding soft tissues. Scrape the elevator both dorsal and plantar to the TIML.
4. Place the slotted cannula/obturator through the same path just plantar to and scraping against the TIML. The slot should face dorsally at the 12 o'clock position.
5. Remove the obturator from the cannula.
6. Remove any fat or fluid from the cannula with absorbent cotton tip applicators.

7. Insert a short 4-mm 30° scope into the cannula.
8. Visualize the entire TIML by advancing the scope. The ligament is dense and white. The lumbrical tendon can often be seen just lateral to the TIML.
9. The intermetatarsal nerve can be visualized by rotating the cannula 180° so that the slot is facing plantar at 6 o'clock. The nerve can often be seen unless obscured by fat. It is often thickened distally, tapers, and becomes normal proximally.
10. Return the cannula back to the 12 o'clock position.
11. Remove the scope from the cannula.
12. Slide the disposable endoscopic knife onto the locking device with the lever in the open position.
13. Insert the knife and locking device assembly into the scope and advance the knife blade until it nearly touches the lens. The blade should also be parallel to the lens. Push the lever of the locking device forward until finger tight.

14. Advance the scope and knife assembly through the cannula. Visualize the knife blade transecting the TIML from distal to proximal. While cutting the TIML, maintain the cannula tight against the ligament. Place more tension on the TIML by placing a finger of the nondominant hand between the adjacent metatarsal necks.

15. Withdraw the scope and knife assembly and remove the knife from the scope. Reinsert the scope to confirm complete transection of the TIML. The divided edge of the ligament can be observed to further separate by applying manual digital pressure between the adjacent metatarsal heads.

16. Irrigate the wound through the cannula.

17. Remove the cannula and insert the elevator into the wound and palpate the interspace. The taut TIML should no longer be palpable.

18. Deflate the tourniquet; irrigate and close the wound with one or two interrupted mattress sutures. Apply a soft compression dressing and postoperative shoe.

19. If the surgeon chooses to perform a neurectomy in cases in which the nerve is very large and bulbous, the incision can be extended proximally 1–2 cm and neurectomy can be performed in routine fashion (Figs. 12.3–12.6).

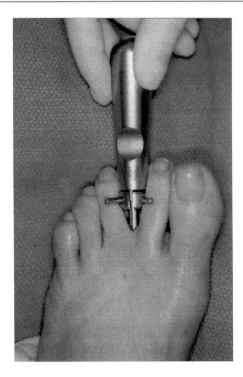

Fig. 12.3 Intraoperative view of insertion of the cannula and obturator into the second webspace, notch at 12 o'clock, positioned to view the TIML

Postoperative Care

Ice and elevation are recommended for the first 48–72 h. Weightbearing as tolerated is permitted in a surgical shoe. Crutches or a walker are provided as needed. Sutures are removed in 12–14 days. A comfortable shoe or sandal may then be worn. Vigorous activities such as running or racket sports should be avoided for 4–6 weeks. Patient should be advised that complete resolution of symptoms may take up to 4 months.

Outcomes

Barrett reported 88% good and excellent results in more than 40 patients [1]. In my first 24 patients, there were 82% good and excellent results at 6 months postoperatively.

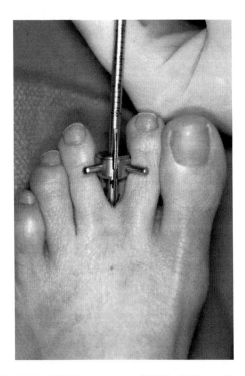

Fig. 12.4 (**a**) Endoscopic view of TIML. (**b**) Normal interdigital nerve. (**c**) Thickened interdigital nerve (neuroma)

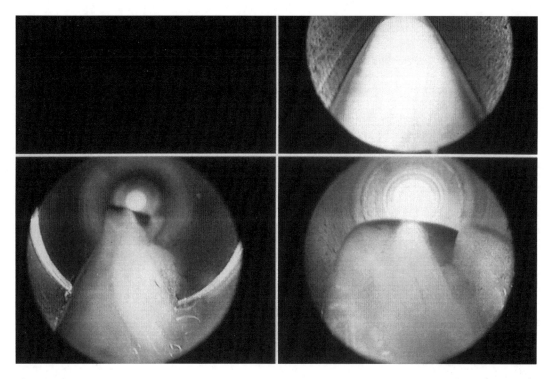

Fig. 12.5 Intraoperative view of knife mounted to scope in position in cannula ready to enter second webspace and transect the TIML

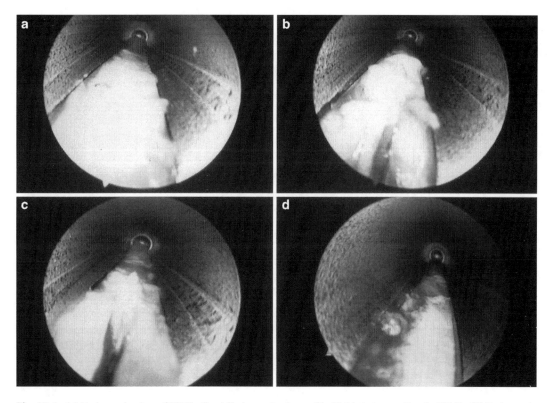

Fig. 12.6 (**a**) Endoscopic view of TIML. (**b**, **c**) Endoscopic views of knife blade transecting the TIML. (**d**) Endoscopic view after release of TIML

Complications

In the first 50 patients, there have been no infections. Two wound dehiscences occurred that healed uneventfully. The postoperative protocol was then changed from suture removal at 10 days postoperative to 14 days postoperative. No further dehiscences have occurred.

Perils and Pitfalls

The key to the procedure is isolating and separating the TIML from the soft tissues. Developing these tissue planes with the elevator is the critical step. Everything else follows. Hugging the TIML with the cannula while cutting is very important. If unable to visualize the TIML, abort the procedure and perform the procedure open.

References

1. Barrett, SL, Pignetti, TT. Endoscopic decompression for routine neuroma: preliminary study with cadaveric specimen: early clinical results. J Foot Ankle Surg 1994;33(5):503–8
2. Dellon, AL. Treatment of Morton's neuroma as a nerve compression; the role for neurolysis. J Am Podiatr Med Assoc 1992;82:399–402
3. Gauthier, G. Thomas Morton's disease: a nerve entrapment syndrome. A new surgical technique. Clin Orthop Relat Res 1979;142:90–2
4. Graham, CE, Graham, DM. Morton's neuroma: a microscopic evaluation. Foot Ankle 1984;5:150–3
5. Shapiro, PS, Shapiro, SL. Sonographic evaluation of interdigital neuroma. Foot Ankle 1995;16:10, 604–606
6. Shapiro, S.L. Endoscopic decompression of the intermetatarsal nerve for Morton's neuroma. Foot Ankle Clin N Am 2004;9:297–304

Percutaneous Z Tendon Achilles Lengthening

13

Bradley M. Lamm and Dror Paley

Achilles tendon lengthening is a delicate procedure whereby the risk of over lengthening (creating calcaneus), rupture, and weakening of the gastrocnemius-soleus muscle is devastating. The Silfverskiöld test is clinically performed to differentiate gastrocnemius equinus from gastrocnemius-soleus equinus. Many surgical techniques have been developed to treat negative results of the Silfverskiöld test. The authors prefer a gastrocnemius-soleus recession in order to preserve muscle strength. However, when a large amount of equinus deformity is present, an Achilles tendon lengthening is performed in order to achieve an adequate amount of length [1]. The authors present a percutaneous technique for Achilles tendon lengthening [2].

Surgical Technique

A longitudinal percutaneous incision is made centrally and just proximal to the Achilles tendon insertion into the calcaneus. This incision is deepened through the Achilles tendon. A Smillie knife is inserted into the split beneath the Achilles tendon sheath and pushed approximately 4 cm proximally. A second percutaneous longitudinal central tendon incision is made over the tip of the Smillie knife. Then each half of the tendon is cut transversely at the level of the incisions, being careful not to injure the tendon sheath. Dorsiflexion of the foot in conjunction with making these transverse cuts allows for the tendon to slide on itself. When a varus hindfoot is present, cut distal medial and proximal lateral. When a valgus hindfoot is present, cut distal lateral and proximal medial. The Achilles tendon fibers spiral distally; therefore, be careful to ensure a complete Z lengthening. In addition, do not cut the tendon sheath. Dorsiflex the foot and observe the tendon lengthening within the sheath, which therefore does not need to be repaired. Because this technique maintains the Achilles tendon sheath, the Thompson's test produces normal plantarflexion. The ankle is then immobilized for 3 weeks postoperatively (Figs. 13.1a–e–13.5).

B.M. Lamm (✉)
International Center for Limb Lengthening,
Rubin Institute for Advanced Orthopedics,
Sinai Hospital of Baltimore, Baltimore, MD, USA
e-mail: blamm@lifebridgehealth.org

D. Paley
Paley Advanced Limb Lengthening
Institute, St. Mary's Hospital,
West Palm Beach, FL, USA

G.R. Scuderi and A.J. Tria (eds.), *Minimally Invasive Surgery in Orthopedics: Foot and Ankle Handbook*,
DOI 10.1007/978-1-4614-0893-2_13, © Springer Science+Business Media, LLC 2012

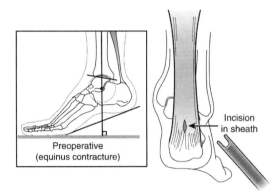

Fig. 13.1 Percutaneous Z tendon Achilles lengthening for correction of equinus. Make a central distal incision through the skin and the Achilles tendon, creating a short split through the tendon longitudinally (From Paley D: *Principles of Deformity Correction*. rev ed, 2005, with kind permission of Springer Science + Business Media)

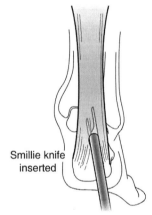

Fig. 13.2 Insert the Smillie knife into the short split (From Paley D: *Principles of Deformity Correction*. rev ed, 2005, with kind permission of Springer Science + Business Media)

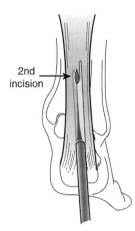

Fig. 13.3 Push the Smillie knife proximally for at least 4 cm and, at the tip of the knife, make a second central longitudinal skin incision (From Paley D: *Principles of Deformity Correction*. rev ed, 2005, with kind permission of Springer Science + Business Media)

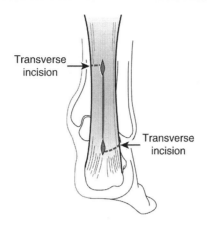

Fig. 13.4 Cut each half of the tendon transversely in one direction proximally and the other direction distally, creating a Z lengthening. The direction of release proximal and distal is performed occurring to the patient's heel position (valgus or varus). Do not cut the tendon sheath (From Paley D: *Principles of Deformity Correction*. rev ed, 2005, with kind permission of Springer Science + Business Media)

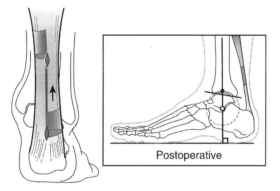

Fig. 13.5 When dorsiflexion of the foot is performed, the tendon sides on itself but maintains tension within the intact sheath. Note the plantigrade foot position (From Paley D: *Principles of Deformity Correction*. rev ed, 2005, with kind permission of Springer Science + Business Media)

References

1. Lamm BM, Paley D, Herzenberg JE. Gastrocnemius soleus recession: a simpler, more limited approach. J Am Podiatr Med Assoc 95:18–25, 2005
2. Paley D. *Principles of Deformity Correction*. 2nd edition, Springer, Berlin, 2003

Percutaneous Distraction Osteogenesis for Treatment of Brachymetatarsia

14

Bradley M. Lamm, Dror Paley, and John E. Herzenberg

A short metatarsal can be acquired or congenital in origin [1]. A congenitally short metatarsal or brachymetatarsia presents unilaterally or bilaterally, typically involving the fourth metatarsal (Figs. 14.1 and 14.2). Congenitally short metatarsals can occur in isolation or in association with systemic syndromes, endocrinopathies, and dysplasias. Syndactyly or polydactyly can occur in combination with congenitally short metatarsals. The cause of brachymetatarsia is thought to be premature closure of the metatarsal epiphyseal growth plate (Fig. 14.3). Acquired short metatarsals are caused by trauma, infection, tumor, Freiberg disease, radiation, and surgery. In addition, acquired short metatarsals can be associated with skeletal and systemic abnormalities (sickle cell anemia, multiple epiphyseal dysplasia, multiple hereditary osteochondromas, and juvenile rheumatoid arthritis). Surgically induced (iatrogenic) shortening of metatarsals are caused by transphyseal fixation, osteotomies of the metatarsals, and internal or external fixation producing a growth arrest or synostoses between metatarsals.

A failed bunionectomy or overly aggressive first metatarsal cuneiform arthrodesis also can result in an acquired short first metatarsal [1, 2].

Patients with brachymetatarsia exhibit a dorsally displaced toe, toe dysplasia, short phalanges, transfer metatarsalgia, cosmetic concerns, and painful corns and calluses. These patients have difficulty wearing shoes because of the high riding toe on the dorsum of the foot, which produces plantar metatarsal head calluses and dorsal digital corns [1, 3]. Surgery to lengthen the short metatarsal can improve cosmesis and shoe wearing and can decrease the pain associated with this deformity.

Acute and gradual lengthening surgical techniques have been described for correction of brachymetatarsia. Acute lengthening of a short metatarsal with autogenous bone grafting was first described in 1969 by McGlamry and Cooper [4]. Since then, many other techniques for acute lengthening (one-stage) have been reported and include interposition of synthetic materials, allograft, and step-cut or oblique osteotomy with distraction and internal fixation [5–8]. Some authors have performed shortening of adjacent metatarsals or proximal phalanxes so as to decrease the amount of metatarsal lengthening needed [9–11].

Gradual lengthening with external fixation (distraction osteogenesis) is preferred for lengthening more than 1 cm [1]. With gradual lengthening, the rate of postoperative lengthening can be adjusted, the patient can bear weight during treatment, and the patient can have input regarding

B.M. Lamm (✉)
International Center for Limb Lengthening, Rubin Institute for Advanced Orthopedics, Sinai Hospital of Baltimore, Baltimore, MD, USA
e-mail: blamm@lifebridgehealth.org

D. Paley
Paley Advanced Limb Lengthening Institute, St. Mary's Hospital, West Palm Beach, FL, USA

J.E. Herzenberg
International Center for Limb Lengthening, Sinai Hospital of Baltimore, Baltimore, MD, USA

G.R. Scuderi and A.J. Tria (eds.), *Minimally Invasive Surgery in Orthopedics: Foot and Ankle Handbook*, DOI 10.1007/978-1-4614-0893-2_14, © Springer Science+Business Media, LLC 2012

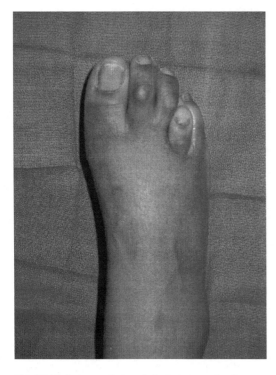

Fig. 14.1 Anteroposterior clinical photograph of a congenitally short fourth metatarsal. Note the underlapping fifth toe

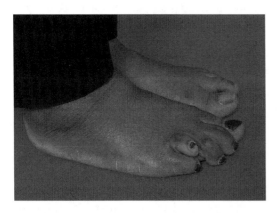

Fig. 14.2 Lateral clinical photograph of a congenitally short fourth metatarsal. Note the dorsal displacement and flexion deformity at the MTPJ of the fourth digit

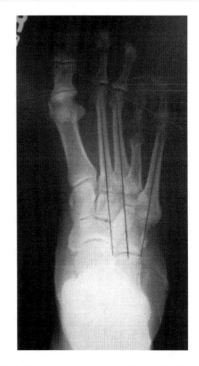

Fig. 14.3 Anteroposterior view radiograph of a congenitally short fourth metatarsal. The metatarsal length is abnormal, with the fourth metatarsal being short of the line formed by drawing the metatarsal parabola angle. Note the slight medial bowing of the short metatarsal. The transverse plane deviation of the adjacent digits converging toward the short metatarsal can be observed

the final length. Gradual lengthening reduces the risk of neurovascular compromise compared with acute lengthening, which can cause severe soft tissue stretch [1, 2]. Gradual lengthening of short metatarsals has been performed with subsequent interpositional bone graft [12, 13] and with distraction osteogenesis alone [14–16]. Various types of external fixation devices (mini-Hoffman, Ilizarov semicircular, and monolateral fixators) have been used to achieve metatarsal lengthening [17–20].

The metatarsal phalangeal joint (MTPJ) is at risk for subluxation during gradual lengthening of a metatarsal [21, 22]. With greater amounts of lengthening, the joint is more susceptible to subluxation. The subluxation forces decrease with distance from the osteotomy to the joint. Soft tissue rebalancing of the digit and pinning of the MTPJ are important adjunctive steps to maintain the MTPJ reduced during lengthening. Traditionally, a separate Kirschner wire is used to stabilize the MTPJ [2]. However, this pin can easily become dislodged during the lengthy treatment time. By connecting the digital pin to the external fixation device, this pin is incorporated into the apparatus to form a more stable ray construct.

At the time of surgery, it might be necessary to perform a release of the dorsal toe contracture to allow for appropriate toe realignment to pin the digit. Pinning the digit to the metatarsal head stabilizes the MTPJ throughout the lengthening. Attaching the pin to the external fixator ensures that this important stabilizing pin will not dislodge. Other potential complications result from inadequate restoration of the metatarsal parabola in the transverse plane. Creating a plantigrade metatarsal head in the sagittal plane provides the necessary realignment for normal pedal function.

We present our percutaneous metatarsal lengthening technique to prevent MTPJ subluxation during metatarsal lengthening. In addition, we present a systematic technique to ensure the proper plane and vector of metatarsal lengthening to maintain anatomic sagittal and transverse plane alignment, respectively.

Surgical Technique

A systematic percutaneous technique to ensure the proper plane and direction of metatarsal lengthening is outlined. Position the patient supine on the radiolucent table with a bump under the left hemisacrum to obtain a foot forward position. Based on the reducibility of the MTPJ contracture, digital surgery (partial or complete MTPJ release with or without arthroplasty or arthrodesis of the proximal interphalangeal joint) should be performed to realign the digit before the metatarsal lengthening procedure is begun. A partial MTPJ release (dorsal capsulotomy) should be performed when the digit is reducible. It is not recommended to perform an arthroplasty or arthrodesis because this will result in shortening of an already short ray. In some cases, it might be necessary to release the dorsal MTPJ capsule or rarely lengthen the combined extensor tendon of the toe. After the appropriate MTPJ release is performed, the toe is pinned with a 0.062-in. -diameter Kirschner wire in the realigned position. Under fluoroscopic guidance, the wire is inserted from the tip of the toe across the MTPJ, stopping at the distal external fixation pins. Preoperative planning with a four-pin Orthofix

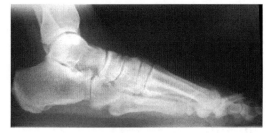

Fig. 14.4 Lateral view radiograph of a congenitally short fourth metatarsal. Note the extension contracture of the toe and increased fourth metatarsal declination at the level of the distal metaphyseal-diaphyseal junction (region of the growth plate). The dorsal cortex of the short metatarsal is parallel to the adjacent metatarsals

Mini-M100 external fixator (Verona, Italy) determines the initial spread and locations of the pins. Insert the half-pins percutaneously, under fluoroscopic control, bicortical and perpendicular to the shaft of the metatarsal.

The first half-pin is placed at the distal-most region of the metaphyseal-diaphyseal junction. A 1.8-mm wire works well to predrill the hole, under fluoroscopic control, perpendicular to the metatarsal on the lateral view. Remove the wire and insert a 3.0- to 2.5-mm tapered half-pin, typically measuring 60 mm in total length and 20 mm of thread length (Fig. 14.4). Because the fixator is mounted perpendicular to this first pin, the first pin determines the plane of lengthening. It is important that the plane of metatarsal lengthening be such that the final position of the metatarsal head is located at the appropriate level in the sagittal plane.

Set the monorail mini external fixator so that the half-pin clamps are at the smallest distance apart, minimizing the pin spread. This ensures maximum lengthening capability and that all of the half-pins are maintained within the short metatarsal. If the metatarsal is very short, it might be necessary for the most proximal half-pin to be placed in the tarsus (cuboid) spanning the Lisfranc joint. Insert the second half-pin, the most proximal of the four half-pins, proximally in the base of the metatarsal, parallel to the first pin and just distal to the adjacent metatarsal cuboid joint. A 1.8-mm wire works well to predrill the hole for half-pin placement and is bent

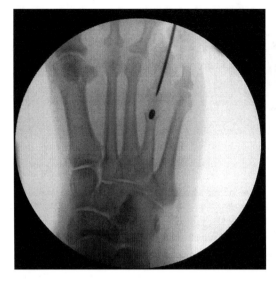

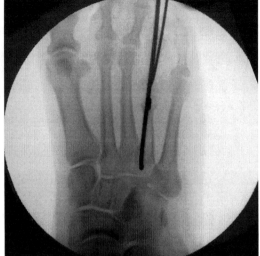

Fig. 14.5 Fluoroscopic anteroposterior view showing that the first pin is placed at the distal most region of the metatarsal metaphyseal-diaphyseal junction. This half-pin is inserted in the center of the metatarsal (bicortical) and perpendicular to the longitudinal bisection of the metatarsal (sagittal plane axis) on the lateral view. The placement of this pin defines the sagittal plane of metatarsal lengthening

Fig. 14.6 Fluoroscopic anteroposterior view showing that the second pin is placed at the most proximal region of the metatarsal. Similar to the first half-pin, it is inserted perpendicular to the sagittal plane axis of the metatarsal on the lateral view (parallel to the first pin). In addition, the exact medial/lateral position of this second half-pin defines the direction or vector of metatarsal lengthening (two points define a line). This second pin defines the vector of metatarsal lengthening and thus the final position of the metatarsal head, compared with the adjacent metatarsal heads in the transverse plane

distally, under fluoroscopic guidance, to check the direction of lengthening (Fig. 14.5). This second half-pin establishes the direction of metatarsal lengthening (two fixed points determine a line) and is important because it determines the final position of the metatarsal head in the transverse plane (Fig. 14.6). Also, this second (most proximal) half-pin determines the position of the most proximal half-pin cluster and thus indirectly determines the osteotomy level. Therefore, the more proximal this second pin is placed, the more metaphyseal the osteotomy level is. Diaphyseal osteotomy requires a longer consolidation phase. According to the preoperative plan, two half-pins are placed in the distal end of the metatarsal and two in the base of the fourth metatarsal adjacent to the metatarsal cuboid joint (Fig. 14.7). Make a percutaneous incision (5 mm in length) lateral to the short metatarsal at the proximal metaphyseal-diaphyseal junction between the two half-pin clusters. Use a small hemostat to dissect down to the metatarsal, and with a periosteal elevator, gently lift the dorsal and plantar periosteum. To begin the osteotomy, a 1.5-mm wire is used to drill multiple orthogonal

holes into the metatarsal under fluoroscopic control. The level of the osteotomy is just distal to the most distal of the proximal half-pin clusters; care needs to be taken not to extend the osteotomy into the half-pin. A small osteotome is then used to complete the osteotomy without producing excessive osteotomy displacement, which can tear the periosteum (Figs. 14.8 and 14.9). The osteotomy is then reduced with the use of fluoroscopy and the Orthofix Mini-M100 external fixator, which is applied and tightened. Next, the toe Kirschner wire is bent 90° outside the skin and again 90° over the dorsum of the toe. A third 90° bend is needed to attach it with an end clamp to the external fixator. It is necessary to have the screw distraction end of the fixator proximal and the tapped end of the fixator distally oriented (Figs. 14.10 and 14.11). Traditionally, a separate Kirschner wire is used to stabilize the MTPJ [2]. However, the pin can easily become dislodged during the lengthy treatment time. By connecting the digital pin to the

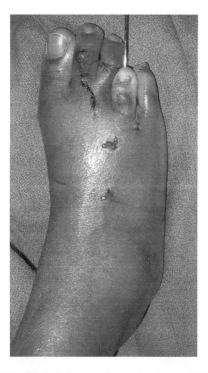

Fig. 14.7 Clinical photograph showing the parallelism of the most distal and proximal half-pins in the fourth metatarsal. Note that the second and third hammertoes have been corrected. To correct the dorsal contracture of the fourth toe, a dorsal capsulotomy was performed through a percutaneous dorsal lateral incision and pinning was then performed. The 0.062-in. Kirschner wire is advanced across the MTPJ after all the half-pins are placed

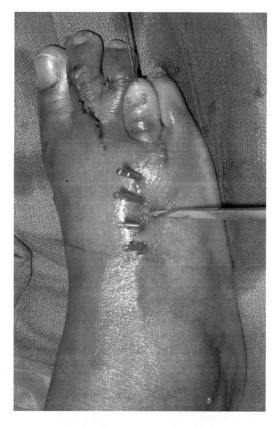

Fig. 14.9 Intraoperative photograph of the percutaneous fourth metatarsal osteotomy. A percutaneous dorsal lateral incision is made, and, under fluoroscopic guidance, a 1.5-mm wire is used to drill multiple orthogonal holes into the metatarsal at the level of metaphyseal-diaphyseal junction. A small osteotome is then used to complete the osteotomy

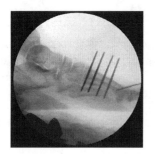

Fig. 14.8 Fluoroscopic lateral view confirms that all four half-pins are parallel to each other and perpendicular to the longitudinal axis of the fourth metatarsal

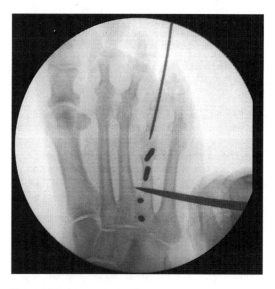

external fixation device, the pin is incorporated into the apparatus to form a more stable construct. Note that the digital pin is attached to the moving segment of the external fixator. The percutaneous osteotomy incision is closed and a compressive dressing applied along with toe dressings. Begin distraction after 5 days, at a rate

Fig. 14.10 Intraoperative fluoroscopy is used to ensure completion of the osteotomy

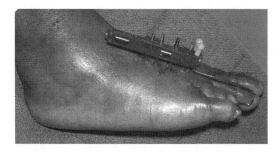

Fig. 14.11 Immediate postoperative lateral view clinical photograph showing parallel half-pins and the fourth digit pinned in a reduced position. The 0.062-in. diameter Kirschner wire is then bent to attach it with an end clamp into the distal aspect of the external fixator

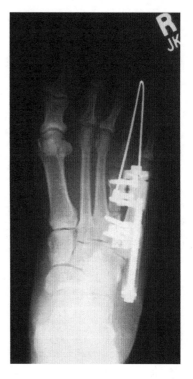

Fig. 14.13 Postoperative anterop/osterior view radiograph showing the fixator in place. The distraction begins after 5 days, at a rate of 0.25 mm twice per day

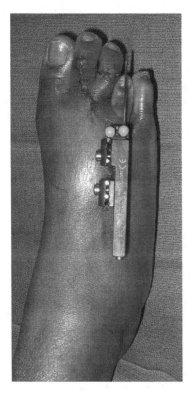

Fig. 14.12 Immediate postoperative anteroposterior view clinical photograph showing that the tapped end of the external fixator should be oriented distally to allow for attachment of the digital Kirschner wire. Note that the lengthening end of the external fixator is oriented toward the patient

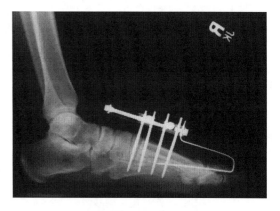

Fig. 14.14 Postoperative lateral view radiograph showing the fixator in place. Note that the pinning of the MTPJ prevents joint subluxation. This method of attaching the digital pin to the fixator prevents dislodgment of the pin during the lengthening and consolidation phases of treatment

Discussion

of 0.25 mm twice per day. When the bone is at the final length and fully consolidated, the frame is removed (Figs. 14.12–14.18).

Preoperative planning is important to identify the amount of metatarsal length necessary to reestablish the metatarsal parabola. For example, if the

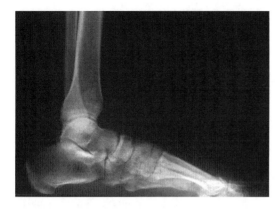

Fig. 14.15 Lateral view radiograph, obtained with the patient in a weight-bearing position after removal of the fixator, showing healed regenerated bone with accurate sagittal plane alignment

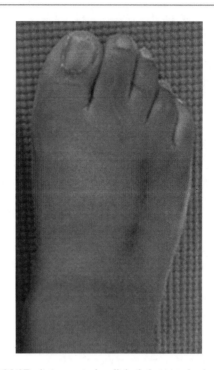

Fig. 14.17 Anteroposterior clinical photograph, obtained with the patient in a weight-bearing position at final follow-up, showing correction of the second and third hammertoes and proper length restoration of the fourth digit

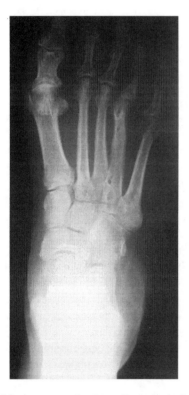

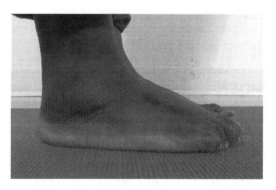

Fig. 14.18 Lateral clinical photograph, obtained with the patient in a weight-bearing position at final follow-up, showing accurate sagittal plane alignment of the second, third, and fourth digits

Fig. 14.16 Anteroposterior view radiograph, obtained with the patient in a weight-bearing position after removal of the fixator, showing healed regenerated bone with accurate transverse plane alignment and proper length restoration

amount of metatarsal length needed to reestablish the metatarsal parabola is 20 mm, the amount of time required to obtain this length would be approximately 45 days, based on the latency period of 5 days and the desired distraction rate of 0.5 mm per day. This is useful information to discuss with the patient preoperatively. The rate of distraction might need to be adjusted during the postoperative period; therefore, appropriate patient education is important. The consolidation period varies depending on a multitude of factors (location of osteotomy, age of patient, whether the patient smokes, rate of lengthening, and amount of lengthening) but typically ranges from 2 to 4 months. Therefore, the prediction of needed metatarsal length provides a time line for the patient's total length of treatment (lengthening phase and consolidation phase).

Intraoperatively, applying four half-pins that are perpendicular to the mid-diaphyseal axis of that metatarsal and parallel to each other is important for accurate sagittal and transverse plane lengthening and thus for the final alignment. Because the fixator is mounted perpendicular to the first half-pin, this half-pin ensures the correct plane for bone lengthening. Almost no room for error exists in transverse placement because of the narrow nature of the bone. It is important that the plane of metatarsal lengthening be such that the final position of the metatarsal head is located at the appropriate level in the sagittal plane. The second half-pin determines the direction or vector of lengthening (two fixed points define a line). Little room for error exists because the fifth and third metatarsals are located a set distance apart in the transverse plane. It is important that the vector of metatarsal lengthening be such that the final position of the metatarsal head is located at the appropriate level in the transverse plane.

Conclusion

Therefore, accurate placement of the most distal half-pin and the most proximal half-pin defines the plane and direction of lengthening in both the sagittal and transverse planes, respectively. The technique of a percutaneous minimally invasive osteotomy in the metaphyseal region of the metatarsal is essential for successful formation of regenerate bone. Pinning of the toe across the MTPJ is important to minimize digital subluxation and digital flexion contracture during lengthening. In addition, our technique of connecting the digital wire to the external fixator prevents dislodgment of this wire during treatment. Currently, the senior author (B.M.L.) has modified the technique to further prevent stiffness of the metatarsophalangeal joint after treatment. Pinning across the MTPJ has been shown to produce stiffness regardless of

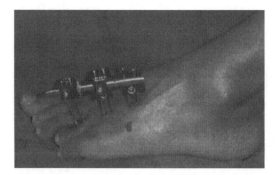

Fig. 14.19 Clinical photograph obtained immediately after surgery shows the senior author's (B.M.L.) modified technique to prevent postoperative MTPJ stiffness. Note the parallelism of the half-pins in the fourth metatarsal and toe. The fourth toe was manually reduced (without MTPJ release) and was maintained in a neutral position with the second fixator. The distal most external fixator (Penning minifixator, Orthofix, Inc., Mckinney, TX) across the MTPJ provides distraction, prevents joint subluxation during lengthening, and maximizes postoperative joint flexibility. In addition, the small percutaneous metatarsal osteotomy incision is seen laterally

the length of time the pin is maintained. Therefore, piggybacking or adding a second fixator to span the MTPJ provides joint distraction and digital realignment thereby protecting the joint. This modification has shown excellent short-term results and maintains MTPJ position and flexibility (Fig. 14.19). Preoperative consultation should include the time prediction for both the lengthening and consolidation phases and a cosmetic discussion of toe length (phalanges also can be short in cases of congenitally short metatarsals) and forefoot width (after lengthening, patients might feel as if the forefoot is wider). Routine biweekly follow-up is critical during the lengthening phase to avoid complications such as under lengthening and over lengthening of the metatarsal, premature consolidation, nonunion, and malunion.

Acknowledgments I thank Alvien Lee for expertise and assistance with the photography.

References

1. Davidson RS. Metatarsal lengthening. Foot Ankle Clin 6:499–518, 2001
2. Levine SE, Davidson RS, Dormans JP, Drummond DS. Distraction osteogenesis for congenitally short lesser metatarsals. Foot Ankle Int 16:196–200, 1995

3. Root ML, Orien WP, Weed JH. Normal and abnormal function of the foot. Clinical Biomechanics, Vol 2. Los Angeles: Clinical Biomechanics Corp. 455, 1977
4. McGlamry ED, Cooper CT. Brachymetatarsia: a surgical treatment. J Am Podiatry Assoc 59:259–264, 1969
5. Choudhury SN, Kitaoka HB, Peterson HA. Metatarsal lengthening: case report and review of the literature. Foot Ankle Int 18:739–745, 1997
6. Page JC, Dockery GL, Vance CE. Brachymetatarsia with brachymesodactyly. J Foot Surg 22:104–107, 1983
7. Mah KK, Beegle TR, Falknor DW. A correction for short fourth metatarsal. J Am Podiatry Assoc 73: 196–200, 1983
8. Handelman RB, Perlman MD, Coleman WB. Brachymetatarsia: a review of the literature and case report. J Am Podiatr Med Assoc 76:413–416, 1986
9. Kim HT, Lee SH, Yoo CI, Kang JH, Suh JT. The management of brachymetatarsia. J Bone Joint Surg 85B:683–690, 2003
10. Kaplan EG, Kaplan GS. Metatarsal lengthening by use of autogenous bone graft and internal wire compression fixation: a preliminary report. J Foot Surg 17:60–66, 1978
11. Biggs EW, Brahm TB, Efron BL. Surgical correction of congenital hypoplastic metatarsals. J Am Podiatry Assoc 69:241–244, 1979
12. Martin DE, Kalish SR. Brachymetatarsia: a new surgical approach. J Am Podiatr Med Assoc 81:10–17, 1991
13. Urbaniak JR, Richardson WJ. Diaphyseal lengthening for shortness of the toe. Foot Ankle 5:251–256, 1985
14. Saxby T, Nunley JA. Metatarsal lengthening by distraction osteogenesis: a report of two cases. Foot Ankle 13:536–539, 1992
15. Magnan B, Bragantini A, Regis D, Bartolozzi P. Metatarsal lengthening by callotasis during the growth phase. J Bone Joint Surg 77B:602–607, 1995
16. Wakisaka T, Yasui N, Kojimoto H, Takasu M, Shimomura Y. A case of short metatarsal bones lengthened by callus distraction. Acta Orthop Scand 59:194–196, 1988
17. Skirving AP, Newman JH. Elongation of the first metatarsal. J Pediatr Orthop 3:508–510, 1983
18. Steedman JT, Peterson HA. Brachymetatarsia of the first metatarsal treated by surgical lengthening. J Pediatr Orthop 12:780–785, 1992
19. Masada K, Fujita S, Fuji T, Ohno H. Complications following metatarsal lengthening by callus distraction for bracthymetatarsia. J Pediatr Orthop 19:394–397, 1999
20. Herzenberg JE, Paley D. Ilizarov applications in foot and ankle surgery. Adv Orthop Surg 16:162–174, 1992
21. Baek GH, Chung MS. The treatment of congenital brachymetatarsia by one-stage lengthening. J Bone Joint Surg 80B:1040–1044, 1998
22. Kawashima T, Yamada A, Ueda K, Harii K. Treatment of brachymetatarsia by callus distraction (callotasis). Ann Plast Surg 32:191–199, 1994

Minimally Invasive Realignment Surgery for the Charcot Foot

15

Bradley M. Lamm and Dror Paley

The aftermath of Charcot, joint subluxation and loss of the bone quality, produces abnormal osseous prominences, which are potential areas for ulceration. Due to the deformed pedal position, the muscle-tendon balance is altered and the resultant aberrant weight-bearing forces increase the risk for ulceration. If ulcers are present, osteomyelitis can ensue, thus, if ulcers are present, they should be eradicated. The best treatment results are achieved when treatment is initiated during the early stages of Charcot neuroarthropathy.

The goal of treatment in the acute Charcot neuroarthropathy is to stabilize the condition. The traditional treatment is total contact casting for immobilizing. However, non-weight bearing in a total contact cast produces osteopenia of the ipsilateral foot and increased weight-bearing forces on the contralateral foot. These resulting sequelae can make it difficult for sequent surgery and can lead to ulceration and Charcot neuroarthropathy in the contralateral foot. Maintaining non-weight-bearing status is difficult for this patient population for multiple reasons (e.g., muscle atrophy, obesity, diminished proprioception).

The goal of treatment in the chronic Charcot neuroarthropathy is to perform Achilles tendon lengthening, ostectomy, débridement, osteotomy, arthrodesis, and open reduction with internal fixation. Acute correction via open reduction with rigid internal fixation or plantar plating are frequently used for reconstruction [1]. In addition, acute correction via open reduction with application of static external fixation has been reported [2]. A recently described method for treating acute Charcot neuroarthropathy is to apply a static external fixator, which acts like a cast by immobilizing the affected joints and bones [3]. A new minimally invasive gradual correction method with the use of external fixation is presented [4, 5].

Clinical Evaluation

Charcot deformities of the foot and ankle are observed at isolated or multiple anatomic locations at various stages (Eichenholtz stages 0, 1, 2, 3) with varying degrees of severity [6, 7]. Plantar ulcers correlate to the anatomic location of the Charcot neuroarthropathy. For example, medial column ulcers of the foot are generally associated with Charcot neuroarthropathy of the tarsometatarsal region and correlate with a medial column collapse. Tarsometatarsal Charcot deformities are typically stable due to the interlocking anatomy

B.M. Lamm (✉)
International Center for Limb Lengthening,
Rubin Institute for Advanced Orthopedics,
Sinai Hospital of Baltimore, Baltimore, MD, USA
e-mail: blamm@lifebridgehealth.org

D. Paley
Paley Advanced Limb Lengthening Institute,
St. Mary's Hospital, West Palm Beach, FL, USA

and are successfully treated conservatively or with a limited surgical approach (ostectomy or acute wedge resection with stabilization) [8, 9]. However, lateral column ulcers are associated with a midfoot Charcot deformity, which typically is not stable. Instability of the lateral column leads to recurrent ulcers, therefore conservative treatment generally fails and surgical reconstruction often becomes necessary [10, 11]. Catanzariti et al. [10] suggested that patients with lateral column Charcot deformity require a more complex surgical reconstruction.

Radiographs of the Charcot foot and ankle can be difficult to decipher; the bones of the hindfoot and midfoot are superimposed because of the subluxation/dislocation of these joints. In addition, bone fragmentation and proliferation of new bone during the early and late stages of Charcot neuroarthropathy, respectively, add to the complexity of radiographic interpretation. Radiographs that show the patient during weight bearing should be obtained in all planes to more easily locate the Charcot deformity. Axial view radiographs are helpful to evaluate hindfoot and ankle deformity [12].

Minimally Invasive Gradual Charcot Foot Reconstruction

The goals of surgical intervention for the Charcot foot and ankle are to restore alignment and stability, prevent amputation, prepare for a shoe or brace, and allow the patient to be ambulatory. Historically, open reduction with internal fixation was the mainstay for treatment of Charcot foot deformities. Large open incisions were made to remove the excess bone and to reduce the fragmented or dislocated bone. In addition, screw fixation or plantar plating was traditionally performed in an attempt to stabilize the Charcot joint. These invasive surgical procedures typically resulted in a nonanatomic correction (e.g., shortening of the foot or incomplete deformity correction) and occasionally resulted in neurovascular compromise, incision-healing problems, infection, and the use of casts or boots for non-weight-bearing patients. Although

performing open reduction has disadvantages, in cases of tarsometatarsal Charcot deformity, it is advantageous. Typically, Charcot neuroarthropathy of the tarsometatarsal joints is associated with mild to moderate deformities because the tarsometatarsal joints are structurally interlocked. Acute realignment achieved by performing a wedge resection and applying internal fixation produces a stable foot.

Gradual deformity correction with external fixation is preferred for large deformity reductions of the dislocated Charcot joint(s). Correction with external fixation allows for gradual, accurate realignment of the dislocated/subluxated Charcot joints. One advantage of using an Ilizarov apparatus to gradually correct the deformity is that the technique is minimally invasive, especially for patients with multiple previous incisions. Gradual correction also allows for anatomic correction without loss of foot length or bone mass. External fixation allows for partial weight bearing and limits neurovascular compromise because the correction occurs slowly over a period of time.

A stable or coalesced foot with Charcot deformity will require an osteotomy for correction of the deformity. The osteotomy can be performed by using the percutaneous Gigli saw technique. Midfoot osteotomies can be performed across three levels (i.e., talar neck and calcaneal neck, cubonavicular osseous level, and cuneocuboid osseous level. Performing a proximal osteotomy across multiple metatarsals is best avoided because of the disturbance of the interossei, the risk of neurovascular injury, and the multiple bones that require stabilization [11].

For an unstable or an incompletely coalesced Charcot foot, correction can be obtained through gradual distraction. Despite the radiographic appearance of coalescence, the majority of Charcot deformities can undergo distraction without ostectomy to realign the pedal anatomy. This first stage consists of osseous realignment is achieved with an external fixator utilizing ligamentotaxis. After realignment, the correction is maintained by creating an osseous fusion with rigid intramedullary metatarsal screws that are inserted percutaneously. This two-stage correction is a new technique that was developed by the senior author (DP). The distraction restores the osseous anatomy and allows for ulcer healing.

Surgical Technique

The first stage consists of osseous realignment achieved by performing ligamentotaxis. A Taylor Spatial Frame (TSF) forefoot 6×6 butt frame construct is applied and provides gradual relocation of the forefoot on the hindfoot. The distal tibia, talus, and calcaneus are fixed with two U-plates joined and first mounted orthogonal to the tibia in both the anteroposterior and lateral planes. The U-plate is affixed to the tibia with one lateromedial 1.8 mm wire and two to three other points of fixation (combination of smooth wires or half-pins). For additional stability, a second distal tibial ring can be added, creating a distal tibial fixation block. It is essential to fix the hindfoot in a neutral position; an Achilles tendon lengthening typically is required to achieve a neutral hindfoot position. We prefer performing percutaneous Z-lengthening of the Achilles tendon. With the hind-foot manually held in a neutral position, the U-plate is fixed to the calcaneus with two crossing 1.8 mm wires. A 1.8 mm medial-lateral talar neck wire also is inserted and fixed to the U-plate. Next, two 1.8 mm stirrup wires are inserted through the osseous segment just proximal and distal to the Charcot joint(s). Stirrup wires are bent 90° just outside the skin to extend and attach but are not tensioned to their respective external fixation rings distant from the point of fixation. These stirrup wires capture osseous segments that are far from an external fixation ring, thereby providing accurate and precise Charcot joint distraction. A full external fixation ring is then mounted to the forefoot with two 1.8 mm crossing metatarsal wires and the aforementioned distal stirrup wire. Digital pinning often is required whereby the digital wires (1.5 or 1.8 mm) are attached to the forefoot ring. Finally, the six TSF struts are placed and final radiographs obtained (anteroposterior and lateral views of the foot to include the tibia). Orthogonal anteroposterior

and lateral view fluoroscopic images are obtained of the reference ring; the images provide the mounting parameters that are needed for the computer planning. The choice of which ring (distal or proximal) to use as the reference ring is per the surgeon's preference; typically, a distal reference is chosen for foot deformity correction. Superimposition of the reference ring on the final films is critical for accurate postoperative computer deformity planning (www.spatialframe. com). TSF planning is critical to fully comprehend before attempting this procedure. In summary, the surgeon enters the deformity and mounting parameters into an Internet-based software that produces a daily schedule for the patient to perform adjustments on each of the six struts. The rate and duration of the patient's schedule is controlled by the surgeon's data entry. The patient is clinically and radiographically followed in the office weekly or biweekly.

Creative frame construction is required because of the small pedal anatomy, which renders it difficult to apply external fixation. When applying the forefoot 6×6 butt frame, it is important to mount the U-plate on the hindfoot and the full ring on the forefoot as posteriorly and anteriorly as possible, respectively. The greatest distance of forefoot and hindfoot ring separation is critical to accommodate the TSF struts. Bone segment fixation is important; otherwise, failure of osteotomy separation or incomplete anatomic reduction occurs. Small wire fixation is preferred in the foot because of the size and consistency of the bones. When treating a patient with neuropathy, construction of extremely stable constructs is of great importance. External fixation for Charcot deformity correction should include a distal tibial ring with a closed foot ring.

After gradual distraction with the TSF has realigned the anatomy of the foot, the second stage is performed. In the second stage, the external fixator is removed while simultaneously performing minimally invasive arthrodesis of the affected joints with percutaneous insertion of internal fixation. Gradual distraction for realignment of the dislocated Charcot joint(s) is obtained in approximately 1–2 months. Before frame removal, small transverse incisions (2–3 cm in

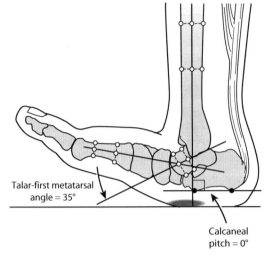

Talar-first metatarsal angle = 35°

Calcaneal pitch = 0°

Fig. 15.1 Illustration of a midfoot (midtarsal joint) Charcot neuroarthropathy with equinus deformity (Eichenholtz stage II or III, with ulceration). Lateral view shows equinus (calcaneal pitch, 0°) and rocker bottom (talar-first metatarsal angle, 35°) (From Paley [11], with kind permission of Springer Science + Business Media)

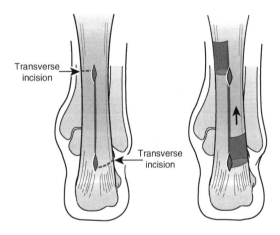

Transverse incision

Transverse incision

Modified with permission from Springer-Verlag © 2002

Fig. 15.2 Percutaneous Achilles tendon Z-lengthening is performed to acutely correct the equinus deformity (*Inset*, modified from Paley [11], with kind permission of Springer Science + Business Media)

length) overlying the appropriate joint(s) are made to perform cartilage removal and joint preparation for arthrodesis. Minimally invasive arthrodesis is easily preformed because the Charcot joint(s) are already distracted. Under fluoroscopic guidance, the guidewires for the

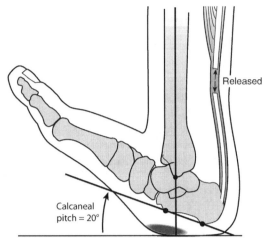

Released

Calcaneal pitch = 20°

Fig. 15.3 After tendon Achilles lengthening, the calcaneal pitch is restored to 20°. Note the resultant forefoot position (From Paley [11], with kind permission of Springer Science + Business Media)

large-diameter cannulated screws are inserted percutaneously through the plantar skin incision into the metatarsal head by dorsiflexing the metatarsophalangeal joint. After the lateral and medial column guidewires are inserted to maintain the corrected foot position, the frame is removed and the foot is re-prepped. Typically, three large-diameter cannulated intramedullary metatarsal screws are inserted: medial and lateral column partially threaded screws for compression of the arthrodesis site and one central fully threaded screw for additional stabilization. These screws span the entire length of the metatarsals to the calcaneus and talus, provide compression across the minimally invasive arthrodesis site, and stabilize the adjacent joints. The intramedullary metatarsal screws cross an unaffected joint, the Lisfranc joint, thereby protecting the Lisfranc joint from experiencing a future Charcot event. The minimally invasive incisions are then closed, and a well-padded U and L splint is applied. Before hospital discharge (length of hospital stay ranges from 1 to 4 days), the patient's operative splint and dressing are removed and a short leg cast applied. A non-weight-bearing short leg cast is maintained for 2–3 months, and then gradual progression to weight bearing is achieved. Thus, the entire treatment is completed in 4–5 months (Figs. 15.1 and 15.8).

a
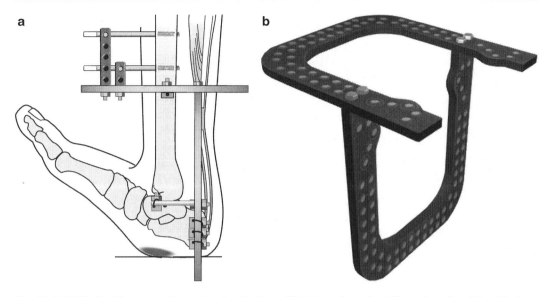

b

Fig. 15.4 (**a**) The hindfoot and ankle are then fixed in the corrected position with the Taylor spatial frame (TSF) (forefoot 6×6 butt). Note the stirrup wires placed adjacent (just distal and proximal) to the midtarsal joint to ensure focused distraction at the Charcot joint.

(**b**) A three-dimensional illustration of two joined U-plates that form the posterior construct for the forefoot 6×6 butt frame (From Paley [11], with kind permission of Springer Science + Business Media)

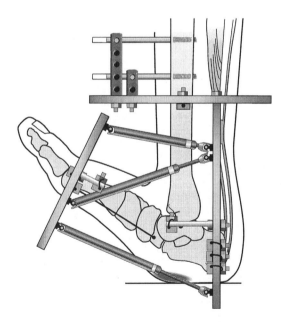

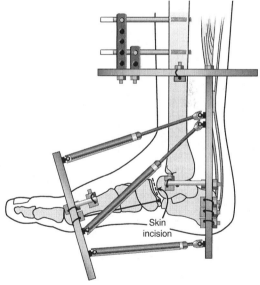

Fig. 15.5 The forefoot ring is mounted perpendicular to the longitudinal axis of the metatarsals. Note that this ring is mounted as distal as possible in order to allow adequate space between the forefoot and hindfoot ring for strut placement (From Paley [11], with kind permission of Springer Science + Business Media)

Fig. 15.6 Gradual distraction (5–15 mm) and realignment of the forefoot to the hindfoot are performed with the external fixator. Just before fixator removal, a minimally invasive fusion of the midtarsal joint is performed through a vertical incision. The plantar ulcer is now healed (From Paley [11], with kind permission of Springer Science + Business Media)

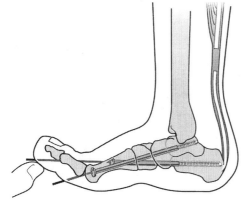

Fig. 15.7 After inserting the percutaneous guidewires for the large-diameter cannulated screws, the fixator is removed. Then, partially threaded intramedullary metatarsal cannulated screws are inserted beneath the metatarsal head percutaneously to compress both the medial and lateral columns of the foot to ensure fusion of the midtarsal joint (From Paley [11], with kind permission of Springer Science + Business Media)

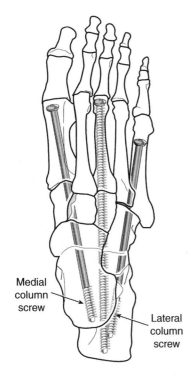

Medial
column
screw

Lateral
column
screw

Fig. 15.8 Anteroposterior view shows a third fully threaded screw inserted to increase midfoot stability. Note the accurate anatomic reduction, fusion of the involved Charcot joint (in this example the midtarsal joint), protection of the adjacent Lisfranc joints (stability via screw fixation), ridged internal stability, restoration of foot length, healed ulceration, and preservation of the subtalar and ankle joints (From Paley [11], with kind permission of Springer Science + Business Media)

Conclusion

We have used this gradual distraction technique during the past 5 years and have achieved good to excellent success. Our short-term results are promising considering that neither recurrent ulceration nor deep infections have occurred. The advantages of our method when compared with the resection and plating method reported by Schon et al. [1] or the resection and external fixation method reported by Cooper [13] are preservation of foot length, soft tissue, and osseous anatomy, and cosmesis. Furthermore, our method is much less invasive.

Acknowledgments I thank Joy Marlowe, BSA, for her excellent illustrative artwork.

References

1. Schon LC, Easley ME, Weinfeld SB. Charcot neuroarthropathy of the foot and ankle. Clin Orthop Relat Res 349:116–131, 1998
2. Jolly GP, Zgonis T, Polyzois V. External fixation in the management of Charcot neuroarthropathy. Clin Podiatr Med Surg 20:741–756, 2003
3. Wang JC, Le AW, Tsukuda RK. A new technique for Charcot's foot reconstruction. J Am Podiatr Med Assoc 92:429–436, 2002
4. Frykberg RG, ed. The High Risk Foot in Diabetes Mellitus. New York, NY: Churchill Livingstone, 1991
5. Trepman E, Nihal A, Pinzur MS. Current topics review: Charcot neuroarthropathy of the foot and ankle. Foot Ankle Int 26:46–63, 2005
6. Eichenholtz SN. Charcot Joints. Springfield, IL: C. C. Thomas, 1966
7. Shibata T, Tada K, Hashizume C. The results of arthrodesis of the ankle for leprotic neuroarthropathy. J Bone Joint Surg 72A:749–756, 1990
8. Brodsky JW, Rouse AM. Exostectomy for symptomatic bony prominences in diabetic Charcot feet. Clin Orthop Relat Res 296:21–26, 1993
9. Simon SR, Tejwani SG, Wilson DL, Santner TJ, Denniston NL. Arthrodesis as an early alternative to nonoperative management of Charcot arthropathy of the diabetic foot. J Bone Joint Surg 82A:939–950, 2000
10. Catanzariti AR, Mendicino R, Haverstock B. Ostectomy for diabetic neuroarthropathy involving the midfoot. J Foot Ankle Surg 39:291–300, 2000
11. Paley D. Principles of Deformity Correction, Rev ed. Berlin: Springer; 2005
12. Lamm BM, Paley D. Deformity correction planning for hindfoot, ankle, and lower limb. Clin Podiatr Med Surg North Am 21:305–326, 2004
13. Cooper PS. Application of external fixators for management of Charcot deformities of the foot and ankle. Foot Ankle Clin 7:207–254, 2002

Percutaneous Supramalleolar Osteotomy Using the Ilizarov/Taylor Spatial Frame

S. Robert Rozbruch

The supramalleolar osteotomy (SMO) can be used to reposition the ankle and foot by correcting deformity about the ankle. Indications for this procedure include malunion of fracture, stiff nonunion, malunion of ankle fusion, arthrosis of the ankle with talar tilt, growth arrest deformity, and congenital or developmental deformity [1, 2].

The SMO can be performed in isolation or can be combined with other procedures such as ankle distraction, ankle fusion, or simultaneous lengthening. In general, SMO can be performed with acute or gradual correction, internal or external fixation, and closing, opening, or neutral wedge technique. While a mild to moderate valgus deformity of the ankle can be corrected with a traditional open surgery using a medial closing wedge technique, acute correction, and internal fixation, this technique has limitations and drawbacks. These include the need for open surgery and implantation of hardware, deformity correction limitations, and no postoperative adjustability.

SMO can be performed using a percutaneous technique in conjunction with an Ilizarov/Taylor Spatial Frame (TSF) (Smith and Nephew, Memphis, TN). The circular frame is percutaneously mounted to match the complete deformity (coronal, sagittal, and axial planes). Then the SMO of the tibia is percutaneously performed. Acute and/or gradual correction can be accomplished by moving the frame-bone complex. All aspects of the deformity can be corrected and there is postoperative adjustability. There is no implantation of internal fixation, making this an attractive option if there is a history of infection. When skin is compromised and the soft tissue envelope is a concern, this technique is advantageous because it avoids open incisions and bulky subcutaneous hardware. Complex deformities in an oblique plane and combined with rotational deformity can be efficiently approached in this manner. Excellent frame stability generally allows the patient to weight bear as tolerated.

This chapter addresses the clinical indications, preoperative assessment, surgical technique, and postoperative care for the technique of percutaneous SMO using the Ilizarov/TSF.

Clinical Indications

Malunion of Fracture

Malunion of a tibia fracture in the distal third of the leg will cause abnormal force transmission across the ankle and lead to posttraumatic arthrosis [1, 3, 4]. While valgus deformities are more easily compensated through inversion of the subtalar joint, the deformity will lead to wear of the ankle joint. A varus deformity is functionally debilitating to the patient because there is limited ability to compensate with hindfoot eversion. Recurvatum deformity leads to uncovering of the

S.R. Rozbruch (✉)
Limb Lengthening and Deformity Service, Hospital for Special Surgery, Weill Medical College of Cornell University, New York, NY, USA
e-mail: rozbruchsr@hss.edu

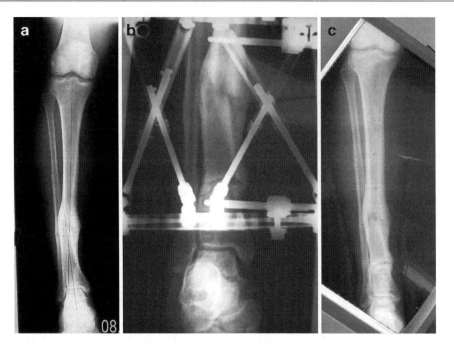

Fig. 16.1 A 35-year-old man with 15-year-old malunion of the tibia who presents with ankle pain and varus deformity. (**a**) Preoperative AP radiograph showing varus deformity at the mid-distal third of the tibia. The apex of the deformity was located in the supramalleolar region because of the translation at the malunion site. (**b**) AP radiograph at end of distraction of the SMO correction. (**c**) One-year follow-up AP radiograph showing a good restoration of the tibial axis

talus and compensatory ankle equines contracture. Procurvatum deformity limits dorsiflexion of the ankle and leads to anterior ankle impingement [4]. Oblique plane deformities and rotation and translation deformities are common in malunions.

A malunion of the mid-distal third of the leg that is composed of varus and translation may have a center of rotation and angulation (CORA) [4, 5] or apex of deformity in the supramalleolar region. The SMO becomes a convenient way to correct this because the supramalleolar bone is metaphyseal, previously uninjured, and has better healing potential than the actual site of the nonunion (Fig. 16.1).

The goal is to correct the deformity in both the coronal and sagittal planes. The goal is to achieve a lateral distal tibial angle (LDTA) of 90° (Fig. 16.2a) and an anterior distal tibial angle (ADTA) of 80° [4, 5] (Fig. 16.2b). The use of the Ilizarov/TSF is particularly useful for a gradual correction of a simple or large oblique plane deformity [6–8].

Associated symptomatic arthritis may be addressed as well. Ankle distraction [9] (Fig. 16.3) or ankle fusion (Fig. 16.4) can be performed distal to the SMO with the addition of another level of treatment.

Stiff Nonunion

The same deformity types mentioned in malunions will be seen in this group. An excellent application of gradual correction is for a hypertrophic stiff nonunion with deformity [8, 10, 11]. This type of nonunion has fibrocartilage tissue in the nonunion site that has the biologic capacity for bony union. It lacks stability and axial alignment. Gradual distraction of this type of nonunion to achieve normal alignment results in bone formation. The nonunion acts like regenerate and bony healing occurs. Modest lengthening of no more than 1.5 cm should be done through the nonunion. If additional lengthening is needed, a second osteotomy for lengthening is performed. Several studies have confirmed Ilizarov's success with this technique [1, 6, 8]. The principle

Fig. 16.2 (**a**) Normal lateral distal tibial angle (LDTA). (**b**) Normal anterior distal tibial angle (ADTA) (From Scuderi GR, Tria AJ Jr, Berger RA (eds.), MIS Techniques in Orthopedics. New York: Springer, 2006, with kind permission of Springer Science + Business Media, Inc.)

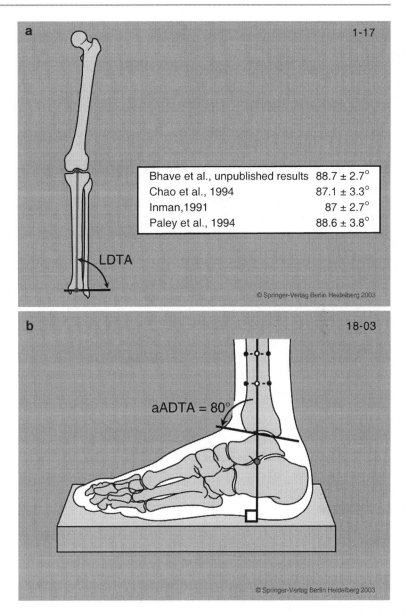

a   1-17

Bhave et al., unpublished results	88.7 ± 2.7°
Chao et al., 1994	87.1 ± 3.3°
Inman, 1991	87 ± 2.7°
Paley et al., 1994	88.6 ± 3.8°

LDTA

© Springer-Verlag Berlin Heidelberg 2003

b   18-03

aADTA = 80°

© Springer-Verlag Berlin Heidelberg 2003

advantages are not having to open the nonunion site in the face of poor skin and widened callus and gaining length through an opening wedge correction. This is particularly beneficial to the region above the ankle where the soft tissue envelope is often compromised. This technique is not useful for mobile atrophic nonunions and less applicable to infected nonunions.

Malunion of Ankle Fusion

An ankle fusion that is malpositioned can be corrected through an SMO [10–12]. In this case, the osteotomy can be done very distally because wire penetration into the ankle joint is not a concern. One can correct all deformities including anterior translation (Fig. 16.5). If some lengthening is needed,

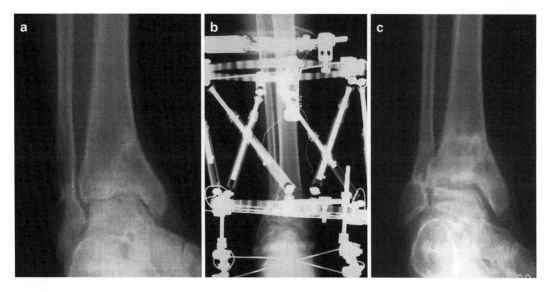

Fig. 16.3 A 20-year-old woman with posttraumatic arthrosis of the ankle. (**a**) Preoperative AP radiograph showing varus tilt of the talus and extensive medial cartilage loss. (**b**) After SMO to put talus in neutral and ankle distraction. (**c**) Two-year follow-up showing normal alignment and improved joint space

it may be done through the same osteotomy or through an osteotomy in the proximal tibia.

Ankle Arthrosis with Deformity

Ankle arthrosis may be associated with an angular deformity of the distal tibia [13]. Tilt of the talus may develop with joint space narrowing on one particular side of the ankle joint. In this situation, the SMO may be used to achieve a neutral talus relative to the axis of the tibia [2, 14, 15]. This can be combined with an ankle distraction [9, 10] (Fig. 16.3).

Ankle and Foot Deformity

A combined deformity consisting of ankle valgus with foot planovalgus and forefoot abduction can be seen in rheumatoid arthritis, as an example (Fig. 16.6). An SMO can be used to correct (and even overcorrect to a small degree) the ankle valgus. In addition, internal rotation at the SMO can be used to compensate for some of the planovalgus and forefoot abduction [14, 16]. Correction of

a foot deformity above the ankle is very powerful in that it effects a large translation change to the foot. One is limited by the desire to avoid an oblique ankle joint line. In cases of ankle fusion or correction of ankle fusion, obliquity of the ankle fusion mass is not a significant problem.

Growth Arrest Deformity

Asymmetric damage to the distal tibial growth plate can occur from trauma or infection. This will lead to deformity and shortening of the leg. The distal tibial growth plate contributes 40% of the tibial growth (Fig. 16.7).

Congenital and Developmental Deformity

Neuromuscular

Asymmetric muscle pull can lead to deformity at the ankle [17]. This is seen in Charcot–Marie–Tooth (CMT) disease with first equinovarus of

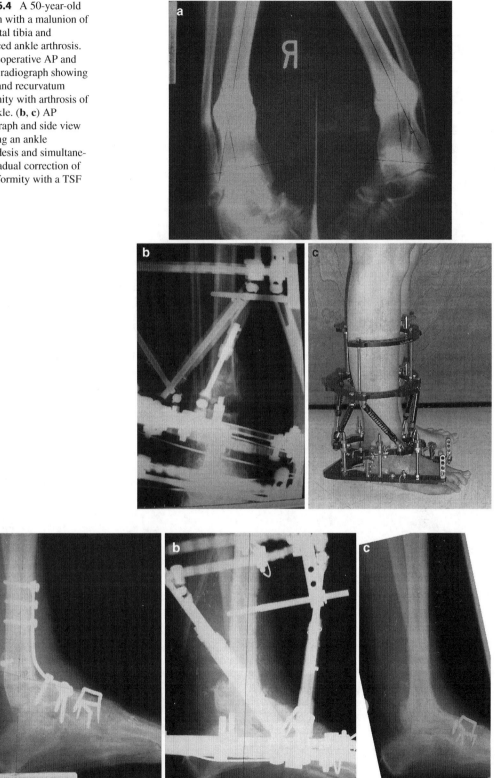

Fig. 16.4 A 50-year-old woman with a malunion of the distal tibia and advanced ankle arthrosis. (**a**) Preoperative AP and lateral radiograph showing varus and recurvatum deformity with arthrosis of the ankle. (**b, c**) AP radiograph and side view showing an ankle arthrodesis and simultaneous gradual correction of the deformity with a TSF

Fig. 16.5 A 40-year-old woman with malunion of ankle fusion. (**a**) Lateral radiograph showing anterior translation deformity. (**b**) After correction with an SMO and gradual correction with a TSF. (**c**) One-year follow-up

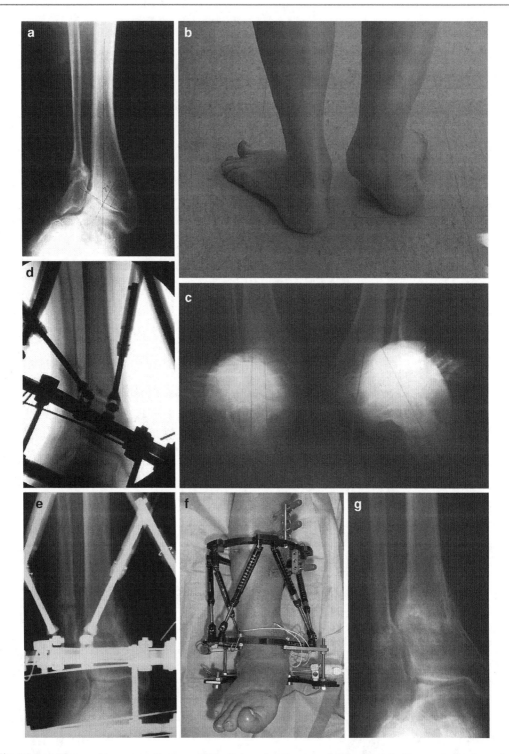

Fig. 16.6 A 77-year-old woman with rheumatoid arthritis who has an ankle/foot deformity. (**a**) Preoperative AP radiograph showing valgus ankle deformity. (**b**) Back view showing ankle/hindfoot valgus and forefoot abduction. (**c**) Saltzman view illustrating the deformity. Note that the apex of deformity is in the supramalleolar region. (**d**) After SMO and application of frame to match the deformity. (**e, f**) After the distraction phase, showing correction of the deformity. (**g**) One year later, showing a healed osteotomy

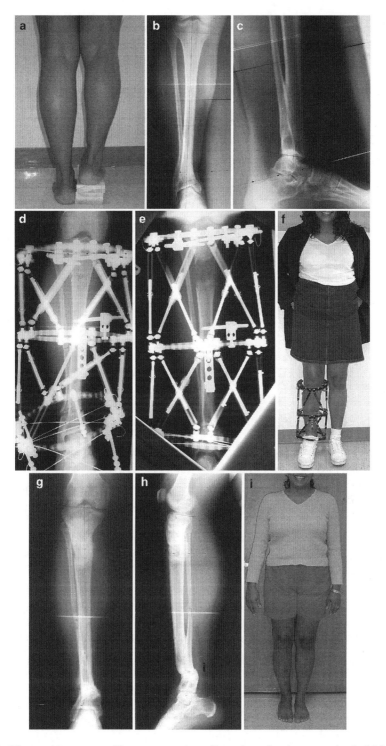

Fig. 16.7 A 25-year-old woman with posttraumatic growth arrest of the distal tibia. (**a**) Back view showing that an LLD of 6-cm ankle varus is compensated by mobile hindfoot eversion. (**b**) Preoperative AP radiograph showing the varus deformity. (**c**) Lateral radiograph showing a procurvatum deformity. The apex of the deformity is periarticular. (**d**) Postoperative radiograph showing non-displaced SMO and proximal tibial osteotomy. (**e**) After distraction, showing a proximal tibial lengthening and distal tibia correction. (**f**) Standing front view at end of distraction. (**g, h**) AP and lateral radiographs 1 year later, showing healed osteotomies. Note the intentional medial and posterior translation of the distal fragment because the osteotomy site was away from the apex of deformity. (**i**) Standing front view showing equal leg lengths and correction of deformity

the foot and later talar tilt, which further increases the varus deformity. This pattern can also be seen after nerve injury. Valgus deformities have been observed in myelomeningocele [18, 19]. External rotation deformities have been observed in patients with cerebral palsy [20] and sacral agenesis.

Fibrous Dysplasia and Ollier's Disease

These tumor-like conditions are associated with deformity. This seems to occur when the lesions affect the growth plate. Deformities of the ankle related to growth disturbance at the distal tibial physis can be corrected with an SMO. When an osteotomy is performed through Ollier's bone, new normal bone will grow.

Achondroplasia

In addition to varus deformities of the proximal tibiae, there are often varus deformities of the distal tibiae as well. Double-level tibial osteotomies including an SMO may be done to correct all deformities and to divide a large lengthening between two sites.

Preoperative Assessment

Clinical Evaluation

In the history, one should obtain information about the type of bony and soft tissue injury, surgical procedures performed, history of infection, and the use of antibiotics. High-energy injuries and open fractures have a higher risk for infection. Information about back pain, perceived leg length discrepancy (LLD), use of a shoe lift, and deformity should be elicited from the patient. The presence of deformity will often lead to the patient's report of a feeling of increased pressure on the medial or lateral part of the foot with a valgus or varus deformity, respectively. A short leg will often lead to complaints of low back pain

and contralateral hip pain. If antibiotics are being used to suppress an infected nonunion, an attempt should be made to discontinue these for 6 weeks prior to surgery in order to obtain reliable intraoperative culture samples. Discontinuation of antibiotics must be done with caution and careful observation, particularly in compromised patients like those with diabetes or on immunosuppressive medications. The current amount of pain, the use of narcotics, and the ability to ambulate with or without support should be noted.

On physical examination, one should look for deformity and LLD with the patient standing still and walking. The inability to bear weight suggests an unstable nonunion. The view from the back is helpful for seeing coronal plane deformity. LLD is evaluated by using blocks under the short leg and by examining the level of the iliac crests. The view from the side is helpful for observing sagittal plane deformity, and equines contracture. The combination of recurvatum deformity above the ankle and equines contracture of the ankle will lead to a foot translated forward position with an extension moment on the knee. Range of motion of the ankle, subtalar, forefoot, and toes should be recorded. Rigid compensation for ankle deformity through the subtalar joint is an important factor. This typically occurs when there is long-standing ankle deformity. If this is present, it must be taken into account when correcting the ankle. The condition of the soft tissue envelope, especially previous surgical wounds and flaps, and neurovascular findings should be recorded. This includes the posterior tibial and dorsalis pedis pulses, foot sensation, and dorsiflexion and plantarflexion motor function of the ankle and toes.

Rotational deformity is best assessed on clinical exam with the patient in the prone position. *Thigh-foot axis* (TFA) is used to assess rotational deformity of the tibia. Rotational profile of the femur is used to assess rotational deformity in the femur. Computed tomographic (CT) scan can also be used for this purpose. CT scan cuts at the proximal femur, distal femur, proximal tibia, and distal tibia allow analysis of rotational deformity [4, 10].

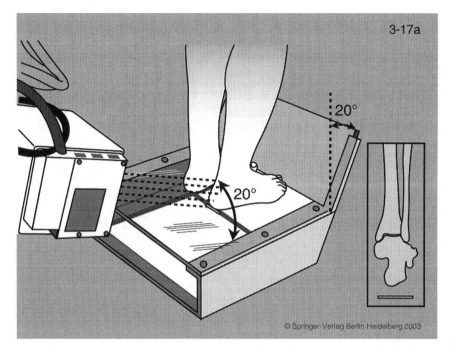

Fig. 16.8 Saltzman view schematic diagram (From Scuderi GR, Tria AJ Jr, Berger RA (eds.), MIS Techniques in Orthopedics. New York: Springer, 2006, with kind permission of Springer Science + Business Media, Inc.)

Radiographic Assessment

Radiographs should include anteroposterior (AP), lateral, and mortise views of the ankle, Saltzman's view of both feet (Fig. 16.8) and a 51″ bipedal erect leg x-ray including the hips to ankles with blocks under the short leg to level the pelvis. LLD as well a limb alignment can be measured from a standing bipedal 51″ radiograph. The short leg is placed on blocks to level the pelvis and the height of the blocks is recorded [4, 5]. This can be done with the patient using crutches if necessary. These radiographs yield crucial information about LLD, deformity, presence of hardware, arthritis, and bony union. A supine scanogram can also be used to measure length discrepancy but this is not useful for alignment analysis. CT scan and magnetic resonance imaging (MRI) can be used for further evaluation as needed. The CT scan can be helpful in getting more information about bony union. The MRI can be helpful for obtaining information about the condition of cartilage in the ankle and subtalar

joints and the presence of infection. Nuclear medicine studies can also be used, but we have not found them to be very helpful in this evaluation.

Laboratory studies including white blood cell count, erythrocyte sedimentation rate, and C-reactive protein can be helpful for diagnosing the presence of infection. Selective lidocaine injections into the ankle and subtalar joints may be helpful for diagnosing the dominant source of pain.

Surgical Planning

The proximal tibial axis is represented with an antegrade mid-diaphyseal tibial line. The coronal plane distal tibial axis is represented with a perpendicular line to the ankle joint drawn retrograde (normal LDTA is 90°) (see Fig. 16.2a). The intersection of these lines is the apex of deformity (Fig. 16.9). In the sagittal plane, the distal tibial axis is drawn 80° to the lateral joint line (remember that normal ADTA is 80°) (see Fig. 16.2b).

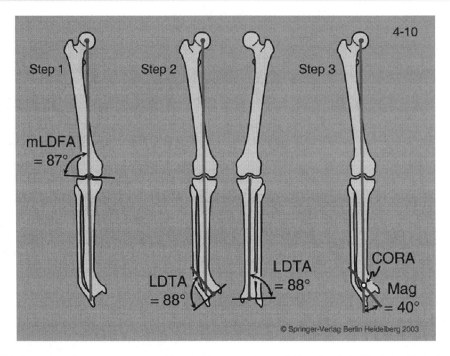

Fig. 16.9 Correction of varus can cause injury to the posterior tibial nerve with stretch and needed medial translation. Correction of procurvatum can cause injury to the posterior tibial nerve with stretch and needed posterior translation (From Scuderi GR, Tria AJ Jr, Berger RA (eds.), MIS Techniques in Orthopedics. New York: Springer, 2006, with kind permission of Springer Science + Business Media, Inc.)

The intersection of these lines is the apex of deformity. The rotational deformity is assessed from the TFA done on physical examination. If the osteotomy is at the level of the CORA, then no translation is needed. If the osteotomy is done at a level that is different from the CORA, then translation at the osteotomy site will be needed to fully correct the deformity [4, 5] (Fig. 16.10).

Treatment Principles

Features of the Ilizarov Method

The Ilizarov method is particularly useful for addressing the full spectrum of posttraumatic ankle pathology. Listed below are versatile features of the Ilizarov method [7, 9–12, 21].

1. Avoid internal fixation in the presence or history of infection
2. Allows a minimal incision technique in setting of poor soft tissue

3. Utilizes acute and/or gradual correction of deformity
4. Utilizes opening wedge correction, avoiding the need for bone resection
5. Useful for large deformity correction
6. Postoperative adjustability for compression or correction
7. Simultaneous lengthening is possible for optimization of LLD
8. Allows multiple-level treatment (a modular approach)
9. Weight bearing and ankle range of motion are encouraged.

Acute Versus Gradual Correction

One can employ either acute or gradual correction of a nonunion or malunion [1, 8]. Acute corrections can be performed in conjunction with all methods of fixation including plates [19, 22], intramedullary (IM) nails, and external fixation frames.

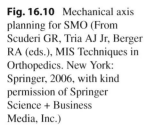

Fig. 16.10 Mechanical axis planning for SMO (From Scuderi GR, Tria AJ Jr, Berger RA (eds.), MIS Techniques in Orthopedics. New York: Springer, 2006, with kind permission of Springer Science + Business Media, Inc.)

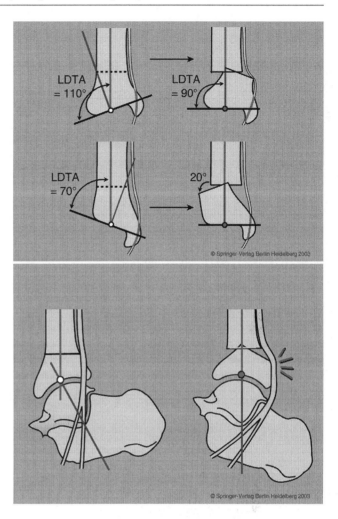

Gradual correction requires the use of specialized frames. The personality of the problems helps guide the surgeon toward the best method. For example, a distal tibial malunion with 15° valgus deformity and 2 cm shortening is best handled with an osteotomy to gradually correct the angular deformity and lengthen the bone with a specialized frame. The Ilizarov method is utilized to gradually correct the complete deformity with distraction osteogenesis. One may choose to perform the deformity correction and lengthening at one level if bone regeneration potential is good. Alternatively, one may choose to perform a double level osteotomy – one level at the CORA [5] for deformity correction, and one level for lengthening in the proximal tibia metaphysis (see Fig. 16.7). Gradual correction achieves treatment of shortening and carries less risk of posterior tibial nerve stretch neuropraxia than if attempted with an acute correction (Fig. 16.10).

The use of plates and IM nails requires an acute correction of angular and translational deformity. Acute corrections are particularly useful for modest deformity correction, mobile atrophic nonunions that are opened and bone grafted, and small bone defects that can be acutely shortened. The principle advantage of acute correction is earlier bone contact for healing and a simpler fixation construct. Acute corrections are generally better tolerated in the femur and humerus and less well tolerated in the tibia and ankle, related to issues of neurovascular insult.

Gradual correction with a specialized frame is useful for large deformity correction [11, 21, 23], associated limb lengthening, bone transport to treat segmental defects [24], and for stiff hypertrophic nonunion repair [8]. Gradual correction employs the principle of *distraction osteogenesis* commonly referred to as the *Ilizarov method* [12, 25]. Bone and soft tissue is gradually distracted at a rate of approximately 1 mm per day in divided increments. Bone growth in the distraction gap is called *regenerate*. The interval between osteotomy and the start of lengthening is called the *latency phase* and is usually 7–10 days. The correction and lengthening is called the *distraction phase*. The *consolidation phase* is the time from the end of distraction until bony union [25]. This phase is most variable and is most affected by patient factors such as age and health. If the *structure at risk* (SAR) is a nerve, such as the peroneal nerve for a proximal tibia valgus deformity or the posterior tibial nerve for an equinovarus deformity of the ankle (Fig. 16.9), gradual correction may be the safer option. The correction can be planned so that the SAR is stretched slowly. If nerve symptoms do occur, the correction can be slowed or stopped. Nerve release can be employed in select situations based on the response to gradual correction [4].

Surgical Technique

Wire and Pin Configuration

Tensioned skinny wires and half-pins lend approximately the same stability to the frame. The proximal ring or ring block is secured with three or four points of fixation. We typically use one skinny wire (1.8-mm wire for adults) as a reference wire from anterolateral to posteromedial for purposes of mounting the ring. Additional fixation is secured with half-pins. Six-millimeter hydroxy-coated pins are our first choice for adult patients. These are inserted after drilling a 4.8-mm tract [7].

The distal tibial ring is usually secured with two or three skinny wires (tensioned to 130 kg) and a half-pin. The reference wire is placed in the tibia alone parallel to the ankle. Next, a fibula-tibia wire is inserted posterolateral to anteromedial to reinforce the syndesmosis and prevent fibula migration. A posteromedial to anterolateral wire can also be added. Finally, an anteromedial (medial to the tibialis anterior tendon) to posterolateral 6-mm half-pin is used to add stability in the sagittal plane. Fixation may be extended across the ankle to the foot if additional stability of the distal segment is needed.

Taylor Spatial Frame

Terminology

Rings are placed on either side of the defect site and the anticipated lengthening site(s) (Fig. 16.10). The rings can be placed independently to optimally fit the leg. This is called the *rings first method*. One ring is chosen as the *reference ring* for each level of movement, and it is important that this ring be placed orthogonal to the axis of the tibia. Mounting parameters are defined by the center of the reference ring and this defines the point in space where the deformity correction will occur. It is important to maintain enough distance between rings so that the struts can fit properly. In this frame, one is limited by the shortest length of strut. The advantages of this frame are that the application is easier and the fit on the leg is better when using the *rings first method*. In addition, residual deformity at the lengthening and docking sites can be addressed by using the same frame to correct angulation and translation simultaneously in the coronal, sagittal, and axial planes without major frame modification. This minimizes angular deformity at the lengthening sites [6, 7].

One ring is chosen to be the *reference ring*. The "virtual hinge" around which the correction occurs is defined by the origin and corresponding point (CP). The *origin* is a point chosen on the edge of one bone segment at the defect site. A *corresponding point* on the other bone segment is chosen with the goal of reducing the CP to the origin. *Mounting parameters* define the location of the origin relative to the reference ring. Mounting parameters are defined by the spatial relationship between the center of the reference ring and the origin in the coronal, sagittal, and axial planes.

This defines a virtual hinge around which the deformity correction will occur. TSF struts are used to connect the rings across the deformity.

Deformity Parameters

There are six deformity parameters that will describe the relationship between the proximal segment and the distal segment (the reference segment has the origin and the moving segment has the corresponding point) (Fig. 16.11a, b). Deformity parameters consist of an angulation and a translation in the coronal, sagittal, and axial planes. In the coronal plane, the angulation is varus or valgus and the translation is medial or lateral. In the sagittal plane, the angulation is apex anterior or apex posterior and the translation is anterior or posterior. In the axial plane, the angulation is internal or external rotation and the translation is short or long.

Mounting Parameters

Because the TSF enables correction around a virtual hinge, one must communicate its location (origin) to the computer program (Fig. 16.11c). A grid projected from the reference ring allows one to specify the location of the origin. The location of the origin relative to the center of the reference ring in the coronal, sagittal, and axial planes is recorded. For example, the center of the reference ring may be 10 mm lateral, 25 mm posterior, and 35 mm distal to the origin.

Structure at Risk

The speed of the correction is determined by the surgeon by choosing a structure that he or she wants to move at a determined rate (Fig. 16.11d). Typically, a structure in the concavity of the deformity is the SAR. For example, if we are correcting a varus deformity, the SAR may be the medial cortex of the tibia or the posterior tibial nerve. If we are correcting a valgus, recurvatum deformity, the SAR will be the anterolateral surface of the tibia. We usually move the SAR at 1 mm per day [25], although, this can be varied.

Fibula Osteotomy

Osteotomy of the fibula is usually performed with the use of a tourniquet at the beginning of the

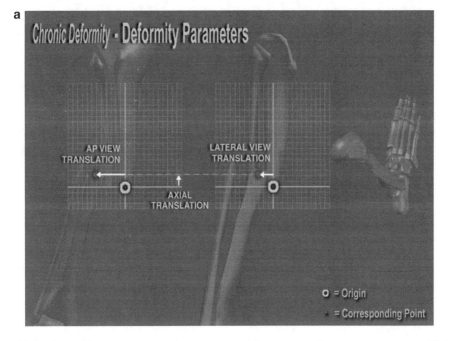

Fig. 16.11 Taylor Spatial Frame concept and language. (**a**) Measurement of translation deformity parameters. (**b**) Measurement of angulation deformity parameters. (**c**) Measurement of mounting parameters. (**d**) Structure at risk relative to origin. (**e**) Before correction. (**f**) After correction

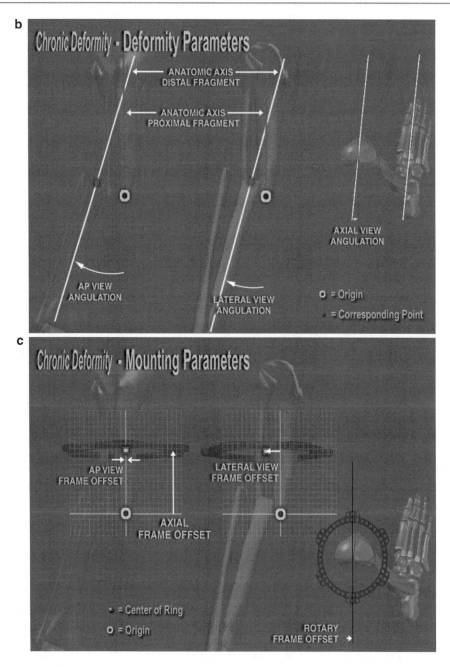

Fig. 16.11 (continued)

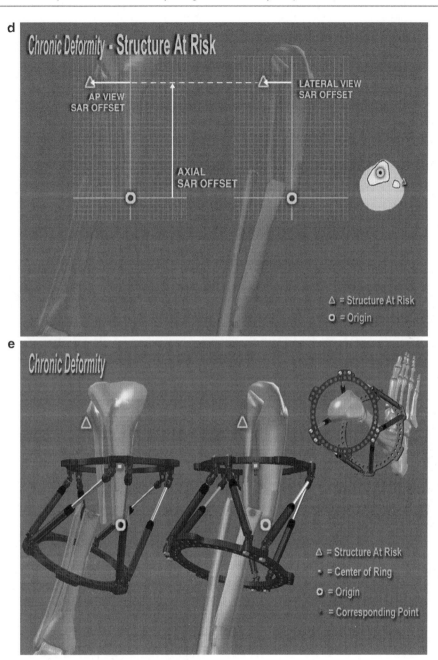

Fig. 16.11   (continued)

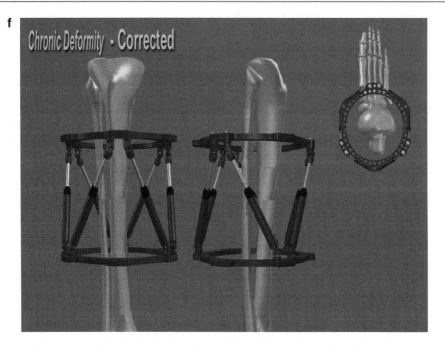

Fig. 16.11 (continued)

procedure prior to frame application. A lateral exposure is a simple and safe way to approach the fibula. It is best to locate the osteotomy at or near the apex of deformity, although osteotomy at exactly the same level of the tibia is avoided. This is done to avoid formation of a synostosis.

The shape of osteotomy may be transverse or oblique. When correcting valgus deformity gradually, a transverse osteotomy is done that will be gradually distracted and the gap will fill in with regenerate. When correcting varus deformity, the fibula will need to shorten [3, 21, 26]. This is accomplished with either fibula resection or an oblique osteotomy where the fragments can overlap.

Supramalleolar Tibial Osteotomy

After the frame has been mounted on the intact bone, the tibial osteotomy is performed. The strut connections between the rings are recorded and then removed. Through a 1-cm skin incision, medial to the tibialis anterior tendon and approximately 1 cm proximal to the distal tibial pins, the SMO is performed. The fluoroscopy is positioned to obtain a lateral x-ray of the distal tibia. A multiple drill hole osteotomy technique is used. This entails three passes of the drill along the planned osteotomy line. The SMO is then completed by passing the osteotome across the medial cortex, lateral cortex, and through the bone center to crack the posterior cortex. Rotation of the osteotome and ultimately rotation of the rings completes the osteotomy [4]. Alternatively, a Gigli saw technique can be used to perform the SMO.

Extension Across the Ankle

If there is an ankle contracture, then a foot ring is placed and gradual correction can be done simultaneously. Hinges are placed at the axis of the ankle as in the situation of an ankle distraction. A pulling rod can be placed anterior or a pushing rod posterior to motor the correction (Fig. 16.12).

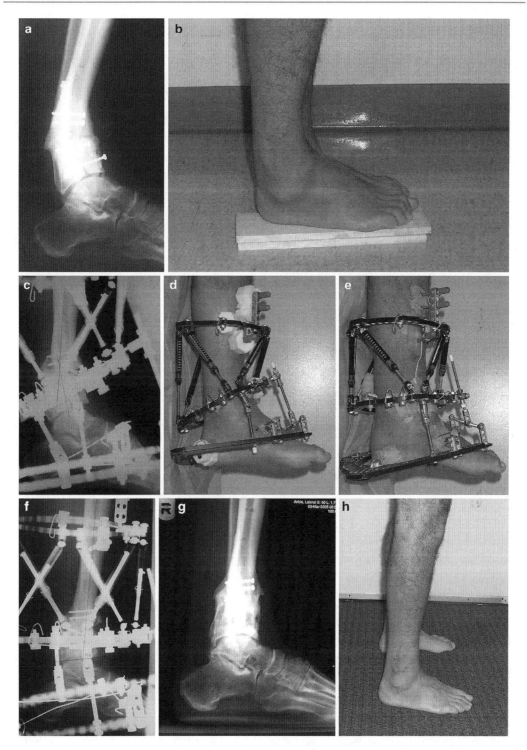

Fig. 16.12 A 48-year-old man with deformity after pilon fracture. (**a**) Preoperative lateral x-ray showing a recurvatum malunion combined with an ankle equines contracture. (**b**) Side view showing foot forward position. (**c**, **d**) Postoperative x-ray and clinical photo showing the frame matching the deformity at the two levels of correction. (**e**, **f**) After correction of the two levels of deformity. (**g**, **h**) Two years later, the patient has minimal pain

Proximal Tibial Osteotomy

If there is shortening of the tibia, this can be addressed at the same time as the deformity correction at the apex of the deformity. An osteotomy at the proximal tibia for lengthening can be done if the bone-healing potential at the apex of deformity is not optimal (see Fig. 16.7).

Postoperative Care

Patients are admitted to the hospital for 2–3 days. Nonsteroidal anti-inflammatory medications are avoided in all osteotomy patients for fear of adverse affects on bone formation. The patients receive intravenous antibiotics for 24 h and are then switched to oral antibiotics. The patients are discharged on oral antibiotics for 10 days and oral pain medication. Patients return to the office 10 days postoperatively where sutures are removed and they are educated on how to perform strut adjustments. Patients are seen every 2 weeks during this adjustment period and then once monthly during the consolidation period.

Deformity Correction

Correction of the deformity begins after a latency period of 7–10 days. The web-based Smith and Nephew program is used to generate a daily schedule for strut adjustments that the patient will perform at home. The computer requires the input of basic information including the side, the deformity parameters, the size of the rings and length of struts used, the mounting parameters measured during frame application, and rate of daily adjustment. Additionally, a SAR is selected and entered into the program to assure the correct speed of gradual correction. For valgus producing osteotomy, the structures at risk are the medial soft tissues because they are in the concavity of the correction and will be stretched the greatest distance. Using this information, a clear and simplified prescription is created for the patient to follow every day. We prescribe that struts 1 and 2 be turned in the morning, struts 3 and 4 in the afternoon, and struts 5 and 6 in the evening for a total movement of 1 mm per day. The duration of the adjustment phase depends on the amount of correction needed and is typically between 14 and 28 days. The length of time in the frame is approximately 3 months.

Pain Management

Transdermal wires and pins can be irritating, and we encourage patients to use appropriate oral pain medications. This is especially true during the adjustment period. Once the correction is complete, the frame is no longer moving, and the pain level decreases. Severe or atypical pain merits an evaluated for infection or deep vein thrombosis (DVT).

Pin Care

The dressings are removed on postoperative day 2. Nurses teach proper daily pin care consisting of a mixture of half normal saline and half hydrogen peroxide applied to the pin sites with sterile cotton swabs. Pins and wires are covered with Xeroform dressings at the skin. Patients are allowed to begin showering on the fourth postoperative day. They are instructed to wash the frame and pin sites with antibacterial soap as an adjuvant form of pin care. Problematic smooth wires can be removed in the office without anesthetic. This is particularly done after the distraction phase or if a wire is painful and infected.

Rehabilitation

Ilizarov stressed the importance of early physical conditioning in conjunction with the application of circular fixators. Early motion increases blood flow to the lower extremity, prevents joint stiffness, and shortens recovery time [25]. Physical therapy assists with weight bearing as tolerated ambulation and range of motion exercises for the knee and ankle joints. Crutches are typically needed for the first 4–6 weeks after surgery. Occupational therapy provides a custom neutral foot splint to prevent equines posturing during sleep. Patients are encouraged to attend outpatient physical therapy where they continue with their rehabilitation programs.

Frame Removal

Fixators are removed when patients are ambulating without pain or the use of an assistive device and when callus is seen on three cortices around the osteotomy site. This is typically 3 months after the index surgery. We prefer to remove the frames in the operating room. The removal of HA coated pin can be painful and is best done under sedation. We choose to curette and irrigated all half pins sites in an effort to keep pin tracts clean. Transfixation wire sites are not debrided unless there is concern over a specific site. At the time of frame removal, bony union and maturation of the regenerate may be evaluated with a routine x-ray or a stress test under C-arm fluoroscopy. If there is a real concern about bony union, then the struts are removed and the rings manually compressed and distracted, looking for motion at the osteotomy site. A lack of consolidation will require replacement of the struts and prolonging the time in the frame. Once the fixator is removed, patients are placed into a short leg cast for 2 weeks. They are allowed 50% partial weight bearing for 2 weeks then progress to full weight bearing thereafter, first in a cam walker boot and then in a regular shoe.

Complications

Pin Infection

Pin-site infection is a common complication that we encounter when using external fixation. Pin infections are marked by erythema, increasing pain, and drainage around the pin or wire. The vast majority of these infections respond well to more aggressive local pin care and oral antibiotics. If the infection does not resolve quickly, then broader spectrum antibiotics are added or the pin or wire is removed. More advanced infections are treated with removal of the pin or wire and local bone debridement in the operating room, and

intravenous antibiotics as needed. Loose pins and wires are removed and the pin sites debrided even in the absence of infection.

Premature Consolidation

Incomplete corticotomy can complicate SMO. A circumferential division of the tibial cortex may be assured by rotating the proximal and distal rings in opposite directions and witnessing uninhibited motion through the corticotomy site. Other methods have been described, including acute distraction and angulation at the osteotomy site, but these techniques are more disruptive to the periosteum and not recommended.

True premature consolidation of the osteotomy is rare in the adult patient. Once the osteotomy is performed, there is a latency period of 7–10 days before any correction is attempted. If the latency period is prolonged, then the osteotomy site will consolidate prematurely. Similarly, if the correction is carried out too slowly, the osteotomy site may heal, preventing further correction.

Patient Related

The success of any gradual correction system is founded in the patients' abilities to participate in their own care. Patients are responsible for performing their own strut adjustment three times daily at the outset of treatment. The TSF has simplified this process through color coordination and a precise numbering system. Even so, patients have made strut adjustment errors. These mistakes are usually quickly acknowledged and remedied. Patients need to be seen frequently (every 10–14 days) during the adjustment period to avoid errors.

Nonunion

Osseous nonunion can complicate any osteotomy procedure. Causes may include inadequate fixation, lack of weight bearing, smoking and other causes of poor blood flow to the extremity, patient comorbidities, too rapid a correction, poor osteotomy technique, and an osteotomy through diaphyseal bone. Nonunions are treated aggressively with a variety of methods including compression across the osteotomy site, percutaneous periosteal and endosteal stimulation, and additional points of fixation. Nonunions are rare when using the TSF technique. In fact, when there is impaired healing, this specialized frame provides ideal circumstances for effective treatment.

Nerve Injury

Direct injury to the nerve can occur during surgery from pin or wire insertion during the osteotomy. A more common mechanism is stretch injury that occurs during distraction. This is discussed above in the section "Acute Versus Gradual Correction."

Deep Vein Thrombosis

Deep vein thrombosis is always a concern with surgery of the lower extremity. Treatment is aimed at prevention. Patients are launched into early rehabilitation programs emphasizing immediate mobility to avoid venous stasis. There is no restriction to movement at the ankle, knee, or hip, and frame stability allows comfortable weight bearing early in the postoperative period. While in the hospital, patients receive subcutaneous low molecular weight heparin. Upon discharge, patients start a 1-month course of aspirin (ASA) despite concerns about its effects on bone healing. With this regimen, we have not had any cases of DVT or pulmonary embolism.

References

1. Pugh K, Rozbruch SR. Nonunions and malunions. In: Baumgaertner MR, Tornetta P (eds.) Orthopaedic Knowledge Update Trauma 3. Rosemont, IL: American Academy of Orthopaedic Surgeons, 2005, pp. 115–130

2. Stamatis ED, Myerson MS. Supramalleolar osteotomy: indications and technique. Foot Ankle Clin 2003;8(2): 317–333

3. Graehl PM, Hersh MR, Heckman JD. Supramalleolar osteotomy for the treatment of symptomatic tibial malunion. J Orthop Trauma 1987;1(4):281–292

4. Paley D. Principles of Deformity Correction, 1st ed. Berlin: Springer, 2005

5. Paley D, Herzenberg JE, Tetsworth K, McKie J, Bhave A. Deformity planning for frontal and sagittal plane corrective osteotomies. Orthop Clin North Am 1994;25(3):425–465

6. Feldman DS, Shin SS, Madan S, Koval KJ. Correction of tibial malunion and nonunion with six-axis analysis deformity correction using the Taylor Spatial Frame. J Orthop Trauma 2003;17(8):549–554

7. Fragomen A, Ilizarov S, Blyakher A, Rozbruch SR. Proximal tibial osteotomy for medial compartment osteoarthritis of the knee using the Taylor Spatial Frame. Tech Knee Surg 2005;4(3):175–183

8. Rozbruch SR, Helfet DL, Blyakher A. Distraction of hypertrophic nonunion of tibia with deformity using Ilizarov/Taylor Spatial Frame. Report of two cases. Arch Orthop Trauma Surg 2002;122(5):295–298

9. Inda JI, Blyakher A, O'Malley MJ, Rozbruch SR. Distraction arthroplasty for the ankle using the Ilizarov Frame. Tech Foot Ankle Surg 2003;2(4):249–253

10. Rozbruch SR. Post-traumatic reconstruction of the ankle using the Ilizarov method. J Hosp Spec Surg 2005;1:68–88

11. Shtarker H, Volpin G, Stolero J, Kaushansky A, Samchukov M. Correction of combined angular and rotational deformities by the Ilizarov method. Clin Orthop Relat Res 2002 Sep;(402):184–195

12. Paley D. The correction of complex foot deformities using Ilizarov's distraction osteotomies. Clin Orthop Relat Res 1993 Aug;(293):97–111

13. Pearce MS, Smith MA, Savidge GF. Supramalleolar tibial osteotomy for haemophilic arthropathy of the ankle. J Bone Joint Surg Br 1994;76(6):947–950

14. Benthien RA, Myerson MS. Supramalleolar osteotomy for ankle deformity and arthritis. Foot Ankle Clin 2004;9(3):475–487, viii

15. Stamatis ED, Cooper PS, Myerson MS. Supramalleolar osteotomy for the treatment of distal tibial angular deformities and arthritis of the ankle joint. Foot Ankle Int 2003;24(10):754–764

16. Sen C, Kocaoglu M, Eralp L, Cinar M. Correction of ankle and hindfoot deformities by supramalleolar osteotomy. Foot Ankle Int 2003;24(1):22–28

17. Fraser RK, Menelaus MB. The management of tibial torsion in patients with spina bifida. J Bone Joint Surg Br 1993;75(3):495–497

18. Abraham E, Lubicky JP, Songer MN, Millar EA. Supramalleolar osteotomy for ankle valgus in myelomeningocele. J Pediatr Orthop 1996;16(6): 774–781

19. Selber P, Filho ER, Dallalana R, Pirpiris M, Nattrass GR, Graham HK. Supramalleolar derotation osteotomy

of the tibia, with T plate fixation. Technique and results in patients with neuromuscular disease. J Bone Joint Surg Br 2004;86(8):1170–1175

20. Inan M, Ferri-de Baros F, Chan G, Dabney K, Miller F. Correction of rotational deformity of the tibia in cerebral palsy by percutaneous supramalleolar osteotomy. J Bone Joint Surg Br 2005;87(10): 1411–1415

21. Rozbruch SR, Blyakher A, Haas SB, Hotchkiss R. Correction of large bilateral tibia vara with the Ilizarov method. J Knee Surg 2003;16(1):34–37

22. Best A, Daniels TR. Supramalleolar tibial osteotomy secured with the Puddu plate. Orthopedics 2006; 29(6):537–540

23. Mangone PG. Distal tibial osteotomies for the treatment of foot and ankle disorders. Foot Ankle Clin 2001; 6(3):583–597

24. Rozbruch SR, Weitzman AM, Watson JT, Freudigman P, Katz H, V, Ilizarov S. Simultaneous treatment of tibial bone and soft-tissue defects with the Ilizarov method. J Orthop Trauma 2006;20(3):197–205

25. Ilizarov GA. Clinical application of the tension-stress effect for limb lengthening. Clin Orthop Relat Res 1990 Jan;(250):8–26

26. Mendicino RW, Catanzariti AR, Reeves CL. Percutaneous supramalleolar osteotomy for distal tibial (near articular) ankle deformities. J Am Podiatr Med Assoc 2005;95(1):72–84

Hallux Valgus Surgery: The Minimally Invasive Bunion Correction

17

Sandro Giannini, Roberto Bevoni,
Francesca Vannini, and Matteo Cadossi

Historical Perspective

The main goal of surgical correction of hallux valgus is the morphologic and functional rebalance of the first ray, correcting all other characteristics of the deformity [1]. Historically, distal metatarsal osteotomies have been indicted in cases of mild or moderate deformity with an intermetatarsal angle as large as 15°. Using certain osteotomies, it is possible to correct intermetatarsal angles as large as 20°. Distal osteotomies may also be used to correct deformities characterized by deviation of the distal metatarsal articular angle (DMAA) or to address concomitant stiffness [2]. Since the first operation published by Revenrdin [3] in 1881, many authors have reported their experience using different operations, each of them characterized by different indications, approaches, designs, and fixation [4–12]. Several comparative studies have been reported comparing radiographic and clinical results among many different techniques, and a review of the literature

reveals the satisfaction with all operations to be in the upper 80% level or higher [2, 13]. In 1983, New (personal communication) reported a percutaneous technique for hallux valgus correction. This technique was then reported by Bosh et al. [14], who perform a Hohmann-type [4] osteotomy fixed by only one K-wire, as described by Lamprecht and Kramer [15] in 1982, and, more recently, Magnan et al. [16] reported a description of his experience. These percutaneous operations reduce the surgical trauma because they are performed without large incisions and soft tissue procedures. They require, on the other hand, the use of particular instrumentation, such as Lindemann's osteotrite, manipulators, or dislocators. Furthermore, with these percutaneous techniques, the correction is performed blindly, and the intraoperative use of fluoroscopy is needed. The minimally invasive bunion correction used by us is not a new technique [17, 18] because it uses an osteotomy and a stabilization method already reported by other authors, making the surgical technique usable in accordance with current concepts in hallux valgus surgery.

Our technique, in fact, consists of a linear distal osteotomy at the metatarsal neck level, as described by Hohmann [4], Wilson [6], and Magerl [9], which is performed through a small medial incision and is stabilized using only one K-wire, as reported by Lamprecht and Kramer [15] and Bosh et al. [14] The characteristics of this technique can be summarized with the abbreviation SERI (simple, effective, rapid, inexpensive). This technique is simple and can be easily

S. Giannini (✉)
School of Orthopaedics, Rizzoli Orthopedic Institute,
Bologna University, Bologna, Italy
e-mail: sandro.giannini@ior.it

R. Bevoni • M. Cadossi
Rizzoli Orthopedic Institute, University of Bologna,
Bologna, Italy

F. Vannini,
Department of Orthopaedics and Traumatology,
Rizzoli Orthopedic Institute,
University of Bologna, Bologna, Italy

G.R. Scuderi and A.J. Tria (eds.), *Minimally Invasive Surgery in Orthopedics: Foot and Ankle Handbook*, 129
DOI 10.1007/978-1-4614-0893-2_17, © Springer Science+Business Media, LLC 2012

repeated, without removal of the eminence and without lateral release. It is minimally invasive and is performed under direct vision and without radiations. The technique is effective because, using different inclinations of the bone cut and different displacements of the head (lateral, dorsal, plantar, medial tilt, or rotation), it is possible to correct the pathoanatomy of each deformity. The surgical time spent is approximately 5 min. This can be reached after an adequate learning curve and permits obtaining a surgical time saving of 12 min compared with the most commonly used techniques (i.e., scarf). Finally, the technique is inexpensive because no particular instrumentation is needed, the hardware is only one K-wire for stabilization, a short surgical time is spent, and fewer complications are reported.

Indications and Contraindications

The SERI technique is indicated to correct mild to moderate reducible deformity when the hallux valgus angle is as large as 40° and the intermetatarsal angle is as large as 20°. The operation is indicated if the metatarsophalangeal joint is either incongruent or congruent, or with modification of the DMAA, and if mild degenerative arthritis is present. The technique is indicated even in cases of recurrent deformity. Specific contraindications of the SERI technique are patients older than 75 years, severe deformity with the intermetatarsal angle larger than 20°, severe degenerative arthritis or stiffness of the metatarsophalangeal joint, and severe instability of the cuneometatarsal or metatarsophalangeal joint.

Preoperative Planning

The preoperative plan includes acquiring a complete history of the patient, and a physical and radiographic examination. The patient's complaints of pain, limitation in the use of footwear, and cosmetic concerns should be considered. Moreover, the severity of the prominent medial eminence and the hallux valgus deformity, as well as the great toe mobility at the metatarsophalangeal

joint and the reducibility of the deformity should be evaluated. The latter is tested by pushing laterally the metatarsal head with one hand, and simultaneously pushing the great toe medially with the other hand. Stability of the metatarsophalangeal and cuneometatarsal joints must be assessed. Combined rotational deformity of the great toe or callosities under the first or second and third metatarsal heads must be considered, as well as any associated deformities of the lesser toes.

A standard radiographic examination, including anteroposterior and lateral weight-bearing views of the forefoot, allows the assessment of the arthritis and congruency of the joint; measurement of the hallux valgus angle, intermetatarsal angle, DMAA, and metatarsal and the digital formula. Therefore, planning of the operation is performed in terms of the obliquity of the bone cut, the extent of the medial-lateral or dorsal-plantar dislocation of the metatarsal head, and the correction of the DMAA.

As with any other technique, during bunion correction, the main concern is the ability to perform precisely and surgically what has been planned preoperatively. To facilitate this, we developed software that, beginning with a scanned, standard weight-bearing anteroposterior view, is able to simulate the correction needed, considering any anatomic variables of each patient. The software is able to state the precise amount of the bone cut inclination and the dislocation of the metatarsal head (Fig. 17.1).

Technique

Before surgery, the patient's foot or feet are scrubbed using disinfectant soap. The operation is usually performed using local or block anaesthesia and 7.5 mg ropivacaine hydrochlorate monohydrate. An Esmarch bandage is used at the ankle level. The patient is placed in the supine position. The foot is kept extrarotated, and the lateral edge is placed on the operating table. Normally, with this technique, soft tissue release is not needed because attenuation is achieved with the lateral offset of the metatarsal head itself.

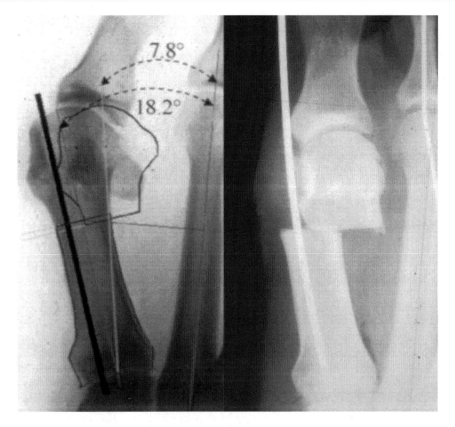

Fig. 17.1   The computerized planning of the osteotomy and the correction obtained on the postoperative x-rays

If a slight stiffness of the metatarsophalangeal joint is present, manual stretching of the adductor hallucis is performed, forcing the big toe into a varus position.

A 1 cm medial incision is made just proximal to the medial eminence through the skin, subcutaneous tissue, and down to the bone (Fig. 17.2a). The soft tissues are separated dorsally and plantarly, and they are divaricated using two retractors that are 5 mm in width (Fig. 17.2b). The medial wall of the metatarsal neck is now evident, and a complete osteotomy is performed using a standard pneumatic saw with a $9.5 \times 25 \times 0.4$ mm blade (Hall Surgical Linvatec Corporation, Largo, FL, USA; Fig. 17.2c). With a small osteotome, the head is mobilized. A 2 mm K-wire is inserted, using a normal drill passing through the incision, into the soft tissue adjacent to the bone in a proximal to distal direction along the longitudinal axis of the great toe (Fig. 17.2d). The K-wire exits at the medial area of the tip of the toe close to the nail, is retaken by the drill (Fig. 17.2e), and is retracted up to the proximal end, reaching the osteotomy line (Fig. 17.2f). Using a small, grooved lever (Fig. 17.3a) to prize the osteotomy, the correction is obtained by moving the metatarsal head depending on the pathoanatomy of the deformity (Fig. 17.3b, c). Stabilization of the correction is obtained by inserting the K-wire into the diaphyseal channel in a distal to proximal direction until its proximal end reaches the metatarsal base (Fig. 17.3d). A slight varus position (approximately 10°) of the toe is necessary and is obtained by forcing the toe after K-wire stabilization. If the proximal stump of the osteotomy is prominent medially, a small wedge of bone is removed. The skin is sutured with one 3–0 reabsorbable stitch (Fig. 17.3e). The distal extremity of the K-wire is curved and cut out of the tip of the toe (Fig. 17.4). This technique can be performed

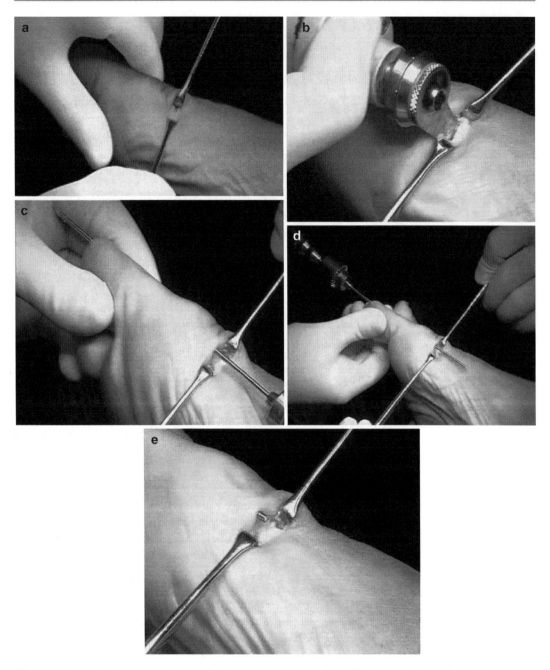

Fig. 17.2 Surgical technique: the skin incision is approximately 1 cm in length. The soft tissues are separated and
divaricated by two retractors 5 mm in width (**a**). The
metatarsal osteotomy performed by a standard saw (**b**).

The insertion of a 2-mm K-wire in the soft tissue of the
great toe along the long axis in a proximal-distal direction
(**c**). The K-wire is retracted (**d**) up to the proximal end
reaching the osteotomy line (**e**)

bilaterally or combined with the correction of any
other associated deformity of the forefoot or hind
foot during the same surgical session. The key
points of the technique are the inclinations of the

osteotomy in the medial-lateral and dorsal-plantar
directions, the displacement of the head vin the
medial-lateral and dorsal-plantar directions, and
the rotation of the metatarsal head and its medial

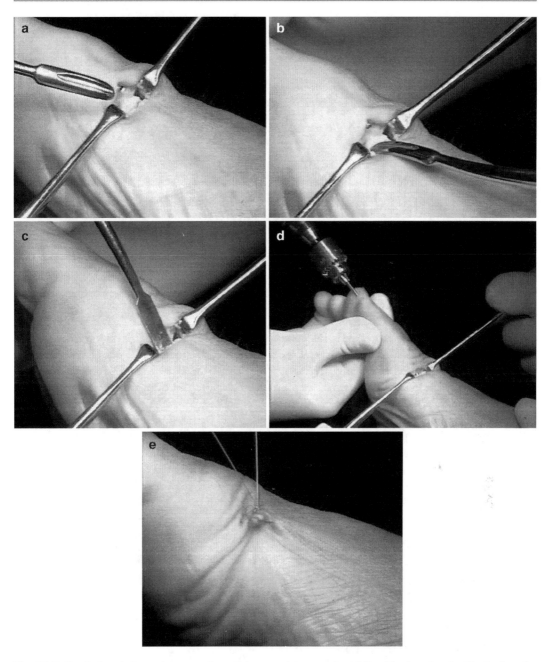

Fig. 17.3 Surgical technique: the grooved small lever (**a**). The correction of the deformity prizing the osteotomy and moving the metatarsal head as necessary (**b**, **c**). The osteotomy is stabilized by inserting the K-wire into the diaphyseal channel in a distal-proximal direction (**d**). The skin is sutured using only one 3–0 reabsorbable stitch (**e**)

tilt according to the correction of the DMAA. The inclination of the osteotomy in the medial-lateral direction is perpendicular to the foot axis (i.e., to the long axis of the second metatarsal bone) if the length of the first metatarsal bone must be maintained (Fig. 17.5a). The osteotomy is inclined in a distal to proximal direction up to 25° if shortening of the metatarsal bone or decompression of the metatarsophalangeal joint is necessary in case of mild arthritis (Fig. 17.5b).

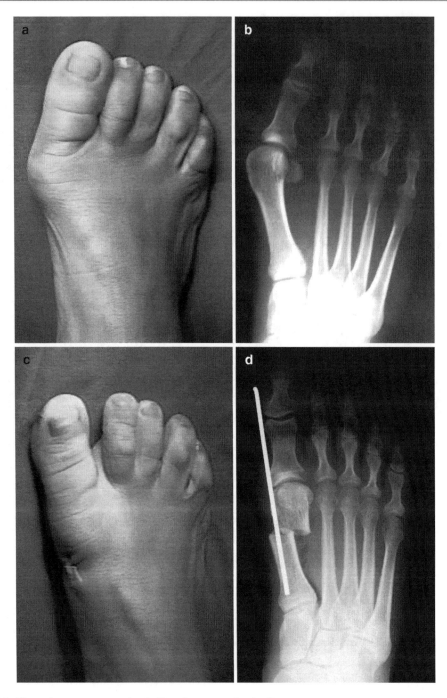

Fig. 17.4 Illustrative case preoperative (**a**, **b**) and postoperative (**c**, **d**)

More rarely, if a lengthening of the first metatarsal bone is necessary (i.e., if the first metatarsal bone is shorter than the second or if laxity of the metatarsophalangeal joint is present), the osteotomy is inclined in a proximal to distal direction as much as 15° (Fig. 17.5c). In a dorsal-plantar direction, the osteotomy is normally inclined approximately 15° in a distal to proximal direction to control the

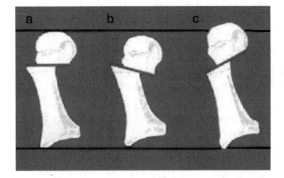

Fig. 17.5 Outline showing the different inclination of the bone cut and dislocation of the metatarsal head allowed by this technique in a mediolateral direction, perpendicular to the long axis of the second metatarsal bone (foot longitudinal axis) (**a**), proximally inclined (**b**), and distally inclined (**c**)

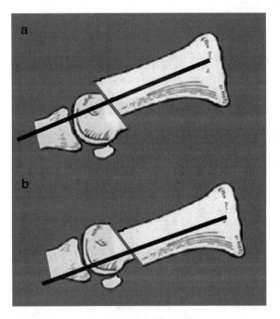

Fig. 17.6 Outline showing the inclination of the osteotomy in a dorsoplantar direction (15° in distal-proximal way) and the plantar (**a**) or dorsal (**b**) dislocation of the metatarsal head. The different position of the K-wire related to the metatarsal head and toe is evident

dorsal dislocation of the metatarsal head under weight bearing (Fig. 17.6). The adjustment of the medial-lateral dislocation of the metatarsal head is performed by introducing the K-wire more or less superficially with regard to the medial eminence. The adjustment of the plantar dislocation

of the metatarsal head, and more rarely of the dorsal dislocation, is obtained by introducing the K-wire in the upper (Fig. 17.6a) or more rarely in the lower (Fig. 17.6b) site, with regard to the long axis of the metatarsal head (Fig. 17.7). If shortening of the metatarsal bone is needed, normally, it is necessary to dislocate the metatarsal head in the plantar direction by several millimeters according to the extent of the shortening performed.

If pronation of the first metatarsal bone is present, the correction is obtained with a derotation of the big toe up to the neutral position (Fig. 17.8). To correct the DMAA, the K-wire is introduced into the soft tissue obliquely in a medial to lateral direction by as many degrees as necessary to obtain the correction (Fig. 17.9).

Results

Results regarding our first consecutive 54 ft in 37 patients (17 bilateral; 34 female patients, 3 male patients; mean age, 48 years; range, 10–70 years) are reported with a mean follow-up of 36 months (range, 22–52 months). The clinical evaluation was carried out postoperatively using the American Orthopaedic Foot and Ankle Society score. The radiographic evaluation preoperatively and postoperatively was carried out considering the hallux valgus angle, intermetatarsal angle, and DMAA measurements. All patients except four (7.4%) declared their satisfaction with the result. Postoperatively, the mean score obtained was 81 points: 35 ft (64.8%) were considered excellent, 10 (18.5%) were good, 5 (9.2%) were fair, and 4 (7.4%) were considered poor. All of the osteotomies healed well, with callus evidence after an average of 3 months. All of the metatarsal bones remodelled themselves over time (Fig. 17.10), even in cases with marked offset at the osteotomy (several millimetres of bony contact). In our experience, the healing of the osteotomy and remodelling capability of the metatarsal bone are not related to the offset at the osteotomy, but it is preferable to obtain a bony contact not less than one third of the metatarsal section.

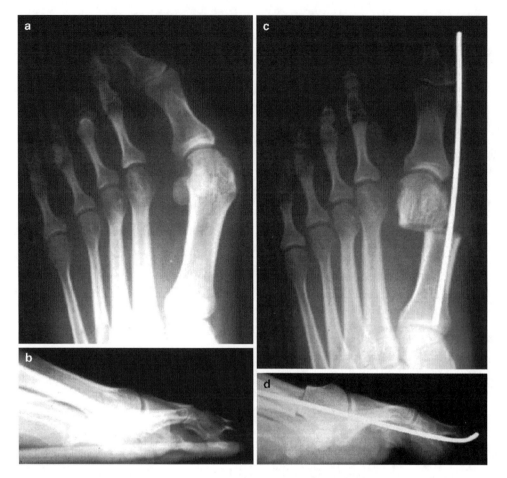

Fig. 17.7 Illustrative case: hallux valgus deformity combined with first metatarsal overloading (**a**, **b**). Postoperative x-ray in which the combined dorsal and lateral dislocation of the metatarsal head is evident (**c**, **d**)

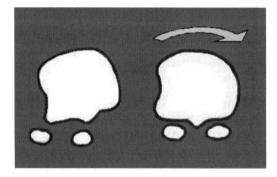

Fig. 17.8 Outline showing the derotation of the metatarsal head to assess the pronation of the metatarsal bone if present

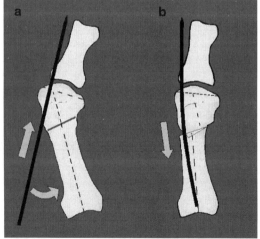

Fig. 17.9 Outline showing the correction of the distal metatarsal articular angle (DMAA). The K-wire is inserted into the soft tissue with a mediolateral inclination according to the correction of the DMAA. (**a**). After the medial tilting of the head, the K-wire is introduced in a distal-proximal direction into the diaphysis (**b**)

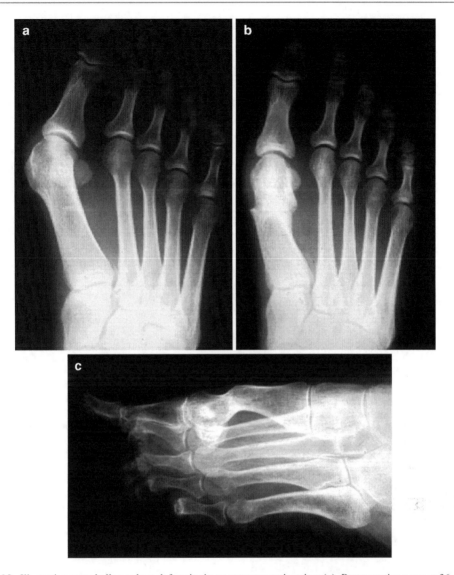

Fig. 17.10 Illustrative case: hallux valgus deformity in an anteroposterior view (**a**). Postoperative x-ray at 36-months follow-up. Good bone remodelling is evident (**b, c**)

Complications

No severe complications, such as avascular necrosis of the metatarsal head or nonunion of the osteotomy, have been reported. In 5 ft (9.2%), the radiographic healing of the osteotomy occurred more than 4 months after surgery. Three feet (5.5%) underwent a skin inflammatory reaction around the K-wire outlet at the tip of the great toe, and one patient sustained a deep vein thrombosis. All fair and poor results are the results of an incorrect indication, such as severe arthritis, or incorrect surgical technique with an incomplete correction. Transfer metatarsalgia with plantar callosities under the second and third metatarsal head are reported in the 4 ft (7.4%) considered poor.

Postoperative Management

After the operation, a gauze compression dressing is applied and a control radiograph (anteroposterior and oblique views) is acquired to confirm the placement of the osteotomy and the correction of any characteristics of the deformity. Ambulation is allowed immediately using "talus" shoes, and foot elevation is advised when the patient is at rest. K-wire fixation resulting from wire bending on insertion produces a very stable and elastic stabilization, maintaining the same position obtained during surgery, and favouring early healing of the osteotomy combined with early weight bearing (Fig. 17.11). After 1 month, the dressing, the suture, and the K-wire are removed. Passive and active exercises such as cycling and swimming are advised, and wearing comfortable, normal shoes, and gradually returning to former footwear is recommended. As a general rule, postoperative swelling does not linger for more than 1 month.

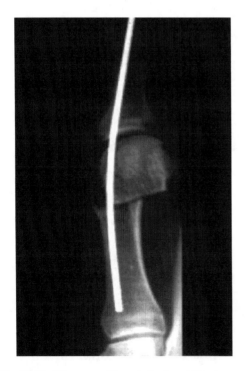

Fig. 17.11 The very stable and elastic stabilization produced by the bent K-wire, combined with early weight bearing, favours an early healing of the osteotomy

Conclusions

This minimally invasive technique enables surgeons to treat approximately 80–90% of all hallux valgus deformities without removal of the eminence and without open lateral release, performing only a manipulation of the big toe, with more than 90% excellent and good results after the learning curve. This technique is simple, and is performed under direct vision and without radiation. It is inexpensive because no particular instrumentation is needed, a short surgical time is spent, and fewer complications are reported.

References

1. Giannini S, Ceccarelli F, Mosca M, et al. Algoritmo nel trattamento chirurgico dell'alluce valgo. In: Malerba F, Dragonetti L, Giannini S (eds.), Progressi in medicina e chirurgia del piede, "L'alluce valgo." Bologna: Aulo Gaggi, 1997:155–65
2. Chang JT. Distal metaphyseal osteotomies in hallux abducto valgus surgery. In: Banks AS, Downey MS, Martin DE, et al (eds.), McGlamry's comprehensive textbook of foot and ankle surgery. Philadelphia: Lippincott, 2001:505–27
3. Revenrdin J. De la deviation en dehors du gros orteil (hallux valgus. Vulg. "oignon" "bunions" "ballen") et de son traitment chirurgical. Trans Int Med Congr 1881;2:406–12
4. Hohmann G. Symptomatische oder Physiologische Behandlung des Hallux Valgus? Munch Med Wochenschr 1921;33:1042–5
5. Mitchell CL, Fleming JL, Allen R, et al. Osteotomy bunionectomy for hallux valgus. J Bone Joint Surg Am 1958;40:41–60
6. Wilson JN. Oblique displacement osteotomy for hallux valgus. J Bone Joint Surg Br 1963;45:552–6
7. Austin DW, Leventen EO. A new osteotomy for hallux valgus: a horizontally directed "V" displacement osteotomy of the metatarsal head for hallux valgus and primus varus. Clin Orthop Relat Res 1981 Jun;157:25–30
8. Youngswick FD. Modifications of the Austin bunionectomy for treatment of metatarsus primus elevatus associated with hallux limitus. J Foot Surg 1982;21:114–6
9. Magerl F. Stabile osteotomien zur Behandlung des Hallux valgus und Metatrsale varum. Orthopade 1982;11:170–80
10. Kalish SR, Spector JE. The Kalish osteotomy: a review and retrospective analysis of 265 cases. J Am Podiatr Med Assoc 1994;84:237–49

11. Lair PO, Sirvers SH, Somdhal J. Two Reverdin-Laird osteotomy modifications for correction of hallux abducto valgus. J Am Podiatr Med Assoc 1988;78:403–5

12. Elleby DH, Barry LD, Helfman DN. The long plantar wing distal metaphyseal osteotomy. J Am Podiatr Med Assoc 1992;82:501–6

13. Grace DL. Metatarsal osteotomy: which operation? J Foot Surg 1987;36:46–50

14. Bosh P, Markowski H, Rannicher V. Technik und erste Ergebnisse der subkutanen distalen Metatarsale -I-Osteotomie. Orthopaedische Praxis 1990;26:51–6

15. Lamprecht E, Kramer J. Die Metatarsale -I-Osteotomie nach Behandlung des Hallux valgus. Orhopaedische Praxis 1982;8:636–45

16. Magnan B, Bortolazzi R, Samaila E, Pezze L, Rossi N, Bartolozzi P. Percutaneous distal metatarsal osteotomy for correction of hallux valgus. Surgical technique. J Bone Joint Surg Am 2006;88 Suppl 1 Pt 1:135–48

17. Giannini S. Indications, techniques and results of minimal incision bunion surgery. Presented at the 32nd Annual Meeting of the American Orthopaedic. Foot and Ankle Society February 16, 2002, Dallas, TX, USA

18. Giannini S, Ceccarelli F, Bevoni R, Vannini F. Hallux valgus surgery: the minimally invasive bunion correction (S.E.R.I.) Tech Foot Ankle Surg 2003;2(1): 11–20

Minimally Invasive Closed Reduction and Internal Fixation of Calcaneal Fractures

J. Chris Coetzee and Fernando A. Pena

Calcaneal fractures are the most common fractures in the foot, but treatment protocols vary significantly depending upon surgeon and institute preference. As far back as 1984, Yuang-Zhang Ma et al. [1] published an approach where they combined manual manipulation of the heel with "percutaneous poking" of the fracture fragments. In 2001, Omoto et al. [2] published their results after just manual manipulation of the heel after a calcaneus fracture. Their results are difficult to interpret because no standardized outcome tool is included on their results.

Buckley et al. showed that without stratification of the groups, the functional results after nonoperative care of displaced intraarticular calcaneal fractures were equivalent to those after operative care [3]. This paper confirmed that not all calcaneal fractures are created equal, and that one should have very specific guidelines on how and when to surgically treat a fracture. With this in mind, there is a subgroup of calcaneal fractures that are best treated with minimally invasive techniques.

The initial indication for percutaneous fixation of calcaneal fractures was a compromise when risks of formal open reduction were moderately high and likely result of nonoperative treatment would be predictably poor, as in the following examples in Figs. 18.1 and 18.2. At the present time, those criteria still hold true, but there are certain fractures that are probably preferentially treated with percutaneous fixation.

Indications

The following fractures lend themselves perfectly to minimally invasive treatment: two-part tongue-type fractures (Essex-Lopresti); two-part joint depression-type fractures; and fracture dislocations with simple joint injury (no more than two-part injuries).

Surgical Technique

Prerequisites

- Percutaneous reduction and limited internal fixation must be performed early, ideally within 3–5 days of the injury. After that time, it will be increasingly difficult, if not impossible to manipulate the fragments.
- Anesthesia must provide complete muscular relaxation. A general anesthetic is preferred.
- Employ indirect reduction techniques; a very good fluoroscope is essential to adequately visualize the reduction.

J.C. Coetzee (✉)
Fairview University Medical Center, Minneapolis, MN, USA

Minnesota Sports Medicine and Twin Cities Orthopedics, Eden Prairie, MN, USA
e-mail: jcc@ocpamn.com

F.A. Pena
Department of Orthopaedic Surgery, University of Minnesota, Minneapolis, MN, USA

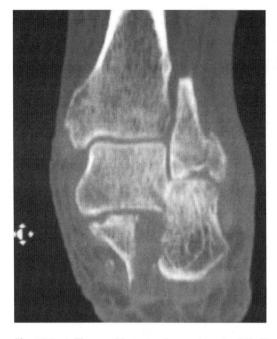

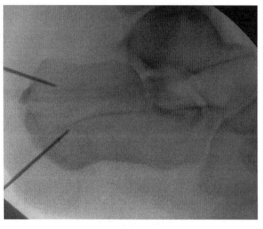

Fig. 18.3 Initial K-wire placement for reduction of a Saunders II fracture with the posterior tuberosity rotated and impacted

Fig. 18.1 A 53-year-old construction worker who fell off a roof. He smokes a pack of cigarettes a day. Note the lateral dislocation of the calcaneus with impaction and impingement of the distal fibula

The patient is placed in a lateral or semilateral position on a beanbag to allow easy and direct access to the lateral aspect of the calcaneus. A semilateral position is preferred. That position allows the surgeon to externally and internally rotate the leg to allow proper fluoroscopy views to evaluate reduction and K-wire placement. The usual sterile prepping and draping is done. A tourniquet is not routinely used. In fact, if the procedure is done very early, it is probably advisable not to use a tourniquet. This might further compromise the blood supply to the skin.

Tongue Type Essex-Lopresti Fracture

Two or three nonthreaded guide wires for 3.5- or 4.5-mm cannulated screws are inserted. One or two into the posterior (tuberosity) fragment, and one in the posterior, plantar fragment. The guide wires should not cross the fracture plain at this point (Fig. 18.3). This is followed by inserting a Steinmann pin from medial to lateral through the posterior, plantar fragment. This will help to dislodge the fracture fragment with longitudinal traction on the pin. A threaded pin or "joystick" is then inserted into the tuberosity fragment. This pin should be somewhat parallel to the fracture plain, and should be deep enough to be close to the hard subchondral bone of the subtalar joint.

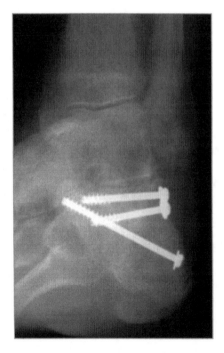

Fig. 18.2 One year after a percutaneous reduction and fixation of the calcaneal fracture dislocation

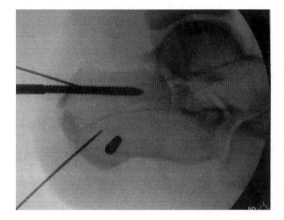

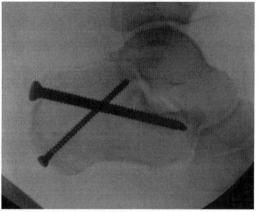

Fig. 18.4 Placement of the Steinmann pin for traction is done from medial to lateral through the plantar aspect of the calcaneus. Placing the screw from the medial aspect limits potential tibial nerve and vascular injuries. The "joystick" for reducing the tuberosity and posterior facet is placed from the posterior aspect just lateral to the Achilles tendon and should be in the lateral (rotated) portion of the posterior facet and tuberosity

Fig. 18.6 Final screw placement, with good reduction of the joint

Significant traction is usually required to disimpact the fragments. Two guide wires are then inserted from lateral into the lateral wall fragment of the posterior facet. While the assistant applies longitudinal traction on the Steinmann pin, the two wires are used as joysticks to reduce the lateral wall to the stable medial portion of the posterior facet. It is especially important to also tilt the fragment out of its "plantar flexed" position. The longitudinal traction could either be done manually, or a Buehler clamp can be applied. I personally find manual traction more reliable because one can apply more traction on one side if the reduction requires that. The guide wires are then advanced into the medial stable portion of the subtalar joint and sustentaculum tali, overdrilled, and short thread cancellous compression screws are inserted (Fig. 18.7a).

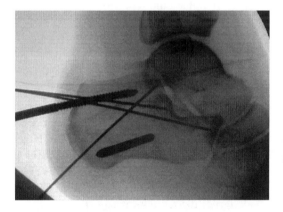

Fig. 18.5 The posterior facet is reduced under fluoroscopy by manipulating the fragments with the joystick while pulling on the transverse Steinman pin that allows disimpaction of the fragments. The guide wires are advanced to cross and immobilize the fragments. A cannulated drill is then used to overdrill, and followed by screw placement

It will be used to lever the tuberosity fragment in place while the assistant applies traction on the Steinmann pin (Figs. 18.4–18.6).

Saunders Type 2b

In this situation, the pin from medial to lateral through the posterior tuberosity is most important.

Complications

In our own series of 57 patients since 2000, the perioperative complications included three patients with sural nerve injury symptoms, and only one minor wound complication. There were no major wound problems. The sural nerve, however, is at risk of being injured because it is not exposed and protected.

We speculate that the long-term complications will be mainly caused by the fact that one seldom gets a true anatomic reduction with an indirect

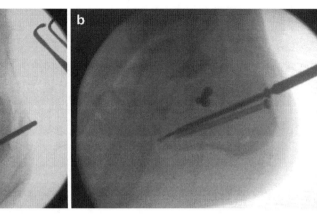

Fig. 18.7 (a) Reduction of the posterior facet with the traction pin still in place. (b) After securing the posterior facet fragment, the calcaneal tuberosity is further immobilized by two screws from posterior both sides of the Achilles to the anterior part of the calcaneus

technique. At a minimum of 2-year follow-up, however, there was not any significant increase in subtalar degenerative joint disease (DJD) or other issues compared with the formal open reduction and internal fixation (ORIF) group.

Discussion

With the minimally invasive technique, the surgeon must be theoretically willing to accept less than an anatomic reduction. Even so, the reported literature shows very satisfactory results with this method. There is no report in the literature comparing a no treatment group with a conventional ORIF group with a percutaneous fixation group.

Forgon [4] reported on a series of 265 cases with 89.8% good and excellent results and 10.2% moderate or poor results. Complications included 4.1% loss of reduction, 3.7% wound-healing problems, and 2% failure of technique.

Schildbauer and Sangeorzan [5] published a technical tip to improve distraction of the calcaneus tuberosity through percutaneous means. Placement of a fully threaded screw through the calcaneus tuberosity, in a similar fashion to the one placed for a subtalar fusion, will provide distraction of the calcaneus tuberosity when the screw is turned forward while being stopped from progressing by placing a hard instrument against the plantar aspect of the posterior talar facet. By turning the screw, the calcaneus tuberosity

can only be transported posteriorly and distally through the threads of the screw. This is a minimally invasive way to accomplish a large amount of distraction that otherwise would require large forces to be applied.

Tornetta [6] published his series of 46 patients who underwent percutaneous reduction and internal fixation (PRIF) of the calcaneus for a tongue-type fracture (Sanders 2C) and Sanders 2B. Only six fractures (three type 2B and three type 2C fractures) could not be successfully reduced. At an average follow-up of 3.4 years, 50% of patients had excellent results and 35% had good results. No patient required another surgical intervention. Early discomfort and drainage from the use of K-wires led the surgeon to substitute the use of K-wires with screws at the time of fixation. The final recommendation of the author is to emphasize the need for a preoperative discussion with the patient regarding the possibility of having to either abort the procedure or convert to an ORIF if a satisfactory reduction cannot be accomplished.

In 2002, Gavlik et al. [7] published their series of 15 calcaneus fractures after PRIF. All fractures were classified as Sanders 2. Fractures were reduced with arthroscopic assistance and subsequently fixed with permanent osteosynthesis after anatomic reduction was accomplished. No complications were reported. The AOFAS score of 10 of the 15 patients at an average of 14 months was 93.7 out of 100. Eighty percent of patients were reported as having no complaints during activities of daily living (ADLs) and work-related activities. All patients used normal footwear and no orthotic devices. Their most outstanding recommendation relates to the use of an arthroscopically assisted technique. They report a 25% incidence of not recognized malreduction of the posterior facet fragments while being examined under fluoroscopy. For those cases, the use of subtalar arthroscopy will help to avoid a step off of the posterior facet fragments.

In 2004, Nehme et al. [8] published the results of 15 fractures treated by arthroscopic- and fluoroscopic-assisted PRIF. The type of fractures included on their series were mixed (Sanders 2B), vertical (Sanders 2A), and horizontal (according to the Utheza classification). After administration of the AOFAS outcome tool, the average score at 20 months from the time of injury was 94.5 out of 100. No signs of osteoarthritis could be observed on the last radiographs. Postoperative motion of the subtalar joint was within 80% of the healthy side. The authors point out the moderate steepness of the learning curve and the obligation of converting to an ORIF if the reduction obtained is not satisfactory.

In 2004, Rammelt et al. [9] reviewed their experience with PRIF of calcaneus fractures. Their first recommendation is to address the fracture as early as possible to avoid bony consolidation and therefore the subsequent difficulties to closely manipulate the fragments. Their limit is 14 days from the time of injury. They also emphasize the importance of patient selection and fracture pattern because there is a direct correlation with the final outcome. The fractures eligible for PRIF were tongue type (Sanders 2C), and Sanders type 2A and 2B. The indications for the remaining fracture types are more dependent on the surgeon's experience. They mentioned an alternative to PRIF for the less skillful surgeon that consists of application of an external fixator in a triangular fashion with points of fixation at the talus, calcaneus, and cuboid. The goal is to maintain the proper alignment but mostly the relative position of the hindfoot bones to each other to improve joint mechanics and muscle strength. They discourage the routine use of a trans-subtalar pin and recommend only thinking about that option

with severe contraindications for ORIF or/and when dealing with an extremely unstable fracture pattern. They recommend the use of arthroscopically assisted reduction for the Sanders 2A and 2B, but not so much for the type 2C. The scope is placed along the posterior or anterolateral portal. For the Sanders 2C, they prefer to rely more on high-definition fluoroscopic examination. Finally, any remaining lack of reduction (beyond 2 mm) should be converted to ORIF because the final outcome will be improved.

One can therefore summarize that, in selected cases, closed reduction and percutaneous internal fixation provides a good option of treatment for calcaneal fractures. It might also be possible to avoid the "high" rate of complications seen with ORIF, and at the same time, improve on the poor outcome of nonoperatively treated calcaneus fractures.

References

1. Ma YZ, Chen Z, Qu K, et al. Os calcis fracture treated by percutaneous poking reduction and internal fixation. Chin Med J 1984;97:105–110
2. Omoto H Nakamura K. Method for manual reduction of displaced intra-articular fractured of the calcaneus: technique, indications and limitations. Foot Ankle Int 2001;22:874–879
3. Buckley R, Tough S, McCormack R, et al. Operative compared with nonoperative treatment of displaced intra-articular calcaneal fractures: a prospective, randomized, controlled multicenter trial. J Bone Joint Surg Am 2002;84-A:1733–1744
4. Forgon M. Closed reduction and percutaneous osteosynthesis: technique and results in 265 calcaneus fractures. In: Tscherne H, Schatzker J, (eds.) Major fractures of the pilon, the talus and the calcaneus. New York, Springer, 1993, pp. 207–213
5. Schildhauer TA, Sangeorzan BJ. Push screw for indirect reduction of severe joint depression-type calcaneal fractures. J Orthop Trauma 2002;16:422–424
6. Tornetta P. Percutaneous treatment of calcaneal fractures. Clin Orthop Relat Res 2000;375:91–96
7. Gavlik JM, Rammelt S Zwipp H. Percutaneous, arthroscopically-assisted osteosynthesis of calcaneus fractures. Arch Orthop Trauma Surg 2002;122:424–428
8. Nehme A, Chaminade B, Chiron P, et al. [Percutaneous fluoroscopic and arthroscopic controlled screw fixation of posterior facet fractures of the calcaneus]. Rev Chir Orthop Reparatr Appar Mot 2004;90:256–264
9. Rammelt S, Amlang M, Barthel Z. Minimally-invasive treatment of calcaneal fractures. Injury 2004;35: S-B55–S-B63

Minimally Invasive ORIF of Calcaneal Fractures

Juha Jaakkola and James B. Carr

Calcaneal fracture fixation can be performed using multiple approaches, methods, and implants. There is no consensus regarding the best approach or method of fixation. Moreover, the end result of calcaneal fractures is unsatisfactory in many cases. Some authors have questioned the necessity of operative intervention, arguing that the risk of surgery may not exceed the benefit it may provide [1]. A procedure that reduces the risk while still providing a benefit over nonoperative treatment would appear to be a reasonable compromise.

Described approaches include use of a lateral approach (Kocher approach [2–5] or extensile lateral [6–12], a medial approach [13–16], and a medial and lateral combined approach [17–19]. The extensile lateral approach is currently popular because it provides excellent exposure to the calcaneus, minimizes peroneal tendonitis, and preserves the sural nerve [7, 20]. However, an association with an elevated rate of soft tissue complications, that include amputation, have raised concerns [6, 8, 21].

In this chapter, we discuss a technique using lateral and medial approaches to the calcaneus through small (mini) incisions. This approach limits surgical dissection, therefore preserving

biology. Since exposure is limited, an excellent understanding of the fracture anatomy is essential. The pathoanatomy of calcaneal fractures and how it relates to the reduction technique will consequently be addressed. The technique also utilizes low-profile Synthes mini-fragment plates and screws to reduce the soft tissue tension and implant bulk.

Review of the Literature

The lateral approach was initially described in 1948 by Ivar Palmer [5]. He described a curved 6-cm incision made beneath the lateral malleolus. Unlike the extensile lateral approach, it does not lift up a large soft tissue flap. Reduction of the fracture was subsequently performed with a downward traction via a transfixion wire through the tuberosity and aided by an elevator to lever the fragments through the lateral incision. However, he did not use internal fixation, rather he placed a block of iliac crest to maintain reduction of the posterior facet fragments. He reported that 23 patients treated with this technique all had "favorable" results and returned to work 4–8 months after surgery [5].

Subsequent authors have described the use of this lateral approach in combination with internal fixation with variable results [2–4, 22, 23]. The largest series have been reported by Letrounel [4] and Bézes et al. [2]. Letrounel [4] reported 99 cases with 56% good to excellent results with no

J. Jaakkola (✉)
Southeastern Orthopedic Center, Savannah, GA, USA
e-mail: juhajaakkola@yahoo.com

J.B. Carr
Lewis Gale Orthopedics, Salem, VA, USA

Department of Orthopedics, University of South
Carolina, Columbia, SC, USA

or occasional pain after longer than 2 years follow-up. Bézes et al. [2] reported 257 cases with 85% good to excellent results with a 2.7% infection rate at a 3-year average follow-up.

McReynolds [16] has reported that he first began using the medial approach for open reduction and fixation of calcaneal fractures in 1958. This technique has been adopted by later authors [17–19], but the most extensive experience has been reported by Burdeaux [13–15]. Burdeaux [13–15] advocated the use of a medial incision because it addresses the sustentacular or superomedial spike, which he thought was the key to reduction. He stated that once the medial wall of the calcaneus was restored, "the length and height of the calcaneus are automatically restored"; the other fragments are then reduced to the sustentacular fragment [15]. Reduction using is performed by pulling the tuberosity fragment downward, backward, and medially to the sustentacular fragment [15]. Once reduced, the interlocking of the bone and the tension of the soft tissues stabilizes the fracture. Burdeaux stabilized the medial wall with a staple [15] or a Steinmann pin [13].

Burdeaux recommended reduction of the lateral fragments with the use of an elevator passed through the medial fracture line and direct digital pressure on the lateral side [14, 15]. When reduction of the lateral fragments is unsuccessful, a lateral incision above the peroneal tendons is added. This is more common with joint depression fractures than tongue-type fractures [13, 15]. His other indications for the lateral approach include fractures treated more than 2–3 weeks after injury, severely comminuted fractures, fracture dislocations, and displaced fractures of the calcaneocuboid joint [14].

Burdeaux reported a series of 61 calcaneal fractures in which 77% were reduced with a single medial incision and 14 fractures (23%) required an additional lateral incision [13]. Using this technique, he reported 75% good to excellent results at a 4.4-year average follow-up. Similarly McReynolds reported 64% good to excellent, 18% good-minus, and 18% fair to poor results in a series of 51 calcaneal fractures [16]. Lateral displacement was treated by bimanual compression of the heel, all cases were approached only from the medial side [16].

Romash [24] also reported a series of cases based on the technique described by McReynolds and Burdeaux. He also began with a medial incision and then would add a lateral incision if the posterior facet was not reduced after fixation of the medial spike. He reported 20 cases of displaced intra-articular calcaneal fractures, of which 8 cases (40%) were treated with a single medial incision and 12 cases (60%) required a combined approach [24]. Using this technique, Romash observed that all of the patients were standing and wearing shoes within 6 months, had subtalar ranges of motion at least 60% of the contralateral side, and 70% of the patients were able to return to a preinjury level of activity at an average follow-up longer than 2 years [24].

Although similar to the previously described approaches, Stephenson initially approached the fracture from the lateral side through an incision similar to Palmer [19]. If the medial wall was not aligned after reduction of the posterior facet, lateral wall, and the tuberosity fragment, then a medial incision was added. Stephenson was able to obtain an average restoration of the tuber-joint angle of 86% in 22 patients treated with this technique; 7 of 22 patients required a medial incision [19]. The average subtalar range of motion was 75% of normal, and he obtained a good result in 77% and a fair result in 4% of the 22 patients.

Johnson and Gebhardt also supported the use of a combined approach when a fracture cannot be reduced by a single approach [21]. They reported nine cases treated with a medial and extensile lateral combined approach. The fractures were approached medially and fixation of the medial wall was achieved with a staple. A lateral extensile incision was subsequently used for reduction of the posterior facet and lateral wall. The authors claimed that medial fixation provided enough stability that lateral fixation could be performed with multiple lag screws or limited plate fixation (3.5-, 2.7-, 2.0-mm plates). Using this technique, the authors were able to obtain a reduction of Böhler's and Gissane's angle within 1° of the contralateral foot. Results were good in six and fair in three patients.

Carr and Scherl reported good results using a combined approach in 38 cases at the OTA annual meeting in 1998 [17]. Their description of exposing and reducing all major fragments prior to fixation forms the basis of the ensuing technique.

Fixation

Definitive internal fixation of calcaneal fractures has been performed using various combinations of 2.7-, 3.5-, or 6.5-mm screws [18, 19, 25–28], staples [19], K-wires and Steinmann pins [14, 22, 25], small fragment plates [2, 3, 7, 9, 10, 29], mini-fragment plates [12, 18], and specialty plates [4, 10, 11, 30, 31]. Proponents of smaller implants suggest that they may reduce wound necrosis and peroneal tendon irritation, and that they are amendable to contouring and placement [12, 18, 29]. In a large study of 120 displaced intraarticular calcaneal fractures fixed with 3.5-mm screws and AO anterior cervical H-plates, Sanders et al. reported an 18% incidence of peroneal tendonitis requiring hardware removal [9]. In comparison, Tornetta reported only two cases (6%) of peroneal irritation, which did not require hardware removal, when using mini-fragment plates and screws [12]. In Tornetta's series of 35 cases, 91% had an anatomic reduction and there were no cases of loss of hardware fixation or loosening.

In addition to clinical studies, biomechanical studies have suggested that the smaller implants provide adequate strength of fixation. Carr et al. compared the biomechanical strength of a flattened 1/3 tubular plate to a thicker 3.5-mm reconstruction plate in a cadaver calcaneal fracture model [29]. They reported no statistical difference between the two in cyclic loading or load to failure testing. They hypothesized that the results were attributed bone-to-bone contact obtained by an anatomic reduction of the fracture.

Arthroscopy

The use of arthroscopy has been described for use in the evaluation of reduction for various different fractures. Authors have found arthroscopy to be useful in conjunction with reduction and fixation of distal radius fractures [32, 33], tibial plateau fractures [34], and ankle fractures [35]. Its use has also been described for the evaluation of reduction of calcaneal fractures [27, 36]. Rammelt et al. reported the use of open subtalar arthroscopy to evaluate fracture reduction in 59 cases of displaced intraarticular calcaneus fractures during surgery [27]. Open reduction was performed using an extensile lateral approach and temporary fixation was performed with K-wires. Then the adequacy of posterior facet reduction was assessed with open subtalar arthroscopy prior to definitive fixation. A minor 1- to 2-mm stepoff was identified in 13 (22%) of the cases and reduction was repeated prior to definitive fixation. The same article described 28 patients evaluated with subtalar arthroscopy while undergoing hardware removal 1 year after fixation of a displaced intraarticular calcaneus fracture [27]. The authors found 23.7% of the patients had steps of 2 mm or more and associated full-thickness articular damage. The authors concluded that the existence of a strong correlation between the functional result and the condition of the posterior facet and that open arthroscopy is superior to fluoroscopic imaging.

Pathoanatomy

An understanding of the anatomy of the calcaneus and the pathoanatomy of calcaneal fractures are especially important when using small incision techniques. Since the exposure is limited and fracture reduction is in part indirect, fracture anatomy and imaging studies play a crucial role in this technique.

The articular anatomy of the calcaneus consists of four articulating facets, the posterior, middle, anterior, and cuboid facets. The three articular facets occupying the superior surface (posterior, middle, and anterior facets) all lie at different angles to one another. Between the middle and anterior facets lies the strong ligamentous complex comprised of the talocalcaneal and cervical ligaments [37, 38]. Relative to the talus, the center of the calcaneus is slightly lateral to center of the talus.

The mechanism of the calcaneal fracture has been previously described [5, 15, 39, 40]. At the time of impact, a shear stress on the subtalar joint fractures the calcaneus into medial and lateral portions. This longitudinal or sagittal split occurs within the subtalar joint more laterally if the foot is in valgus and more medially if it is in varus at the time of injury [40]. This primary fracture line runs longitudinally and often includes the cuboid and anterior facets. If this longitudinal fracture line runs posteriorly the length of the tuberosity, a tongue-type fracture as described by Essex-Lopresti is created; and if it does not, a joint depression fracture pattern occurs [14, 40]. Multiple longitudinal fracture lines can also occur, which accounts for comminuted Sanders type 3 and 4 fracture patterns [20]. The medial (or superomedial) fragment containing the strong talocalcaneal ligaments remains attached to the talus and moves downward and medially, leaving the tuberosity fragment forward and lateral [14]. The talus then recoils upward with the superomedial fragment and leaves the lateral fragment imbedded in the body of the calcaneus producing and intraarticular stepoff. A second primary fracture line, created by the talar process, runs in the coronal plane to divide the calcaneus into anterior and posterior fragments. This fracture line extends laterally to create an inverted "Y" pattern and accounts for lateral wall outward displacement (i.e., blow out) [40]. It can also course medially to divide the superomedial fragment in half. The end effect is that the calcaneus is widened and shortened and the articular surface has a stepoff.

The fracture fragments produced by this mechanism include the superomedial fragment, anterolateral fragment, posterior facet, and the tuberosity fragment (Fig. 19.1). The superomedial fragment is attached to the talus as previously described. The anterolateral fragment displaces superiorly. The posterior facet is fractured into two, three, or multiple fragments. The tuberosity fragment is translated laterally, tilted into varus or valgus, and has migrated up in between the superomedial fragment and the posterior facet fragment. It is the restoration of the tuberosity fragment to its original length that is most critical during reduction.

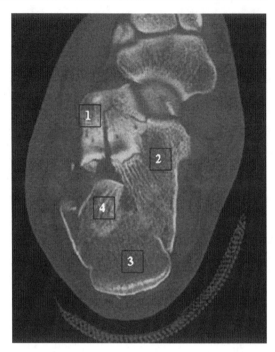

Fig. 19.1 Computed tomography scan depicting the four major fragments produced by a displaced intraarticular calcaneal fracture. (1) anterolateral fragment, (2) superomedial fragment, (3) tuberosity, (4) posterior facet fragment

Technique

Preoperative Planning

Patient evaluation begins with thorough history and a physical examination. Although the mini-open technique reduces the risk of wound complications, the vascular status and skin condition must be addressed preoperatively. Severe peripheral vascular disease and an elevated medical or cardiac risk may be prohibitive for a surgical procedure. The physical examination must assess for associated injuries, the presence of a compartment syndrome, and skin condition of the extremity. Associated injuries have been reported in up to 25% of cases [1] and may preclude surgery or modify the approach. The skin must be assessed for the presence of fracture blisters. Previous studies have suggested that skin blistering, especially blisters with bloody fluid, may increase wound infections [41]. If fracture blisters are very large or cover the area for the surgical approach, surgery should be delayed until they have resolved.

The patient should also be evaluated using plain radiographs. Plain radiographs should include an axial (Harris), dorsoplantar, lateral, and oblique view of the foot. In addition, biplanar computed tomographic (CT) scanning is imperative when using mini-open techniques. CT scans will provide detailed information regarding the pathoanatomy of the fracture and will aid in facilitating the reduction.

Timing

Surgery should be performed within the first week or when the soft tissue condition of the foot and the medical condition of the patient allows. If surgery cannot be performed within 2–3 weeks after injury, then an extensile lateral technique or conservative treatment should be considered. Three to five working days are typically required to obtain the appropriate imaging and schedule operative time.

Surgery

Surgery should be performed with the patient under general anesthesia with muscular relaxation. The patient is placed on the operative table in the supine position with a bump placed under the ipsilateral hip to compensate for the external rotation of the extremity. A tourniquet is placed on the thigh and will be inflated prior to incision.

Equipment needed for the procedure includes a 1.9-mm arthroscope and arthroscopy tower, a large C-arm fluoroscope, Steinmann pins and traction bows, an AO mini-fragment set with extra long screws, a number 15 scalpel, a Jocher elevator, a ball spike pusher, and a drill system.

Surgery typically begins with the lateral approach, but it can also be initiated from the medial side. Irrespective of the initial approach, the reduction of the calcaneal fracture should follow a systematic order (Fig. 19.2). Reduction should first assess the superomedial fragment, which, when reduced, will restore the height, length, and width of the calcaneus. Occasionally the superomedial fragment is relatively well reduced preoperatively, or it may be reducible from the lateral side with a Jocher elevator and calcaneal traction. If the medial wall is reduced, a medial incision may not be necessary.

The lateral approach starts with a 4- to 5-cm incision made 1 cm distal to the lateral malleolus and carried in line with the fourth metatarsal base (Fig. 19.3). The incision is carried down with sharp or blunt scissor dissection. Care must be

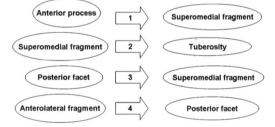

Fig. 19.2 Sequence for reduction of displaced intraarticular calcaneal fractures

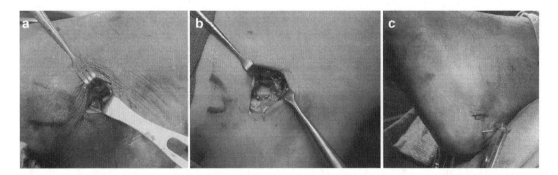

Fig. 19.3 Illustrative cases showing typical lateral (**a** and **b**) and medial (**c**) incisions. Typical lateral plate and subarticular screw positions are also demonstrated (**b**)

observed because the peroneal tendons are more laterally and proximally displaced by the fractured calcaneus than normally encountered. The tendons are identified and plantarly retracted. The peroneal tendon sheath and lateral soft tissue is elevated off of the lateral wall of the calcaneus using a Cobb elevator. Proximal dissection is performed using a 15 blade scalpel to release the calcaneofibular ligament from its calcaneal attachment, and the posterior facet of the calcaneus should be identifiable. A thin threaded Steinmann pin is then drilled medial to lateral through the posterior aspect of the calcaneal tuberosity and attached to a tensioned traction bow. Traction is then pulled to visualize the posterior facet.

A medial approach is usually necessary to reduce the superomedial fragment. The incision is made vertically approximately 2–3 cm distal to the posterior edge of the heel, beginning at the edge of the plantar and dorsal skin (Fig. 19.3). The approach is completed using blunt dissection down to bone. The medial calcaneal sensory nerve branch, which lies immediately below the flexor retinaculum, should be identified and protected. A blunt elevator or hemostat is then passed distally and proximally to elevate the soft tissues off of the medial tuberosity and superomedial fragment. The major neurovascular bundle is located within the soft tissue flap anterior to the incision and is protected with a small retractor. A four- or five-hole 2.7-mm mini-fragment plate can be placed along the superomedial spike and used as an anti-glide plate. If the superomedial fragment is not reducible with traction and manipulation, an anterior process fracture fragment may be preventing reduction. This fracture may be recognized on preoperative CT scans and should be addressed by reduction from the lateral aspect with a leverage "shoehorn" maneuver [42]. Once reduced, it is provisionally pinned with a K-wire from the anterior process into the superomedial fragment. If recognized, the surgeon should address this relationship first.

Once the medial wall has been reduced and fixed, the posterior facet is reduced by elevating the lateral fragment up to the superomedial fragment. Placing an elevator under the fragment, and derotating it up should achieve reduction.

A carefully applied ball spike pusher can assist with this reduction. While it is easy to get a close facet reduction, it is difficult to get an exact reduction. The arthroscope best displays the anterior portion of the facet, while the C-arm best visualizes the posterior portion. After provisional pinning with K-wires, the reduction should be assessed with arthroscopy and fluoroscopic imaging. Definitive fixation is performed with 2.0- or 2.7-mm screws placed subchondrally and directed toward the sustentaculum. The anterolateral fragment is addressed by derotating it medially and plantarly. A 2.0- or 2.7-mm mini-fragment plate is used to fix the anterolateral fragment and can be extended across the lateral wall fragment to the tuberosity fragment (Fig. 19.4).

After the reduction and fixation, wound closure is completed with absorbable subcutaneous sutures and nylon skin sutures. The foot is protected in a bulky splint for 2 weeks. At 2 weeks, the wounds are assessed, radiographs are obtained, and the patient is placed into a nonweightbearing cast for another month. At 6-week follow-up, gentle range of motion exercises are instituted and the foot is placed into an off-the-shelf boot walker nonweightbearing. At 10 week follow-up, if radiographs are stable, partial weightbearing advancing to full weightbearing is initiated. The boot walker is discontinued and a slow progressive increase in activity is introduced at 12–14 weeks.

Conclusion

A combined medial and lateral approach using small incisions and low-profile mini-fragment AO plates and screws is an effective technique for addressing most displaced intraarticular calcaneal fractures. The technique may reduce the incidence of soft tissue complications reported using extensile lateral techniques, reduce the tendon irritation from using more bulky implants, and improve range of motion (Fig. 19.5). However, limited-exposure techniques also require a thorough understanding of the fracture pathoanatomy and the methods for its reduction. Experienced surgeons should be able to utilize this technique, especially in conjunction with

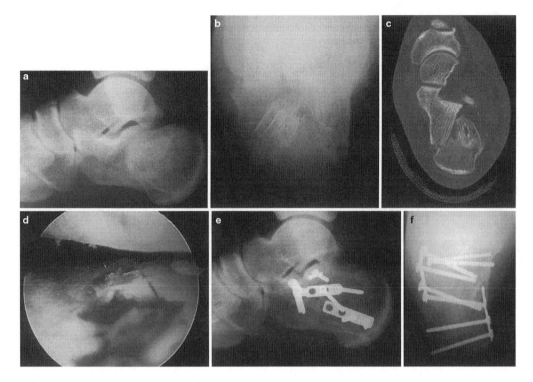

Fig. 19.4 A clinical example of a medial lateral approach used for a joint depression fracture (Sanders type 2). Preoperative radiographs (**a** and **b**) and a CT scan (**c**) show depression of Böhler's angle and an intraarticular stepoff. Postoperative arthroscopic image (**d**) and radiographs (**e** and **f**) showing correction of intraarticular stepoff and restoration of Böhler's angle

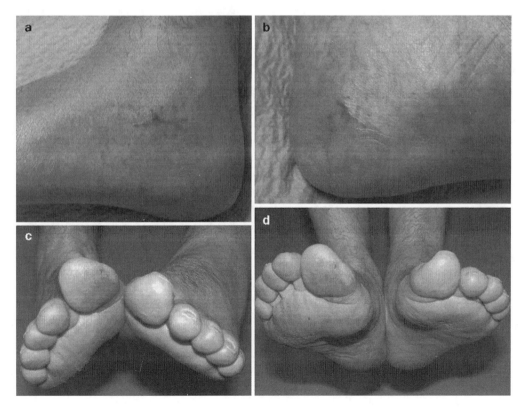

Fig. 19.5 Clinical photographs of the same patient illustrating the lateral (**a**) and medial (**b**) incisions and range of motion (**c** and **d**) at 6-month postoperative follow-up

previous training in calcaneal fracture treatment and when utilizing it initially on less complex fracture patterns.

References

1. Buckley R, Tough S, McCormack R, Pate G, Leighton R, Petrie D, Galpin R. Operative compared with non-operative treatment of displaced intra-articular calcaneal fractures. A prospective, randomized, controlled multicenter trial. J Bone Joint Surg Am 2002;84(A):1733–1744
2. Bézes H, Massart PL, Delvaux D, Fourquet J, Tazi F. The operative treatment of intraarticular calcaneal fractures. Indications, technique and results in 257 cases. Clin Orthop Relat Res 1993;290:55–59
3. Gupta A, Ghalambor N, Nihal A, Trepman E. The modified Palmer lateral approach for calcaneal fractures: wound healing and postoperative computed topographic evaluation of fracture reduction. Foot Ankle Int 2003;24:744–753
4. Letrounel E. Open treatment of acute calcaneal fractures. Clin Orthop Relat Res 1993;290:60–67
5. Palmer I. The mechanism and treatment of fractures of the calcaneus: open reduction with the use of cancellous grafts. J Bone Joint Surg 1948;30(A):2–8
6. Abidi N, Dhawan S, Gruen G, Vogt M, Conti S. Wound-healing risk factors after open reduction and internal fixation of calcaneal fractures. Foot Ankle Int 1998;19:856–861
7. Benirschke S, Sangeorzan B. Extensive intraarticular fractures of the foot: surgical management of calcaneal fractures. Clin Orthop Relat Res 1993;290:128–134
8. Folk J, Starr A, Early J. Early wound complications of operative treatment of calcaneus fractures: analysis of 190 fractures. J Orthop Trauma 1999;13:369–372
9. Sanders R, Fortin P, DiPasquale T, Walling A. Operative treatment in 120 displaced intraarticular calcaneal fractures: results using a prognostic computed tomography scan classification. Clin Orthop Relat Res 1993;290:87–95
10. Thordarson D, Krieger L. Operative vs. nonoperative treatment of intra-articular fractures of the calcaneus: a prospective randomized trial. Foot Ankle Int 1996;17:2–9
11. Thordarson D, Latteier M. Open reduction and internal fixation of calcaneal fractures with a low profile titanium calcaneal perimeter plate. Foot Ankle Int 2003;24:217–221
12. Tornetta P. Open reduction and internal fixation of the calcaneus using minifragment plates. J Orthop Trauma 1996;10:63–67
13. Burdeaux B. Fractures of the calcaneus: open reduction and internal fixation from the medial side a 21-year prospective study. Foot Ankle Int 1997;18:685–692
14. Burdeaux B. The medial approach for calcaneal fractures. Clin Orthop Relat Res 1993;290:97–107
15. Burdeaux B. Reduction of calcaneal fractures by the McReynolds medial approach technique and its experimental basis. Clin Orthop Relat Res 1983;177:87–103
16. McReynolds I. The case for operative treatment of fractures of the os calcis. In: Leach RE, Hoaglund FT, Riseborough EJ (eds.) Controversies in Orthopaedic Surgery. Philadelphia, WB Saunders, 1982, pp. 232–254
17. Carr J, Scherl J. Small incision approach for intraarticular calcaneal fractures. Presented at *Orthopaedic Trauma Association Annual Meeting*; 1998; Toronto, ON, Canada
18. Johnson E, Gebhardt J. Surgical management of calcaneal fractures using bilateral incisions and minimal internal fixation. Clin Orthop Relat Res 1993;290:117–124
19. Stephenson J. Surgical treatment of displaced intraarticular fractures of the calcaneus: a combined lateral and medial approach. Clin Orthop Relat Res 1993;290:68–75
20. Sanders R. Displaced intra-articular fractures of the calcaneus. J Bone Joint Surg 2000;82(A):225–250
21. Koski A, Koukkanen H, Tukiainen E. Postoperative wound complications after internal fixation of closed calcaneal fractures: a retrospective analysis of 126 consecutive patients with 148 fractures. Scand J Surg 2005;94:243–245
22. Ebraheim N, Elgafy H, Sabry F, Freih M, Abou-Chakra I. Sinus tarsi approach with trans-articular fixation for displaced intra-articular fractures of the calcaneus. Foot Ankle Int 2000;21:105–113
23. Wiley W, Norberg J, Klonk C, Alexander I. "Smile" incision: an approach for open reduction and internal fixation of calcaneal fractures. Foot Ankle Int 2005;26:590–592
24. Romash M. Calcaneal fractures: three-dimensional treatment. Foot Ankle Int 1988;8:180–197
25. Fernandez D, Koella C. Combined percutaneous and "minimal" internal fixation for displaced articular fractures of the calcaneus. Clin Orthop Relat Res 1993;290:108–116
26. Levine D, Helfet D. An introduction of the minimally invasive osteosynthesis of intra-articular calcaneal fractures. Injury 2001;32:S-A51–S-A54
27. Rammelt S, Gavlik J, Barthel S, Zwipp H. The value of subtalar arthroscopy in the management of intra-articular calcaneus fractures. Foot Ankle Int 2002;23:906–916
28. Tornetta P. Percutaneous treatment of calcaneal fractures. Clin Orthop Relat Res 2000;375:91–96
29. Carr J, Tigges R, Wayne J, Earll M. Internal fixation of experimental calcaneal fractures: a biomechanical analysis of two fixation methods. J Orthop Trauma 1997;11:425–429
30. Raymakers J, Dekkers G, Brink P. Results after operative treatment of intra-articular calcaneal fractures with a minimum follow-up of 2 years. Injury 1998;29:593–599

31. Zwipp H, Tscherne H, Therman H, Weber T. Osteosynthesis of displance intraarticular fractures of the calcaneus. Results in 123 cases. Clin Orthop Relat Res 1993;290:76–86

32. Edwards C2nd, Haraszti C, McGillivary G, Gutow A. Intraarticular distal radius fractures: arthroscopic assessment of assessment of radiographically assisted reduction. J Hand Surg (Am) 2001;26: 1036–1041

33. Geissler W. Intra-articular distal radius fractures: the role of arthroscopy? Hand Clin. 2005;21:407–416

34. Lubowitz J, Elson W, Guttmann D. Part I: arthroscopic management of tibial plateau fractures. Arthroscopy 2004;20:1063–1070

35. Ono A, Nishikawa S, Nagao A, Irie T, Sasaki M, Kouno T. Arthroscopically assisted treatment of ankle fractures: arthroscopic findings and surgical outcomes. Arthroscopy 2004;20:627–631

36. Rammelt S, Amlang M, Barthel S, Zwipp H. Minimally-invasive treatment of calcaneal fractures. Injury 2004;35:S-B55–63

37. Hall R, Shereff M. Anatomy of the calcaneus. Clin Orthop Relat Res 1993;290:27–35

38. Sarrafian S. Biomechanics of the subtalar joint complex. Clin Orthop Relat Res. 1993;290:17–26

39. Carr J. Mechanism and pathoanatomy of the intraarticular calcaneal fracture. Clin Orthop Relat Res 1993;290:36–40

40. Carr J, Hamilton J, Bear L. Experimental intra-articular calcaneal fractures: anatomic basis for a new classification. Foot Ankle Int 1989;10:81–87

41. Giordano C, Koval K, Zuckerman J, Desai P. Fracture blisters. Clin Orthop Relat Res 1994;307:214–221

42. Carr J. Surgical treatment of intra-articular calcaneal fractures. A review of small incision approaches. J Orthop Trauma 2005;19:109–117

Minimal Dual-Incision ORIF of the Calcaneus

20

Michael M. Romash

The treatment of calcaneal fractures continues to evolve. In the past 25 years, a great deal of information about the mechanism of injury, the fracture patterns, and treatment have been *rediscovered*, confirmed, and instituted. This progress has established the principles that are applied in open reduction and internal fixation (ORIF) of these fractures. The techniques by which these principles are applied continue to advance and change. What was done through a large exposure can be done with smaller incisions and less tissue disruption without diminishing the end result. The dual-incision approach to the heel fracture is an example of this change.

Mechanism of Injury

The calcaneus fails when it is suddenly axially loaded [1–5]. The tuberosity of the calcaneus is lateral to the axis of the leg. When the fracturing force is applied, a shear stress occurs in the bone. The plane of this stress is directed obliquely from superior lateral to inferior medial, anterior lateral to posterior medial (Fig. 20.1). The calcaneus fractures along this plane producing the primary fracture line. The tuberosity displaces laterally, proximally, and angles into some varus. (A patient described this as a shifting of tectonic plates when

M.M. Romash (✉)
Orthopedic Foot and Ankle Center of Hampton Roads,
Chesapeake Regional Medical Center, Chesapeake,
VA, USA
e-mail: orthofoot@cox.net

his fracture was discussed with him.) While this is occurring, the lateral aspect of the posterior facet impacts the talus. This drives this portion of the posterior facet down into the calcaneus. It rotates forward while it is pushed down. If the facet fractures within the posterior limit of the subtalar joint, it is a *joint depression* fracture. If this fragment continues back and exits through the tuberosity, it is a *tongue* fracture. The anterior body of the talus then continues to drive into the calcaneus at the angle of Gissane, causing another fracture involving the anterior calcaneus (Fig. 20.2).

These fractures produce four major fragments, the sustentacular fragment, the tuberosity fragment, the posterior lateral fragment, and the anterior fragment. These major fragments may further comminute into smaller fragments. The number of smaller fragments in the posterior facet correlates with the success of treatment.

The sustentacular fragment is referred to as the constant fragment. This stays in its anatomic position relative to the talus. During reduction, all fragments are reduced to the sustentacular fragment.

Principles of Reduction

The displacements and angulations described above must be reversed. Motion of the hindfoot complex depends upon the smoothness of the articular surfaces of the calcaneus and the three-dimensional (3D) spatial relationships that result

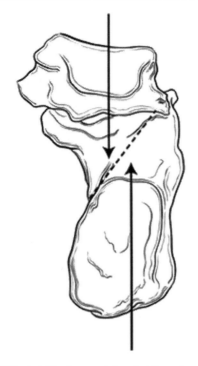

Fig. 20.1 Axial load causes internal oblique shear stress along plane of primary fracture line

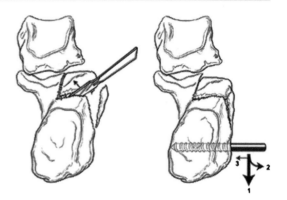

Fig. 20.3 Reduction of the tuberosity to the sustentaculum. Reduction of the posterior lateral fragment to the tuberosity

between the talus, calcaneus, and cuboid due to the proper shape length and height of the calcaneus. Carr [2] has described the concept of the medial and lateral columns of the calcaneus. It is necessary to reconstruct both columns.

Disimpaction of the fragments must be accomplished. Then reduction of the tuberosity to the sustentaculum reestablishes the medial wall of the calcaneus. This establishes the height by reconstructing the medial column. The posterior lateral facet fragment can then be elevated, derotated, and fixed to the sustentacular fragment. After this is accomplished, the lateral wall can be molded into its anatomic position.

In the process of derotating the posterior facet fragment, its anterior margin provides the landmarks for the reduction of the anterior lateral fragment to the remainder of the construct, thus reestablishing the length of the lateral column. The articular surface of the anterior process may then be reduced (Fig. 20.3).

Preoperative Assessment

The medical history must be obtained. Specifically, a history of smoking, diabetes, neuropathy, and vascular disease must be sought. These presence of these conditions may effect the decision-making process. These are relative contraindications to surgery, but do not exclude surgical intervention.

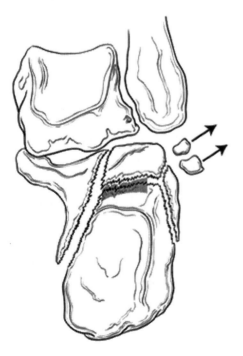

Fig. 20.2 Resultant secondary fractures in the posterior aspect of the heel

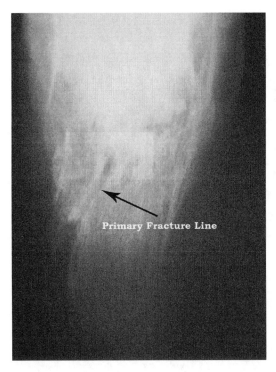

Fig. 20.4 Axial heel view of acute fracture, the primary fracture line is apparent

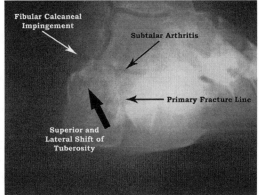

Fig. 20.5 Broden's view of an acute fracture, primary fracture line, shift of tuberosity, and intraarticular component

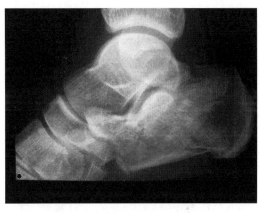

Fig. 20.6 Lateral view demonstrating loss of Bohler's angle and depression of the subtalar facet

The standard physical examination parameters are to be observed. These are the evaluation of the vascular and neurological status of the foot. The possibility of compartment syndrome must be considered. Specific findings to look for are skin "tenting" over boney prominences and fracture blisters [6, 7]. Skin tented over the posterior prominence of a tongue-type fracture or the spike of bone that marks the inferior margin of the sustentacular fragment carry the risk of skin necrosis. If this situation exists, a reduction must be accomplished quickly to relieve the tenting.

X-ray assessment is mandatory. Plane films include the axial heel view, lateral view, Broden's oblique view, and anteroposterior (AP) view of the foot [8–10]. A lateral view of the uninjured foot is recommended. What appears to be a minimally displaced fracture can be shown to have significant displacement when compared with the healthy heel. Measure Bohler's angle of the injured as well as the uninjured heel (Figs. 20.4–20.7) [11, 12].

Computed tomographic (CT) examination provides the best evaluation of the fracture [3]. Axial, coronal, sagittal, and 3D volumetric reconstructions of the heel provide the surgeon with a blueprint of the internal and external architecture of the fracture [13]. The 3D volumetric reconstruction is particularly helpful because it shows the surgeon what will be seen through the portal of exposure during the procedure [9] (Figs. 20.8–20.12).

Timing of Surgery

Unless there is tenting of the skin or another forcing factor, the ORIF is not performed immediately. These patients often are referred a few days

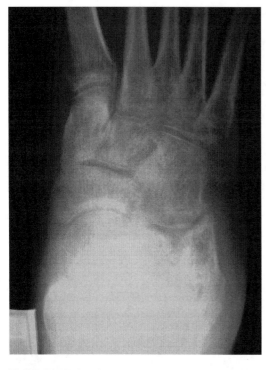

Fig. 20.7 AP view demonstrating calcaneocuboid involvement in a primary fracture of an anterolateral fragment

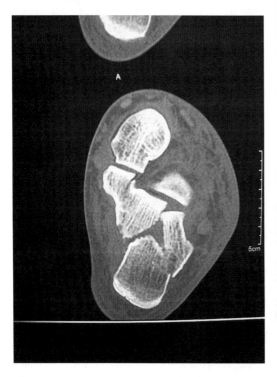

Fig. 20.8 Semicoronal CT scan clearly shows fracture pattern and displacement

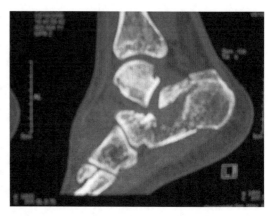

Fig. 20.9 Sagittal CT of acute fracture

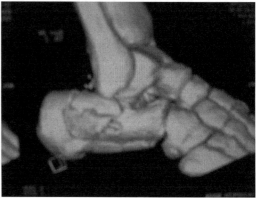

Fig. 20.10 3D volumetric CT, lateral side showing joint depression and lateral wall injury

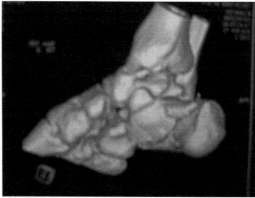

Fig. 20.11 3D volumetric CT, medial side showing displacement of tuberosity, sustentacular fragment, and "shingle" effect medially

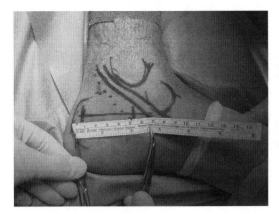

Fig. 20.12 Medial incision

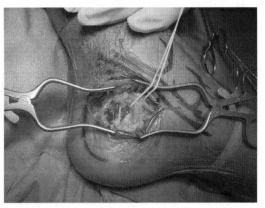

Fig. 20.13 Exposure of the neurovascular bundle medially

after their injury. The foot is often swollen and fracture blisters may be present. I advise waiting until the swelling has diminished and the skin wrinkles are visible. This is the positive wrinkle sign. Blisters may be unroofed and sterilely dressed. Be aware that the blisters often signal significant underlying soft tissue injury.

Technique of Small Dual-Incision ORIF

Patient Positioning

The patient is placed in the supine position with a bolster under the hip on the involved side. An elevated workstation for the foot is created under the drapes from pads. A radiolucent operating table is mandatory and the patient's foot should be placed close to the end of the table so that an intraoperative axial heel view can be seen with the fluoroscope.

Exposure

Medial and lateral exposure of the fracture will be accomplished. The order of exposure is not critical and may be dictated by the preoperative assessment of the fracture. The area requiring the most disimpaction should be approached first. This exposure is much as described by Ian McReynolds [1, 14].

The medial incision is three to four fingerbreadths below the medial malleolus, parallel to the sole centered over the tuberosity fragment. The anterior aspect of the incision just crosses the neurovascular bundle area (Fig. 20.12). Dissect through the abductor hallucis. The fascia under the muscle will be encountered and sectioned. This is entering the tarsal tunnel through the "side door." The neurovascular bundle will be in the anterior aspect of the wound. The neurovascular bundle is mobilized superiorly and inferiorly and generally retracted toward the toes (Fig. 20.13). The short flexors may then be elevated from the medial wall of the calcaneus using a small key elevator. It is important to have a good visual image and orientation to the fracture pattern at this point. The 3D volumetric reconstruction CT scan is quite helpful. The tuberosity fragment shifts lateral and superiorly. The sustentacular fragment then overlays the medial wall of the tuberosity much as roofing shingles overlay each other. The medial wall of the sustentacular fragment may be encountered initially. The surgeon must be aware of this, and be prepared to expose the tuberosity more plantarly and define any Z collapse or minor fragments that may be present (Fig. 20.14).

The lateral incision starts just below the tip of the fibula and extends forward in the line between fourth and fifth ray to the calcaneocuboid joint (Fig. 20.15). The peroneal tendons (often displaced) are mobilized. The extensor digitorum brevis is mobilized with the extensor retinaculum.

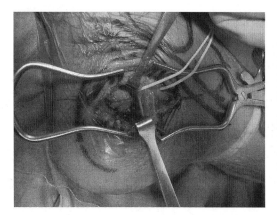

Fig. 20.14 Medial wall of the calcaneus exposed

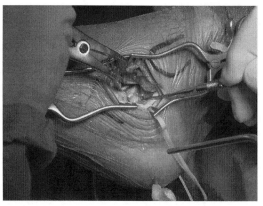

Fig. 20.16 Lateral exposure through the sinus tarsi

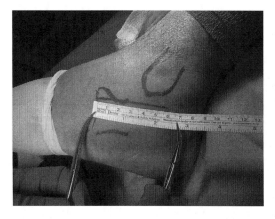

Fig. 20.15 Lateral incision

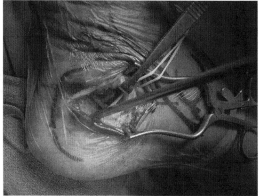

Fig. 20.17 Steinman pin placed through the tuberosity fragment from the medial side

The sinus tarsi region is cleared and the subtalar joint opened. The includes incision of the anterior as well as the lateral capsular structures. The lateral wall of the calcaneus in the area of the incision is exposed. The view into the subtalar joint is enhanced by placing a baby Inge lamina spreader in the sinus tarsi. At this juncture, the lateral and dorsal aspect of the anterior calcaneus is exposed (Fig. 20.16).

The Reduction

Disimpaction

The fragments have been impacted into each other by the injuring force; therefore, the first task is to mobilize them to permit the reduction. Through the medial incision, a large Steinmann pin is placed through the tuberosity fragment from medial to lateral. This is best placed toward the posterior and plantar margin of the fragment (this keeps the area for fixation clear). This pin protrudes 2–3 in. out the lateral side of the heel. A joker elevator, ¼-in. curved Lambotte osteotome, or other instrument is insinuated along the primary fracture plane and in conjunction with pressure on these instruments lifting the posterior lateral facet fragment (blindly), rocking the tuberosity with the Steinman pin and placing traction on the Steinman pin, the tuberosity may be freed (Fig. 20.17). If progress toward this end is not apparent, the lateral incision is used and, through the lateral wall (there is often some comminution here), a boney trapdoor is used to allow a joker elevator to be placed under the depressed and rotated posterior

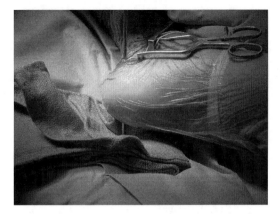

Fig. 20.18 Steinman pin through to the lateral side acting as the point of application of reduction force and the pivot point

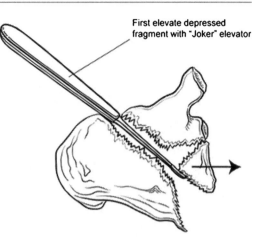

Fig. 20.20 Diagram of the disimpaction of fragments through medial entry point to primary fracture plane and posterolateral fragment

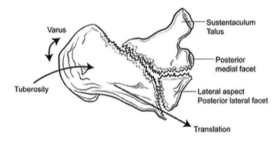

Fig. 20.19 Diagram of initial deformity as viewed with the patient's leg in a figure four position, lateral side down

lateral facet fragment to lift and derotate it. The primary fracture plane may also be disimpacted obliquely across the calcaneus from here.

Reduction and Fixation

I usually rebuild/reduce the heel medially first. The patient is placed in a figure four position. The tip of the Steinman pin that protrudes through the lateral heel is supported on towels placed on the contralateral tibia (Fig. 20.18). This provides a pivot point and reaction point to help with the reduction. This pivot is placed laterally away from the heel. As the medial lever arm of the pin is pulled plantarly and posteriorly, motion about this distant hinge point guides the tuberosity out of varus and translates it into proper position. This is the same principle of the offset hinge used in external fixators to effect angular and translational correction. The reaction force pushes the tuberosity medially, accomplishing the reduction (Figs. 20.19–20.22).

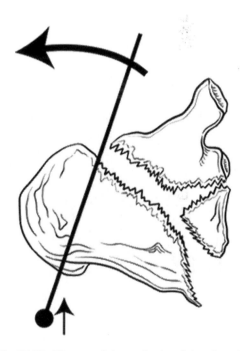

Fig. 20.21 Diagram of the mechanics of the tuberosity reduction maneuver. The point of the Steinman pin acts as the point of application for a medial directed vector of reduction force. The lateral position of the point acts as an offset hinge to permit correction of varus and translational displacement

Once disimpaction and reduction have been accomplished (Fig. 20.23), fixation may be delayed until the posterior facet reduction and internal fixation have been accomplished. I usually choose this sequence.

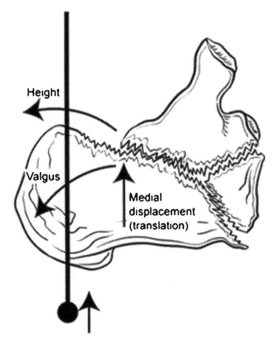

Fig. 20.22 Diagram of position after reduction

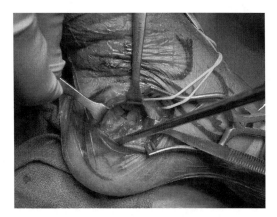

Fig. 20.23 Medial wall reduction after the described maneuver

Alternatively, medial fixation can now be introduced. Staples or a hindfoot plate (Ascension) may be used. If staples are used, one or two 3/32 Steinman pin bone staples of appropriate width to bridge the fracture site (there may be a segment of intercalary comminuted fragments) from the tuberosity fragment to the sustentacular fragment are placed. These do not compress the fracture; rather, they maintain the height and position

of the reduction. Predrill the holes for the staples. Use a 3/32 Steinman pin or drill bit for this. Impact the staples only half way (50%) so that they do not interfere with any lateral fragments (Fig. 20.24). The staples will be seated fully at the completion of the procedure.

If a hindfoot plate is used, the hindfoot plate is "turned over" so that the convex side curve of the plate lays on the concave surface of the medial calcaneus. Further contouring of the plate is done with a bending vise grip. Temporary fixation can be accomplished with short screws. The short screws will not interfere with manipulation of the posterior lateral fragment and will be replaced by appropriate-length screws at the end of the procedure (Fig. 20.24a).

Now address the lateral side. Introduce a baby Inge lamina spreader in the sinus tarsi and use it to lengthen the calcaneus and push the anterior lateral fragment forward. The posterior facet is elevated and derotated, reducing it to the sustentacular fragment. This can be observed anteriorly and posteriorly (Fig. 20.25). Ensure that the posterior aspect of the facet is not *over reduced*, i.e., elevated higher than the medial side. Temporary fixation is done with 0.62-in. K wires from lateral to medial (Fig. 20.26). As the wires are placed, aim slightly plantarly as the joint falls away medially. What appears to be a *transverse shot* may pierce the subchondral bone and go intraarticularly. Usually a significant lateral wall surface is present on the posterior lateral facet fragment. This is often buried behind other fragments of the lateral wall that have been displaced laterally. It is this area of the bone that it is of good quality and best able accept the fixation. The lamina spreader is then eased and the anterior fragment reduced to the posterior fragment.

Intraoperative x-rays are then taken. Use a good quality C-arm fluoroscope. Image the foot in three or four views: axial heel, Broden's oblique view [10], lateral view, and AP foot view. The AP foot view will show the calcaneocuboid joint and may not be needed routinely. The other three views are needed in all cases. The axial heel view shows the medial wall reduction, and Broden's view shows the subtalar joint and permits assessment of the joint surface reduction. The lateral view allows

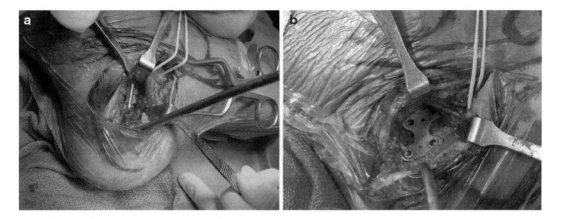

Fig. 20.24 (**a**) Placement of initial medial staple. (**b**) Medial hindfoot plate

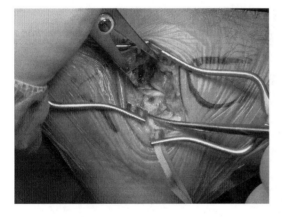

Fig. 20.25 Lateral reduction

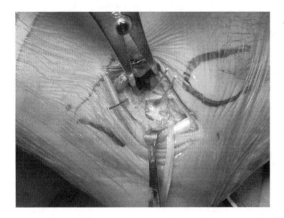

Fig. 20.26 K wires temporarily fixing the lateral reduction

assessment of the height of the heel and the orientation of the medial plate or staple fixation.

If the position is proper, lateral fixation is continued. Cancellous bone graft may be placed

under the posterior facet at the surgeon's discretion. This is done before applying the plate. The "mini calc" plate (Ascension) or anterolateral plate (Synthes, Paoli, PA) is applied. Some shaping of the plate at its distal flange is usually necessary to conform it to the anterior calcaneus. Bending the proximal plate is not always necessary because it will conform to the bone. Locking or nonlocking 3.5-mm screws are used with the mini calc plate, 4.0-mm cancellous screws are used with the Synthes anterolateral plate. The most lateral fragments can be over drilled. The plate is designed to lay along the good quality bone of the posterior facet just inferior to the joint, cross the fracture at the angle of Gissane, and then engage the anterior fragment. It serves as a "washer" laterally, allowing compression from lateral to medial. It keeps the posterior facet and construct elevated and reduced to the anterior fragment (Figs. 20.27 and 20.28).

The medial plate is now applied. A hindfoot plate (Ascension) is turned over so that the convex side curve of the plate lays on the concave surface of the medial calcaneus. Further contouring of the plate is done with a bending vise grip. Temporary fixation can be accomplished with short screws. The short screws will not interfere with manipulation of the posterior lateral fragment and will be replaced by appropriate length screws at the end of the procedure. If staples are used, they are now fully seated (Fig. 20.29a, b).

Final x-rays are made (Figs. 20.30–20.32). The wounds are closed in layers. The muscle over

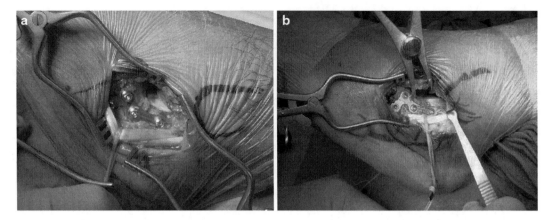

Fig. 20.27 (**a**, **b**) Anterolateral plate applied

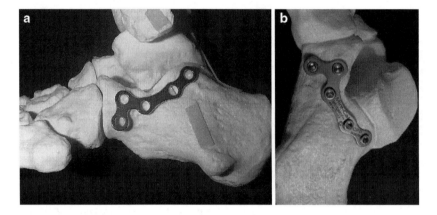

Fig. 20.28 (**a**, **b**) Anterolateral plate on sawbones model

the neurovascular structures on the medial side is approximated. The skin may be closed with simple or running suture (Figs. 20.33 and 20.34).

Special Situations

A Sander's three- or four-fracture pattern usually requires more work to reduce the facet fragments. I have found success by reducing the mid fragment to the sustentaculum with 0.45-in. K wires. These wires are placed from lateral to medial, exiting the skin on the medial side. They are then withdrawn from the medial side until the wire just disappears into the minor fragment. The lateral portion of the posterior facet is then reduced to the construct, held with K wires, and the procedure goes on as described above. After final fixation has been placed, these K wires are removed from the medial side.

It is possible to use this fixation pattern and do a primary subtalar arthrodesis if desired in the case of a destroyed joint. If the medial "zone of injury" has caused considerable change in the muscle layer with noted discoloration and unhealthy appearance, more advanced treatment may be necessary. This is seen and may be anticipated if there has been blistering of the skin in the area [6, 7]. We have had success by excising the questionable tissue and performing an abductor hallucis flap with a split thickness skin graft (STSG) to close and cover the medial side [15] (Fig. 20.35).

Postoperative Management

The foot is placed in a well-padded short leg cast with an A-V impulse bladder under the cast [16]. The foot is in a neutral position. The cast is

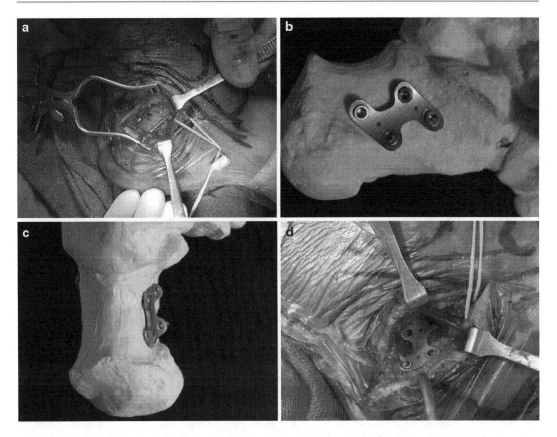

Fig. 20.29 (**a**) Medial staples impacted, final fixation. (**b**, **c**) Hindfoot plate on sawbones model. (**d**) Hindfoot plate fixed to medial wall

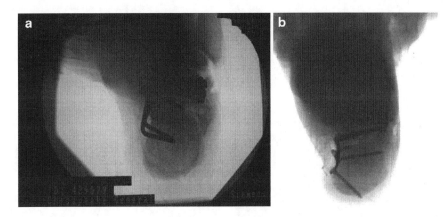

Fig. 20.30 (**a**) Intraoperative axial heel view after ORIF. (**b**) Intraoperative axial after ORIF with mini calc and medial hindfoot plate

bivalved within the first 24 h. Anticipate blood staining on the cast. This dressing is changed 3–7 days postoperatively. A new cast is applied. Sutures are removed 14 days postoperatively. The foot is held in a cast with the patient non-weightbearing (NWB) for 6 weeks. The cast is then exchanged for a fracture boot and the patient encouraged to perform non-weightbearing active

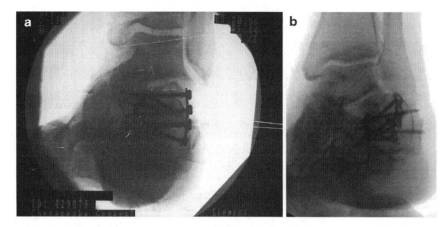

Fig. 20.31 (**a**) Intraoperative Broden's view after ORIF. (**b**) Intraoperative Broden's view after ORIF with mini calc and medial hindfoot plate

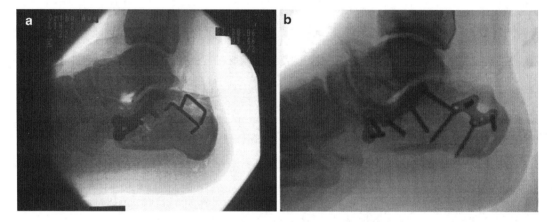

Fig. 20.32 (**a**) Intraoperative lateral view after ORIF. (**b**) Intraoperative lateral view after ORIF with mini calc and medial hindfoot plate

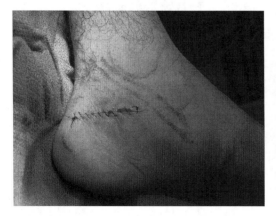

Fig. 20.33 Medial wound closed

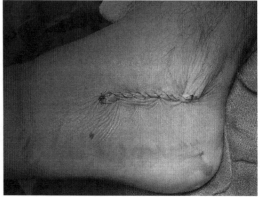

Fig. 20.34 Lateral wound closed

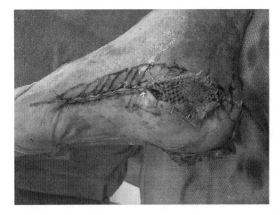

Fig. 20.35 Extended medial incision for abductor hallucis flap

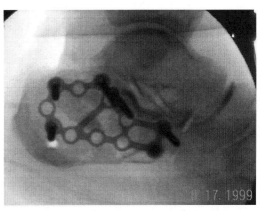

Fig. 20.38 Perimeter plate applied through a lateral incision, note the diagonal bar placed to reinforce plate

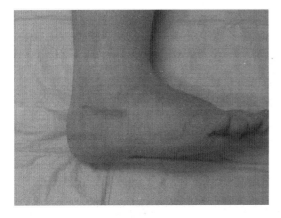

Fig. 20.36 Healed lateral incision

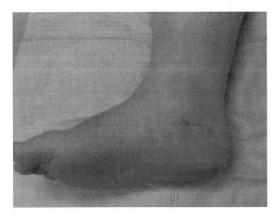

Fig. 20.37 Healed medial incision

and passive motions of the ankle and subtalar complex (Figs. 20.36 and 20.37).

At 8 weeks postoperatively, weightbearing is encouraged. Progression from the fracture boot to a postoperative shoe with rubber or gel heel cup helps this transition. Physical therapy is initiated. This includes calf-strengthening exercises, ankle and subtalar range of motion exercises, and a balance board program. As the patient progresses, exercise bicycle, ski machine, and elliptical trainer use are encouraged. Improvement plateaus approximately 4 months postoperatively. Maximum improvement can be expected at a year from surgery.

Results

One hundred and twenty-nine fractures have been treated in this fashion from 1996 to 2008. The results have been encouraging. Reduction has been accomplished in all cases. Wound problems have been minimal and limited to delayed wound healing in four cases. This occurred with smokers. There have been no sloughs of flaps.

There was one deep infection in a poly traumatized patient who had initial stabilization of the Sander' four-fracture dislocation by a Steinman pin placed percutaneously through the plantar heel into the talus before being referred. He was treated by ORIF with subtalar arthrodesis. He responded to wound café to include wound vacuum and parenteral antibiotics.

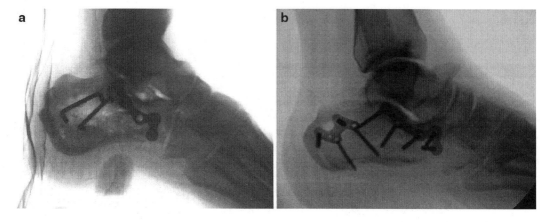

Fig. 20.39 (**a**) ORIF with anterolateral plate and staples. Note that the staples approximate the line and direction of oblique bar of perimeter plate. (**b**) ORIF with mini calc plate and medial hindfoot plate. Note that the medial plate approximates the line and direction of the oblique bar of the perimeter plate

One patient, a heavy recalcitrant heavy smoker, sustained a collapse of the lateral aspect of the posterior facet, which demonstrated osteonecrosis at revision to subtalar arthrodesis. One elderly man bore full weight immediately postoperatively and lost the reduction of the tuberosity fragment. The posterior facet remained flat and he desired no further treatment. The patients have been able to return to normal shoes with a plantigrade foot. They maintain approximately 50% of their subtalar motion. This is comparable with other modes of ORIF. There have been no deep infections or osteomyelitis. Eight subtalar arthrodeses have been performed for posttraumatic arthritis. Four lateral plates have been removed for peroneal tendon irritation. These were plates using standard screws with prominent screw heads. The advance to the low-profile locking mini calc plate without prominent screw heads may diminish the incidence of this procedure. One patient had a screw penetrate the subtalar joint. This was a technical error. His symptoms resolved after the screw was removed. Three patients have had neurological residuals due to the medial approach. Two of these cases were heel hypoesthesia. One patient who had an abductor flap at his index surgery had dysesthesia in the sphere of the lateral plantar nerve. Three patients had hypoesthesia in the sphere of the sural nerve.

When all things are considered, including patient satisfaction, there was greater than 85% "success" rate defined as a united fracture, ability to walk comfortably in standard shoes and maintain half of their subtalar motion centered on the neutral position.

Discussion

This technique has proven to be reliable in treating comminuted intraarticular calcaneal fractures. It is a modification of the principles and technique described by Ian McReynolds [14]. The modification is the addition of the anterolateral plate that connects the posterior to anterior constructs. Use of a small plate in this area in conjunction with subarticular screws outside the plate has been used [17]. The specially shaped anterolateral plate provides a larger washer and more purchase in the anterior fragment.

The fracture pattern creates four fragments and the fixation pattern stabilizes all fragments, reducing them to the "constant fragment" of the sustentaculum. This satisfies the principles of reduction and internal fixation of the calcaneus.

No large flaps are raised. The salvage procedure of subtalar or triple arthrodesis is done through the same lateral approach used for internal fixation, avoiding lifting a large flap for a second procedure.

The procedure allows direct visualization and direct reduction of both the medial and lateral columns of the calcaneus. There is no indirect reduction. The pattern of internal fixation stabilizes all of the fracture fragments. The staples or medial hindfoot plate resist redisplacement of the tuberosity while the plate and screws stabilize the posterior articular facet and the anterior lateral fragment. All fragments are reduced to the constant fragment.

When lateral x-rays are compared of the dual-incision fixation pattern with the present lateral plate fixation, there is similarity in the constructs resisting collapse. The reinforcing bar that goes obliquely across the tuberosity portion of the peripheral plates parallels and overlays the staple fixation of the dual incision construct (Figs. 20.38 and 20.39a, b). The results of this technique are comparable to those reported by other techniques.

Conclusion

The minimal dual-incision technique of open reduction and internal fixation of comminuted intraarticular calcaneal fractures is appropriate and yields satisfactory results. It should be in the foot surgeon's repertoire.

References

1. Burdeaux, B.D. Reduction of calcaneal fractures by the McReynolds medial approach technique and its experimental basis. Clin Orthop, 177:87–103, 1983
2. Carr, J.B., Hamilton, J.J., Bear, L.S. Experimental intra-articular calcaneal fractures: anatomic basis for a new classification. Foot Ankle, 10(2):81–87, 1989
3. Carr, J.B. Three dimensional CT scanning of calcaneal fractures. Orthop Trans 13:266, 1989
4. Romash, M.M. Open reduction and internal fixation of comminuted intra articular fractures of the calcaneus using the combined medial and lateral approach. Oper Tech Ortho, 4(3):157–164, 1994
5. Sangeorzan, B.J. Open reduction and internal fixation of calcaneal fractures. In: Kitaoka, H. (ed.), Master Techniques in Orthopaedic Surgery, The Foot and Ankle. Chapter 30, Lippincott Williams and Wilkons, Philadelphia, pp. 425–447, 2002
6. Giordano, C.P., Koval, K.J. Treatment of fracture blisters: a prospective study of 53 cases. J Orthop Trauma, 9:171, 1995
7. Giordano, C.P., Koval, K.J., Zuckerman, J.D., Desai, P. Fracture blisters. Clin Orthop, 292:214, 1994
8. Atones, W. An oblique projection for roentgen examination of the talocalcaneal joint, particularly regarding intra articular fractures of the calcaneus. Acta Radiol, 24:306, 1943
9. Broden, B. Roentgen examination of the subtaloid joint in fractures of the calcaneus. Acta Radiol, 31:85, 1949
10. Sanders, R., Dipasquale, T. Intra-operative Broden's views in the operative treatment of calcaneus fractures. Orthop Trans, 13:26–267, 1989
11. Bohler, L. Diagnosis, pathology and treatment of fractures of the os calcis. J Bone Joint Surg, 13:75, 1931
12. Bohler, L. The Treatment of Fractures. Vol. 3, Grune and Stratton, New York, pp. 2045–2108, 1958
13. Sanders, R., Fortin, P., Di Pasquale, T., Walling, A. Operative treatment in 120 displaced intra articular calcaneal fractures: results using a prognostic computed tomography scan classification. Clin Orthop, 290:87, 1993
14. McReynolds, S. Trauma to the os calcis and heel cord. In: Jahss, M. (ed.), Disorders of the Foot and Ankle, WB Saunders, Philadelphia, p. 1497, 1984
15. Levin, L.S., Nunley, J.A. The management of soft tissue problems associated with calcaneal fractures. Clin Orthop, 290:151–156, 1993
16. Myerson, M.S., Henderson, M.R. Clinical applications of a pneumatic intermittent impulse compression device after trauma and major surgery to the foot and ankle, Foot Ankle, 14:198, 1993
17. Johnson, E.E., Gebhardt, J.S. Surgical management of calcaneal fractures using bilateral incisions and minimal internal fixation. Clin Orthop, 290:117–124, 1993

Percutaneous Screw Fixation of Hallux Sesamoid Fractures

Geert I. Pagenstert, Victor Valderrabano, and Beat Hintermann

Total sesamoid excision is a powerful tool to cure recalcitrant sesamoid pain, but it has its shortcomings: excision of the lateral sesamoid led to a hallux varus, and excision of the medial sesamoid to a hallux valgus deformity in 10–20% of cases [1–5]. Excision of both sesamoids may cause cock up deformity of the hallux [2, 4, 6, 7]. Each sesamoid is invested in the corresponding tendon sheath of the flexor hallucis brevis. The attachment of the tendon to the base of the proximal phalanx is crucial for the balance of the first metatarsophalangeal (MTP) joint. Injuries to these structures during total excision cause hallucal deviation. In addition, loss of preloading and elevation of the first metatarsal head due to sesamoid excision may lead to transfer metatarsalgia and loss of big toe push off [8, 9].

Alternative procedures have been invented to reconstruct the anatomy [10–14]. The following technique of percutaneous screw fixation of sesamoid bone fractures is one of these procedures. Moreover, the skin incisions used to approach the two sesamoid bones have been connected with adverse effects: the lateral plantar approach was reported to be associated with painful plantar scar formation, and the lateral dorsal approach with accidental harm to the intrinsic hallucal muscles and interdigital nerve neuroma. The medial approach is only useful to reach the medial sesamoid

bone [2–4, 6]. The percutaneous technique needs only a stap incision distal to the weight-bearing area of the sesamoid bone. Sterile strips are used for wound closure.

Indications and Contraindications

Indications for percutaneous screw fixation are a transverse sesamoid fracture, transverse nonunion, or transverse symptomatic bipartite sesamoid. Fragments have to be at least bigger than 3 mm to ensure screw fixation.

In a typical patient history, no trauma is remembered and the development of pain is insidious and chronic in character. Often these conditions are associated with endurance sports and repetitive loading of the first MTP joint as in running or dancing [1, 11, 15]. These symptoms may respond to activity modification alone, but generally 6–8 weeks in custom-made insoles to unburden the painful sesamoid is advised as primary treatment. However, in chronic fractures, to our experience [11, 16] and in most reported cases in literature, conservative therapy is very likely to fail and further treatment will be necessary [1, 5, 15].

The patient has localized pain at one sesamoid bone that exacerbates with passive dorsal extension of the hallux. To document clinical findings of unloading of the first metatarsophalangeal joint (MTP 1), pedobarography is a useful tool (Fig. 21.1) [16]. On examination, conditions that stress the sesamoid complex such as cavus foot

G.I. Pagenstert • V. Valderrabano • B. Hintermann (✉)
Department of Orthopaedic Surgery,
University of Basel, Basel, Switzerland
e-mail: beat.hintermann@ksli.ch

G.R. Scuderi and A.J. Tria (eds.), *Minimally Invasive Surgery in Orthopedics: Foot and Ankle Handbook*,
DOI 10.1007/978-1-4614-0893-2_21, © Springer Science+Business Media, LLC 2012

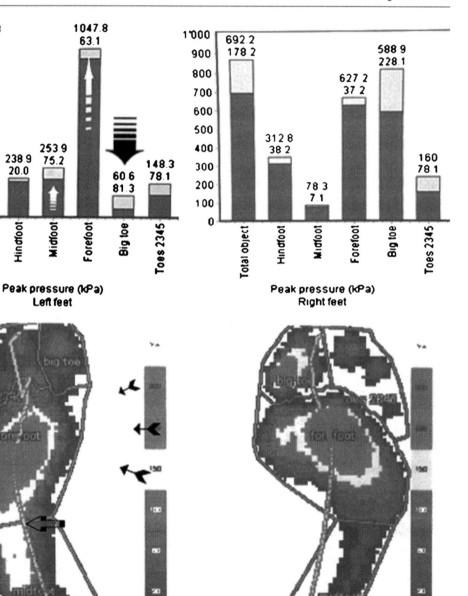

Fig. 21.1 Pedobarography. Left foot with debilitating pain at the first metatarsophalangeal joint caused by sesamoid nonunion. Elevation of the first ray has occurred with lateral drift of the central line of pressure (*arrows* on picture). Big toe push off is markedly reduced compared with the healthy contralateral side (*arrows* on chart)

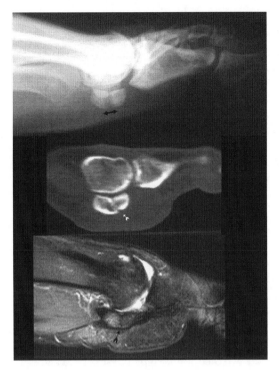

Fig. 21.2 Radiological features. Conventional x-ray shows fracture dislocation, CT scan shows sharp fracture edges, and MRI shows joint effusion, bone edema, and additional tendon and capsular injuries

with a plantar-flexed first ray or splay foot with hallux valgus formation should be included in the surgical plan [16].

Full weight-bearing radiographs of the whole foot and ankle are needed to assess the architecture of the foot. Special sesamoid oblique and tangential views are useful to evaluate sesamoid fracture displacement. Additional features of sesamoid pain can be visualized with magnetic resonance imaging (MRI), computed tomography (CT), and bone scan (Fig. 21.2). MRI results may show bone edema, soft tissue effusion, osteomyelitis, and tendon or ligament injuries. With the CT scan, sharp edges of sesamoid fractures can be displayed but may be absent in old fracture nonunions or bipartite sesamoids. Bone scan results adds little to find the pathology because increased uptake is unspecific [11, 12]. Bone scan results are positive in asymptomatic sesamoid bones [17], fractures, traumatized congenital bipartite bones, osteomyelitis, or tumors.

Contraindications include longitudinal sesamoid fractures, comminuted fractures with multiple fragments too small for screw fixation, and infection.

Preoperative Planning

The preoperative planning for sesamoid fracture screw fixation should include treatment of the possible underlying foot deformity [16]. A metatarsus primus flexus is treated with a dorsal-extension osteotomy, a metatarsus primus varus and hallux valgus is addressed with appropriate osseus and/or soft tissue procedures. Reducing mechanical stress to the sesamoid bone osteosynthesis is thought to improve healing. However, surgical stress reduction alone may cause fracture healing even without sesamoid osteosynthesis in marked foot deformities [16].

Technique

For percutaneous cannulated screw fixation of the sesamoid fracture, the patient is placed in the supine position. A tourniquet is not needed. A stap incision is made and a 1.5-mm K-wire is inserted to the distal pole of the sesamoid with the hallux fixed in hyperextension (Fig. 21.3). Under fluoroscopy, the wire is guided perpendicular to the fracture line through the distal fragment. With the surgeon's thumb, the hallux is held in neutral and pressure is put on the proximal pole and the whole sesamoid bone against the metatarsal head. This procedure levels out the joint surfaces of the sesamoid fragments with the metatarsal joint surface of the metatarsal-sesamoid joint. This constant pressure is continued until the cannulated compression screw is in place to enhance the compressive forces (Fig. 21.3). The authors used 10- to 14-mm compression screw lengths (e.g., Bold-Screw, New Deal, Lyon, France). Both corticalices should be held by the screw to assure compression and fixation of the fragments. Wound closure is achieved with a sterile strip.

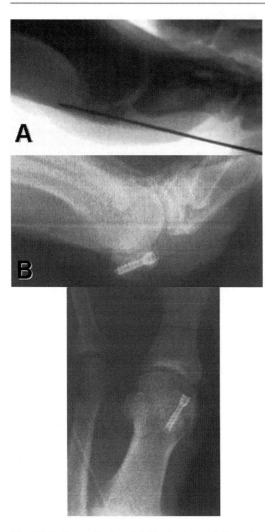

Fig. 21.3 Screw fixation. (**a**) K-wire inserted from distally; (**b**) cannulated compression screw in place

Complications

Improper screw placement may not deliver compression and stability to the fracture and nonunion or dislocation may occur and need sesamoid bone excision. Persistent sesamoid stress caused by unrecognized foot deformity (hallux valgus, pes cavus) may maintain sesamoid bone symptoms and may need further treatment [16].

Postoperative Management

Full weight bearing as tolerated is allowed right after surgery at the heel in a stiff-soled shoe to prevent dorsiflexion of the first MTP joint. No suture removal or wound care is needed since the stap incision was closed by a sterile strip. At 6–8 weeks after surgery, conventional shoes and gradual return to previous activity is allowed.

Results

Blundell and colleagues [12] fixed nine sesamoid fractures in athletes with percutaneous cannulated screws and revealed excellent results. All athletes went back to their previous level of activity. No complication was reported. They concluded that percutaneous screw fixation is a safe and fast procedure. They pointed out that discerning between traumatized bipartite sesamoid and fractured sesamoid bones was not performed because treatment was the same anyway.

The authors performed percutaneous screw fixation in seven athletic patients and had excellent results with full athletic recovery. All patients were endurance athletes (running, dancing), and five were female and two were male. One lateral and six medial sesamoid bone nonunions have been treated. In two patients, the concomitant hallux valgus deformity was corrected in the same surgery and fracture compression of sesamoid screw fixation was controlled under vision [12]. Local anesthesia only was sufficient for percutaneous surgery in the most recent case. All patients went back to sports 8 weeks after surgery.

Conclusion

Percutaneous screw fixation for sesamoid bone nonunion is a safe and fast procedure that can be performed with local anesthesia. In contrast to the standard treatment of total sesamoid bone excision, the percutaneous screw fixation preserves anatomy and function of the hallux sesamoid complex.

References

1. Brodsky JW, Robinson AHN, Krause JO, and Watkins D. Excision and flexor hallucis brevis reconstruction for the painful sesamoid fractures and non-unions: surgical technique, clinical results and histopathological findings. J Bone Joint Surg (Br) 2000 82-B:217
2. Grace DL. Sesamoid problems. Foot Ankle Clin 2000 5:609–627
3. Inge GAL and Ferguson AB. Surgery of sesamoid bones of the great toe. Arch Surg 1933 27:466–489
4. Richardson EG. Hallucal sesamoid pain: causes and surgical treatment. J Am Acad Orthop Surg 1999 7:270–278
5. Saxena A and Krisdakumtorn T. Return to activity after sesamoidectomy in athletically active individuals. Foot Ankle Int 2003 24:415–419
6. Jahss MH. The sesamoids of the hallux. Clin Orthop Relat Res 1981 Jun;(157):88–97
7. McBryde AM, Jr. and Anderson RB. Sesamoid foot problems in the athlete. Clin Sports Med 1988 7:51–60
8. Aper RL, Saltzman CL, and Brown TD. The effect of hallux sesamoid resection on the effective moment of the flexor hallucis brevis. Foot Ankle Int 1994 15:462–470
9. Aper RL, Saltzman CL, and Brown TD. The effect of hallux sesamoid excision on the flexor hallucis longus moment arm. Clin Orthop Relat Res 1996 Apr;(325): 209–217
10. Anderson RB and McBryde AM, Jr. Autogenous bone grafting of hallux sesamoid nonunions. Foot Ankle Int 1997 18:293–296
11. Biedert R and Hintermann B. Stress fractures of the medial great toe sesamoids in athletes. Foot Ankle Int 2003 24:137–141
12. Blundell CM, Nicholson P, and Blackney MW. Percutaneous screw fixation for fractures of the sesamoid bones of the hallux. J Bone Joint Surg (Br) 2002 84:1138–1141
13. Riley J and Selner M. Internal fixation of a displaced tibial sesamoid fracture. J Am Podiatr Med Assoc 2001 91:536–539
14. Rodeo SA, Warren RF, O'Brien SJ, Pavlov H, Barnes R, and Hanks GA. Diastasis of bipartite sesamoids of the first metatarsophalangeal joint. Foot Ankle 1993 14:425–434
15. Van Hal ME, Keene JS, Lange TA, and Clancy WG, Jr. Stress fractures of the great toe sesamoids. Am J Sports Med 1982 10:122–128
16. Pagenstert GI, Valderrabano V, and Hintermann B. Medial sesamoid nonunion combined with hallux valgus in athletes: a report of two cases. Foot Ankle Int 2006 27:135–140
17. Chisin R, Peyser A, and Milgrom C. Bone scintigraphy in the assessment of the hallucal sesamoids. Foot Ankle Int 1995 16:291–294

Proximal Percutaneous Harvesting of the Plantaris Tendon

Geert I. Pagenstert and Beat Hintermann

For decades, in a variety of surgical specialties, the plantaris longus tendon has been used as a free autologous tendon graft [1]. The plantaris is a tendon of a rudimentary developed muscle and harvesting leaves no functional donor site morbidity. However, even foot and ankle surgeons frequently use other autografts because of difficulties finding the tendon with the established harvesting procedure at the medial calcaneus [2, 3]. Enlargement of the incision, multi incisions, and painful scar formation at the level of footwear have been described [4].

Difficulties finding the plantaris distally are explained by its inconstant insertion at the ankle joint capsule, bursa calcanei, flexor retinaculum, blending with the Achilles tendon or intermuscular septum a few centimeters above its insertion at the calcaneus [5, 6]. In different reports, surgeons were able to find the tendon in only 807 to 88% [8] of cases, while cadaver sections and magnetic resonance imaging (MRI) or ultrasound studies have proved its prevalence in 93–98% of cases [5, 9, 10]. In the following discussion, we present an easy and reproductive procedure to harvest at least 30 cm of plantaris tendon over a 2-cm single incision at the medial calf.

G.I. Pagenstert • B. Hintermann (✉)
Department of Orthopaedic Surgery,
University of Basel, Basel, Switzerland
e-mail: beat.hintermann@ksli.ch

Indications and Contraindications

In orthopedic surgery, autografts are used for reconstruction of ligaments or tendons providing mechanical function. If local tissue is absent or too weak, free grafts are indicated. The best graft tissue is located within the surgical field (no enlargement of the surgical field necessary) and provides the greatest mechanical stability, which means that it has aligned strong and elastic collagen fibers. Among autograft tissues, tendons have the highest concentration of aligned collagen fibers. However, only the plantaris tendon at the leg has no crucial function [10]. Harvesting of other tendons can be associated with significant donor site morbidity [11–15]. A biomechanical study of Bohnsack and colleagues [16] compared tensile strength (in newtons per square millimeter) with load to failure of the peroneus longus (61 N/mm^2), peroneus brevis (41 N/mm^2), split peroneus brevis (52 N/mm^2), split Achilles tendon (36 N/mm^2), fascia lata (27 N/mm^2), periostal flap (2 N/mm^2), anterior talofibular ligament (8 N/mm^2), corium (12 N/mm^2), and plantaris tendon (94 N/mm^2) and found that the plantaris tendon had the highest tensile strength per square millimeter [16]. Therefore, especially in the field of foot and ankle surgery, the use of the plantaris tendon is indicated.

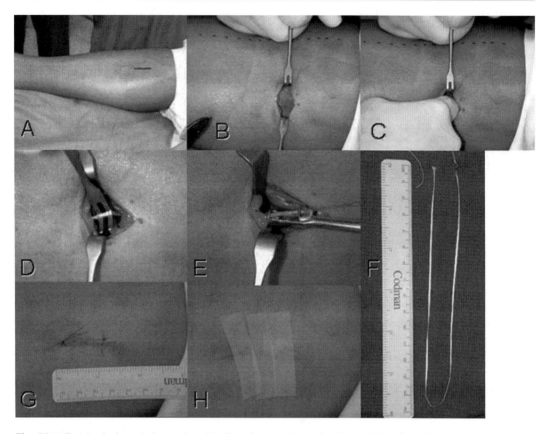

Fig. 22.1 Proximal plantaris harvesting. (**a**) Overview and skin incision to harvest the plantaris longus tendon. (**b**) Blunt dissection to the crural fascia has been made. (**c**) The only palpable tubular structure here is the plantaris tendon. (**d**) The tendon developed. (**e**) The tendon stripper is advanced distally with the tendon under tension. (**f**) The average length of the harvested tendon is 30 cm. (**g**) A small and cosmetic scar is achieved by subcuticular running suture and (**h**) sterile strips

Preoperative Planning

Magnet resonance imaging can prove existence of the plantaris tendon but should not be ordered for this purpose alone [9, 17]. Ultrasound visualization is adequate [18].

Technique

The plantaris longus tendon runs at the medial boarder of the triceps between the muscle bellies of gastrocnemius and soleus [1, 19]. A 2-cm longitudinal incision 30 cm proximal to the

medial malleolus is made (Fig. 22.1a). Subcutaneous blunt dissection to the fascia is performed with respect to the saphenous nerve and vein (Fig. 22.1b). Again, a 2-cm longitudinal incision is made in the fascia to enable the surgeon's finger to enter the intermuscular space (Fig. 22.1c). The only rigid tubular structure that is palpable at this location is the plantaris tendon. The tendon is developed with the finger or a nerve retractor (Fig. 22.1d). With a blunt tendon stripper, the plantaris tendon is dissected in the distal direction. The tendon stripper is advanced, keeping the tendon under tension (Fig. 22.1e). At the calcaneus level, the inner cylinder of the stripper is rotated, which cuts the tendon.

The tendon is stored in a wet sponge for later use (Fig. 22.1f). Fascia is closed with interrupted sutures, and wound closure is done with a subcuticular running stitch (Fig. 22.1g). Wound tension is neutralized with sterile strips to achieve a favorable cosmetic result (Fig. 22.1h).

Complications

The authors performed proximal plantaris harvesting in more than 100 cases and had one case of mild dysesthesia at a broadened scar that did not bother the patient. No saphenous nerve or vein injury has been experienced despite anatomic nearness.

Postoperative Management

Sterile strips can reduce skin tension and broadening of the scar. After wound healing, the patient may use friction massage in case of subcutaneous adhesions.

Results

The harvesting procedure of the plantaris tendon had been controlled in the context of a clinical study that used plantaris tendon autograft for lateral ligament reconstruction of chronic ankle instability. In three (5.3%) of 56 ankle reconstructions, the plantaris tendon could not be located with the previously described harvesting procedure. In one case (1.7%), the plantaris tendon was too weak to serve as proper donor material. In 52 cases (93%), a strong 25- to 35-cm-long tendon graft was harvested [19].

Conclusions

The proximal plantaris harvesting procedure has a higher success than has the traditional distal harvesting procedure. It is associated with no donor site morbidity or complications and may be recommended for all procedures that need strong autograft tissue, especially in the field of foot and ankle surgery.

References

1. White WL. The unique, accessible and useful plantaris tendon. Plast Reconstr Surg 25:133–141, 1960
2. Coughlin MJ, Matt V, Schenck RC, Jr. Augmented lateral ankle reconstruction using a free gracilis graft. Orthopedics 25:31–35, 2002
3. Sammarco GJ, Idusuyi OB. Reconstruction of the lateral ankle ligaments using a split peroneus brevis tendon graft. Foot Ankle Int 20:97–103, 1999
4. Weber BG. Die Verletzungen des oberen Sprunggelenks, 2nd edn, 193–196. Bern, Stuttgart, Wien: Huber, 1972
5. Daseler EH, Anson BH. The plantaris muscle. An anatomical study of 750 specimens. J Bone Joint Surg. 25:822–827, 1943
6. Harvey FJ, Chu G, Harvey PM. Surgical availability of the plantaris tendon. J Hand Surg (Am). 8:243–247, 1983
7. Weber BG, Hupfauer W. Zur Behandlung der frischen fibularen Bandruptur und der chronischen fibularen Bandinsuffizienz. Arch Orthop. Trauma Surg 65: 251–257, 1969
8. Segesser B, Goesele A. [Weber fibular ligament-plasty with plantar tendon with Segesser modification]. Sportverletz Sportschaden 10:88–93, 1996
9. Saxena, A. and Bareither, D. Magnetic resonance and cadaveric findings of the incidence of plantaris tendon. Foot Ankle Int. 21:570–572, 2000
10. Tillmann B, Töndury G. Flexorengruppe der unteren Extremität. In: Leonhardt H, Tillmann B, Töndury G, Zilles K (eds.), Bewegungsapparat, pp. 584–793. Stuttgart, New York: Thieme, 1987
11. Attarian DE, McCrackin HJ, Devito DP, McElhaney JH, Garrett, WE, Jr. A biomechanical study of human lateral ankle ligaments and autogenous reconstructive grafts. Am J Sports Med 13:377–381, 1985
12. Bahr R, Pena F, Shine J, Lew WD, Tyrdal S, Engebretsen L. Biomechanics of ankle ligament reconstruction. An in vitro comparison of the Brostrom repair, Watson-Jones reconstruction, and a new anatomic reconstruction technique. Am J Sports Med 25:424–432, 1997
13. Brunner R, Gaechter A. Repair of fibular ligaments: comparison of reconstructive techniques using plantaris and peroneal tendons. Foot Ankle 11:359–367, 1991
14. Hintermann B. [Biomechanical aspects of muscle-tendon functions]. Orthopade 24:187–192, 1995

15. Hintermann B. Biomechanics of the unstable ankle joint and clinical implications. Med Sci Sports Exerc 31:S459–S469, 1999
16. Bohnsack M, SurieB, Kirsch IL, Wulker N. Biomechanical properties of commonly used autogenous transplants in the surgical treatment of chronic lateral ankle instability. Foot Ankle Int 23:661–664, 2002
17. Wening JV, Katzer A, Phillips F, Jungbluth KH, Lorke DE. [Detection of the tendon of the musculus plantaris longus – diagnostic imaging and anatomic correlate]. Unfallchirurgie 22:30–35, 1996
18. Simpson SL, Hertzog MS, Barja RH. The plantaris tendon graft: an ultrasound study. J Hand Surg (Am). 16:708–711, 1991
19. Pagenstert GI, Valderrabano V, Hintermann B. Lateral ankle ligament reconstruction with free plantaris tendon graft. Tech Foot Ankle Surg 4:104–112, 2005

Percutaneous Fixation of Proximal Fifth Metatarsal Fractures

23

Jonathan R. Saluta and James A. Nunley

Classification

Fractures of the proximal fifth metatarsal can be divided into three general patterns: avulsion of the tuberosity (type 1), Jones fractures (type 2), and diaphyseal stress fractures (type 3) [1]. Tuberosity fractures can be extraarticular or may involve the metatarsocuboid joint (Fig. 23.1). Jones fractures involve the metaphyseal-diaphyseal junction and extend transversely and medially into the 4–5 intermetatarsal joint (Figs. 23.1 and 23.2). Unlike tuberosity fractures, which reliably heal, Jones fractures have a nonunion rate between 7% and 28% [2, 3]. In addition, one third of Jones fractures treated conservatively may go on to closed refracture [4]. Diaphyseal stress fractures occur distal to the 4–5 intermetatarsal joint (Fig. 23.1) and are usually associated with prodromal symptoms. Torg [5] divides diaphyseal stress fractures into three types: acute fractures with sharp margins, delayed unions with a widened fracture line and intramedullary sclerosis, and established nonunions with complete obliteration of the canal.

Treatment

For the majority of tuberosity fractures, conservative management is recommended. A rare indication for surgery would be a large articular stepoff in the metatarsocuboid joint. Depending on symptoms, patients are treated weightbearing in either a hard-soled shoe, removable boot, or cast for 3 weeks. Jones fractures are treated similarly to diaphyseal stress fractures. Nonsurgical management usually consists of nonweightbearing in a short leg cast for 6–8 weeks. However, conservative management is not as reliable in this group, and in most cases surgery is recommended. Surgical candidates include patients engaged in regular athletic activity, patients with high occupational demands, and informed patients who decline conservative treatment.

Surgical Technique

Fixation of minimally to nondisplaced fifth metatarsal base fractures is possible through a percutaneous technique. The first step is to template the fracture because choosing the proper screw is critical to the success of the surgery. Generally the largest diameter screw that will fit the canal should be used. We recommend using a 4.5-mm solid shaft screw for intramedullary canal diameters of 3.5–4.0 mm, a 5.5 screw for canal diameters of 4.1–5.0 mm, and a 6.5 screw for canal diameters of 5.1 mm or greater [6]. A commercially available

J.R. Saluta (✉)
Los Angeles Orthopedic Center, Los Angeles, CA, USA
e-mail: salutaj@yahoo.com

J.A. Nunley
Division of Orthopaedic Surgery, Department of Surgery,
Duke University Medical Center, Durham, NC, USA

G.R. Scuderi and A.J. Tria (eds.), *Minimally Invasive Surgery in Orthopedics: Foot and Ankle Handbook*, 183
DOI 10.1007/978-1-4614-0893-2_23, © Springer Science+Business Media, LLC 2012

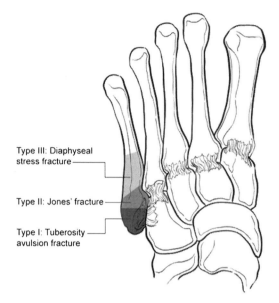

Type III: Diaphyseal stress fracture

Type II: Jones' fracture

Type I: Tuberosity avulsion fracture

Fig. 23.1 Classification of proximal metatarsal fractures

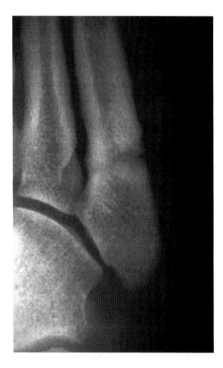

Fig. 23.2 Plain radiograph of a Jones fracture

screw set designed specifically for these fractures contains shaft screws of all three diameters (Fig. 23.3a, b). In addition to proper screw width, an appropriate screw length should be calculated as well. Generally a screw measuring 50% of the

length of the bone is a good place to start. Because the fifth metatarsal has a plantar and lateral bow, a straight screw of greater than 60% of the overall length of the metatarsal may straighten the bow and displace the fracture [7, 8]. Compression is advantageous to help heal this fracture, so if a cancellous lag screw is chosen, one must be certain that all of the threads will cross the fracture site.

Surgery is generally performed under ankle block anesthesia and in an outpatient surgical suite. The patient is positioned supine and the body shifted toward the side of the operating room table that corresponds with the affected foot. It is important that the ipsilateral knee can be flexed and the affected foot can be placed plantigrade on the edge of the table or a sterile operating room fluoroscopy unit. Proper positioning is important because it will keep the working instruments clear of the operating room table. A tourniquet is generally used to provide a bloodless field. Before an incision is made, a K wire is placed upon the lateral aspect of the foot, and fluoroscopy is used to position the pin parallel to and overlapping the proximal metatarsal shaft. This position should correspond to the target screw placement on both the anteroposterior (AP) and lateral images. Two lines are traced in ink on the skin that approximate the pin alignment in both views (Fig. 23.4).

A 2-cm longitudinal incision is made 2 cm proximal to the base of the fifth metatarsal. In our experience, displacement of the fracture commonly consists of mild angulation, and exposure of the fracture site is usually unnecessary. The reduction is accomplished with compression from screw insertion. An important step is to identify and protect the sural nerve and peroneus brevis tendon during screw preparation and insertion. The sural nerve is either overlying or slightly dorsal to the skin incision and can be retracted superiorly (Fig. 23.5). Anatomic studies have shown the sural nerve to lie within 5 mm of the proximal tuberosity [9]. The peroneus brevis tendon is usually retracted inferiorly. A commonly described technique involves partially elevating the attachment of the peroneus brevis in order to gain better exposure of the entry point for the

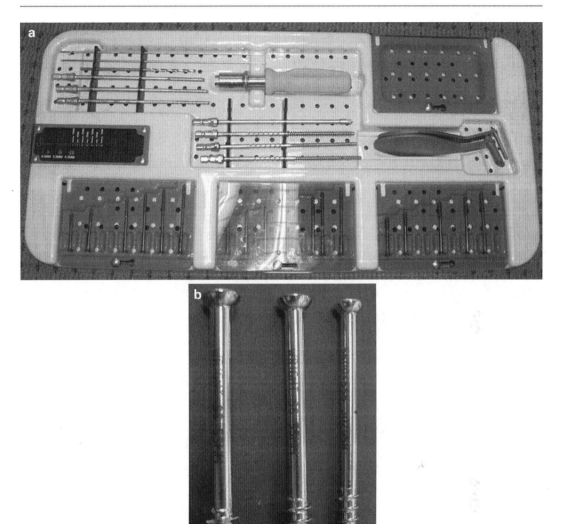

Fig. 23.3 (**a**) Specialty Jones set of screws and instrumentation for fixation of proximal fifth metatarsal fractures (Photo courtesy of Wright Medical). (**b**) 4.5-, 5.5-, and 6.5-mm screws with low-profile heads (Photo courtesy of Wright Medical)

guide wire, but, in our experience, simple retraction of the tendon is adequate. A guide pin is now placed through the incision toward the "high and inside" starting point at the base of the fifth metatarsal. Fluoroscopy is used to place the tip of the pin in a center-center position relative to the intramedullary canal on AP, lateral, and oblique views (Fig. 23.6). The medial edge of the pin should abut the cuboid. The pin is advanced two thirds of the length of the shaft through the center of the medullary canal. In order to keep the guide pin from deviating medially in the fifth metatarsal shaft, the pin should lie almost directly on the lateral calcaneal skin when being advanced.

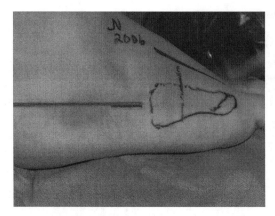

Fig. 23.4 Skin markings for guidewire placement

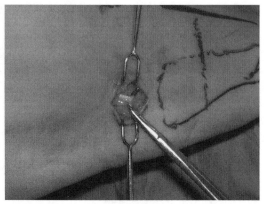

Fig. 23.5 A branch of the sural nerve

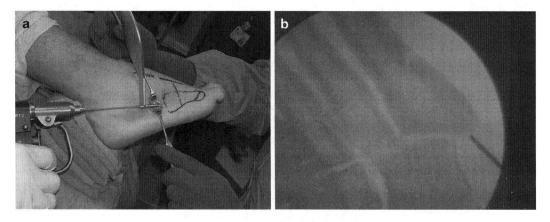

Fig. 23.6 (**a**) Guidewire inserted distally. (**b**) Starting point for guidewire

The pin is next overdrilled with a cannulated drill under fluoroscopic guidance to avoid penetration of the fifth metatarsal cortex (Fig. 23.7). Next, the bone is carefully tapped to the proper size and length corresponding to the intended screw. Countersinking the head has not been necessary in our experience. Using a screw that is longer than the distance tapped can either distract the fracture site or explode the lateral cortex and should be avoided. The appropriate screw is finally advanced under fluoroscopy to make sure that all of the screw threads have just crossed the fracture site. The screw should compress the fracture site, which usually results in an adequate reduction (Fig. 23.8). In our experience, drilling the canal even in sclerotic bone promotes fracture healing, which makes extensile incisions and supplemental bone

grafting usually unnecessary. The incision is irrigated and closed with interrupted nylon sutures.

A technique for avoiding excessive fluoroscopy exposure during pin placement was described by Johnson [9]. His technique requires a slightly longer skin incision that exposes the plantarmost aspect of the proximal tuberosity and part of the peroneus brevis insertion. Without the use of fluoroscopy, a guide pin is placed at the starting point 1 cm dorsal to the palpable inferior margin of the tuberosity and medial to the peroneus brevis insertion (Fig. 23.9). A predetermined plantarflexion angle of 7° is marked on the skin using a goniometer (Fig. 23.10). The guide pin is advanced, overdrilled, and tapped, and the screw is inserted as previously described. A fluoroscan is used to check the final screw placement.

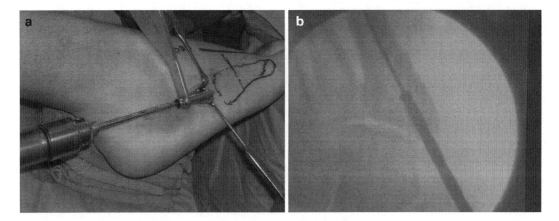

Fig. 23.7 (**a**) Drill inserted with protector. (**b**) Guidewire overdrilled

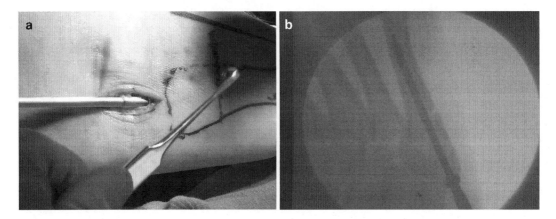

Fig. 23.8 (**a**) Large diameter screw inserted. (**b**) Screw advanced across fracture

Fig. 23.9 Illustration
showing the starting point
in relation to the lateral
and plantar portions of the
fifth metatarsal tuberosity
(From Johnson et al. [9]
Copyright © 2004 by the
American Orthopaedic
Foot & Ankle Society
[AOFAS], reproduced here
with permission.)

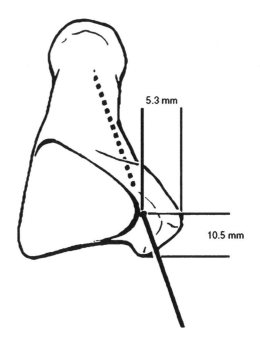

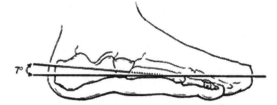

Fig. 23.10 Illustration showing the 7° plantarflexion angle with the ankle dorsiflexed to neutral. The pin would always project along the lateral aspect of the calcaneus after antegrade placement through the starting point (From Johnson et al. [9] Copyright © 2004 by the American Orthopaedic Foot & Ankle Society [AOFAS], reproduced here with permission.)

Postoperative Management

Postoperatively, the patient is splinted and kept touchdown-weightbearing for 2 weeks. At the end of 2 weeks, the patient is allowed to begin progressive weightbearing in a removable boot and with a custom molded orthosis. By the fourth week, the orthosis is maintained, and the patient is transitioned to regular shoes with a stiff sole to reduce motion. Athletes are usually allowed to jog on a track by the fifth to sixth week, and most are back to sports by the seventh to eighth week.

References

1. Quill G Jr. Fractures of the proximal fifth metatarsal. Orthop Clin North Am 1995;26:353–361
2. Torg J, Balduini F, Zelko R, Pavlov H, Peff T, Das M. Fractures of the base of the fifth metatarsal distal to the tuberosity: classification and guidelines for non-surgical and surgical management. J Bone Joint Surg Am 1984;66:209–214
3. Clapper M, O'Brien T, Lyons P. Fractures of the fifth metatarsal: analysis of a fracture registry. Clin Orthop Relat Res 1995;315:238–241
4. Quill G Jr. Fractures of the proximal fifth metatarsal. Orthop Clin North Am 1995;26:353–361
5. Torg J, Balduini F, Zelko R, Pavlov H, Peff T, Das M. Fractures of the base of the fifth metatarsal distal to the tuberosity: classification and guidelines for non-surgical and surgical management. J Bone Joint Surg Am 1984;66:209–214
6. Mall N, Queen R, Glisson R, Nunley JS. Patterns and risk factors of screw failure in intramedullary fixation of fifth metatarsal Jones fractures: a biomechanical study. Unpublished data, 2006
7. Horst F, Gilbert B, Glisson R, Nunley J. Torque resistance after fixation of Jones fractures with intramedullary screws. Foot Ankle Int 2004;25(12):914–919
8. Nunley J. Fractures of the base of the fifth metatarsal: the Jones fracture. Orthop Clin North Am 2001;32(1):171–180
9. Johnson J, Labib S, Fowler, R. Intramedullary screw fixation of the fifth metatarsal: an anatomic study and improved technique. Foot Ankle Int 2004;25(4):274–277

Percutaneous ORIF of Periarticular Distal Tibia Fractures

24

Michael P. Clare and Roy W. Sanders

Periarticular fractures of the distal tibia remain among the more challenging of fractures for the orthopedic surgeon. Traditional methods of treatment have included functional bracing, external fixation with or without limited internal fixation (hybrid fixation), intramedullary nailing, and formal open reduction internal fixation (ORIF). Cadaveric studies have previously described the somewhat tenuous vascular supply to the distal metaphysis, which, combined with inherent limitations in the surrounding soft tissue envelope, pose a risk of nonunion and have led to increasing interest in "biologic" fixation techniques [1].

These techniques are based upon the principles of limited soft tissue stripping, maintenance of the osteogenic fracture hematoma, and preservation of vascular supply to the individual fracture fragments while restoring axial and rotational alignment, and providing sufficient stability to allow progression of motion, uncomplicated fracture healing, and eventual return to function. As such, the evolution of percutaneous plating techniques has led to the development of

M.P. Clare
Division of Foot and Ankle Surgery, The Florida
Orthopaedic Institute, Tampa, FL, USA

R.W. Sanders (✉)
Tampa General Hospital, The Florida Orthopaedic
Institute, Tampa, FL, USA
e-mail: OTS1@aol.com

low-profile, precontoured implants specifically intended for subcutaneous/submuscular application in the distal tibia.

Indications and Contraindications

Percutaneous ORIF techniques are ideal for unstable distal-fourth, extraarticular fractures of the distal tibia with periarticular metaphyseal comminution or distal fracture lines precluding use of a locked intramedullary nail (OTA types 43A1-A3; 43B1) [2]. Other indications include simple two-part, nondisplaced or minimally displaced intraarticular fractures (OTA type 43C1) in which the articular fragments can be anatomically reduced by an abbreviated open reduction, and the remainder completed through percutaneous means [2].

Percutaneous ORIF is also particularly attractive in the event of open fractures, which account for up to 20% of these injuries; overlying fracture blisters, or other significant soft tissue compromise; fractures in patients who are heavy smokers (≥2 packs/day); and fractures in patients with diabetes mellitus, peripheral neuropathy, or other significant medical comorbidities.

We think that complex, comminuted intraarticular fractures of the tibial pilon require an anatomic articular reduction for optimum results,

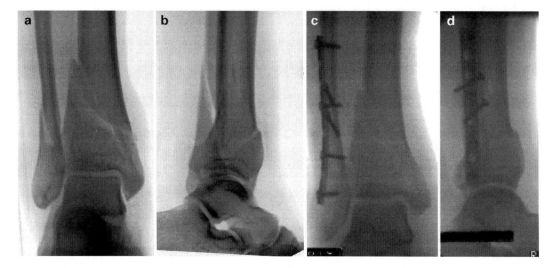

Fig. 24.1 (**a, b**) Preoperative radiographs of a periarticular distal tibia fracture; (**c, d**) intraoperative radiographs after stabilization of fibula – note the indirect reduction of the distal tibia

which thus necessitates a true open reduction and internal fixation. Percutaneous techniques in these instances are therefore contraindicated.

Surgical Technique

Depending on the extent of soft tissue injury, periarticular fractures in the distal tibia typically require temporary stabilization with a spanning external fixator, which maintains axial length and provides provisional stability until soft tissue swelling and/or fracture blisters have sufficiently resolved to allow definitive stabilization. We utilize the "wrinkle test," originally described for calcaneal fractures, as a simple means to determine soft tissue suitability for surgery [3]. The test involves gentle passive ankle dorsiflexion, paying close attention to the skin overlying the area of intended dissection; alternatively, in the presence of a prohibitive external fixator frame, the skin overlying the planned area of dissection can be gently pinched. The presence of skin wrinkles is considered a positive test, indicating that soft tissue swelling has adequately dissipated to proceed with definitive fracture stabilization.

The patient is placed supine on a radiolucent operating table with a bolster beneath the ipsilateral hip, and a pneumatic tourniquet is placed.

We prefer utilizing the tourniquet for any articular reduction, as well as for open stabilization of the fibula, where necessary, in order to provide a bloodless surgical field. The percutaneous plating may then be performed with the tourniquet deflated, depending on the clinical situation. Because of the need for biplanar image intensification, standard fluoroscopy is also required. In the presence of prior external fixation, we typically remove the external fixator frame (still assembled) prior to skin preparation while leaving the Schanz pins in place for assistance with indirect fracture reduction intraoperatively; the frame is then resterilized and preserved on the back table for use where needed.

In the event of an associated fibula fracture, we prefer to first stabilize the fibula to confirm axial length and rotational alignment. In most cases, and particularly with extraarticular fractures of the distal tibia, restoring fibular length and rotation will indirectly reduce the distal tibia, such that only minimal further manipulation is required with tibial stabilization (Fig. 24.1a–d).

Medial Plating of the Distal Tibia

Subcutaneous medial plating is the most common of the percutaneous stabilization techniques

Fig. 24.2 Small medial incision for percutaneous medial plating – note the saphenous nerve (*white arrows*)

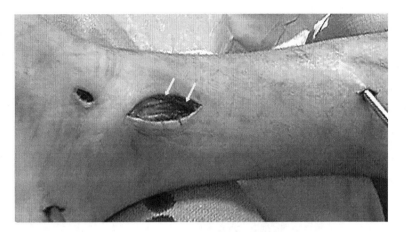

in the distal tibia, and is especially well suited for extraarticular distal-fourth or supramalleolar fractures (OTA types 43A1–3) [2]. A small (2–3 cm) vertical incision is made in line with the medial malleolus, and the underlying saphenous nerve is identified and protected (Fig. 24.2). Alternatively, an oblique or transverse incision may be utilized. Deep dissection then continues down through the extensor retinaculum, but superficial to the underlying periosteum. The full thickness soft tissue envelope is then gently mobilized to facilitate easy passage of the plate, and a subcutaneous tunnel is then developed with a blunt periosteal elevator along the medial border of the tibia in extraperiosteal fashion.

The provisionally selected plate is placed directly on the skin overlying the medial distal tibia and assessed under fluoroscopy for adequacy of length (Fig. 24.3). The required plate length is variable depending on the fracture pattern and extent of comminution, bone quality of the patient, and screw purchase (for nonlocking implants), among other factors. As a general rule, however, four to six screw holes with two to four screws proximal to the main fracture line should provide sufficient stability. The plate is then rotationally contoured where necessary (Fig. 24.4) and gently passed in retrograde fashion under fluoroscopic guidance, specifically avoiding the saphenous nerve (Fig. 24.5). At the present time, most commercially available implants for the medial distal tibia do not have an associated outrigger for assistance with plate passage.

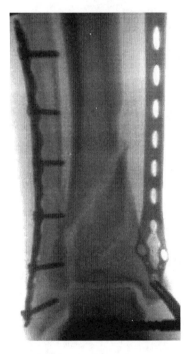

Fig. 24.3 Intraoperative radiograph with a provisionally selected plate – note the length of the plate relative to the apex of the fracture line, allowing four screw holes for the proximal fragment

Sagittal plane alignment of the plate relative to the tibial shaft is then confirmed fluoroscopically. A secondary incision is made at the proximal tip of the plate for manipulation where necessary until the plate is appropriately positioned.

Depending on the fracture pattern and extent of residual displacement, pointed reduction forceps are then used through separate stab incisions

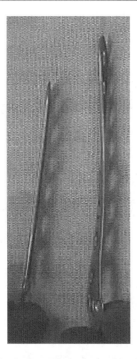

Fig. 24.4 Contouring of the selected plate prior to placement – note the rotational bend through the proximal portion of the plate to match the triangular contour of the distal diaphysis

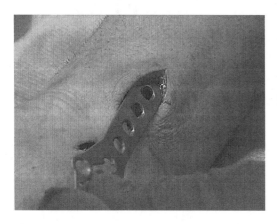

Fig. 24.5 Subcutaneous placement of the plate

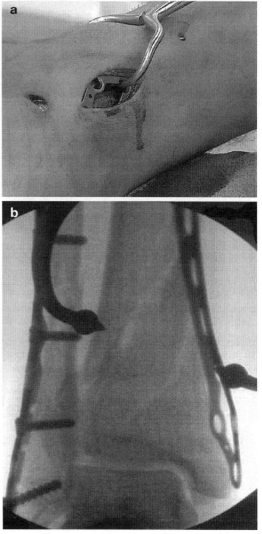

Fig. 24.6 (**a**, **b**) Provisional reduction of the distal tibia with a pointed reduction clamp

to further reduce the proximal fragment to the distal fragment(s) through the plate (Fig. 24.6a, b). In the absence of a fibula fracture, or in the event of significant residual shortening, restoration of axial length may be facilitated through a variety of indirect reduction techniques, including longitudinal traction through the previous external fixator Schanz pins, use of a femoral distractor,

or an articulated tensioning device. Lag screws may be placed outside the plate through separate stab incisions to stabilize additional fracture lines where necessary.

Because of the proximity of the ankle joint, we generally prefer initially stabilizing the distal fragment to the plate, using the distal-most and proximal-most screw holes overlying the distal fragment. Typically, the distal-most screw holes are easily visualized through the small medial incision, while the more proximal screw holes are isolated under fluoroscopy and accessed

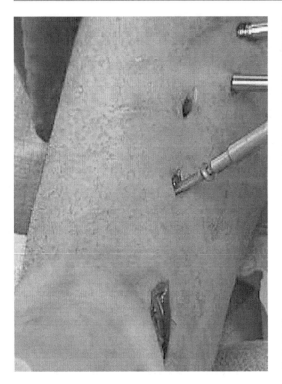

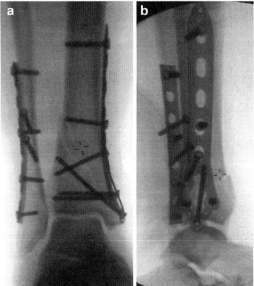

Fig. 24.8 (**a**, **b**) Intraoperative radiographs after definitive stabilization of a distal tibia fracture – note the three screws within the distal fragment, in addition to the cortical lag screw across the primary fracture line

Fig. 24.7 Stabilization of a proximal fragment – note the small stab incisions

through small stab incisions (Fig. 24.7). In general, three to four screws within the distal fragment should provide sufficient stability (Fig. 24.8a, b). With simple, oblique fracture patterns, lag screws may first be placed through the plate across the primary fracture line, thereby securing the distal fragment to the proximal fragment (Fig. 24.9). Additional lag screws may be placed through the plate where necessary for stabilization of vertically oriented fracture lines distally.

The proximal fragment is then secured, utilizing (as a minimum) the proximal-most and apex screw holes within the plate, respectively, which, when combined with the distal screw pattern creates an "internal external fixator" construct (Fig. 24.10a, b). Other screw holes may additionally be filled within the proximal fragment, again depending on the clinical situation, quality of screw purchase, and overall fracture and construct stability (Fig. 24.11a, b).

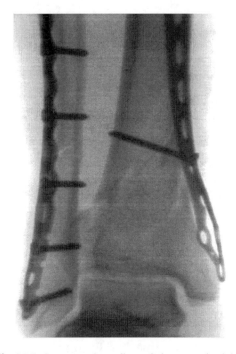

Fig. 24.9 Intraoperative radiograph demonstrating initial lag fixation (through the plate) across the primary fracture line

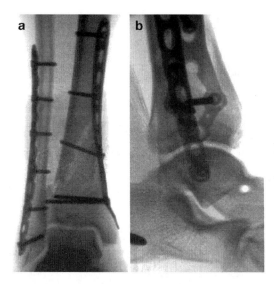

Fig. 24.10 (**a**, **b**) Intraoperative radiograph demonstrating "internal external fixator" construct

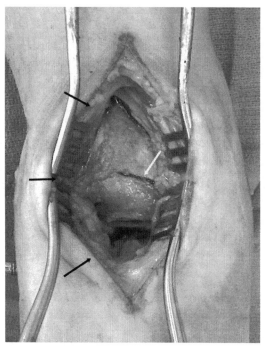

Fig. 24.12 Anterior approach – note the tibialis anterior maintained within the tendon sheath (*black arrows*) and the intraarticular fracture line (*white arrow*)

fragments are reduced through an abbreviated open reduction, and with open fractures in which the traumatic laceration is extended and used for passage of the plate. In these instances, the incision or traumatic laceration itself affords visualization and mobilization of the underlying neurovascular structures. The location of the intraarticular extension, as determined on computed tomographic (CT) evaluation, determines whether an anterior or anterolateral approach is used.

Anterior Approach

A 6-cm incision is made overlying the ankle joint in line with a point approximately one finger-breadth lateral to the tibial crest. Deep dissection continues through the extensor retinaculum, utilizing the interval between the tibialis anterior and extensor hallucis longus tendons. Every effort is made to preserve the continuity of the tibialis anterior tendon sheath to minimize potential wound complications (Fig. 24.12). The underlying anterior tibial/dorsalis pedis artery

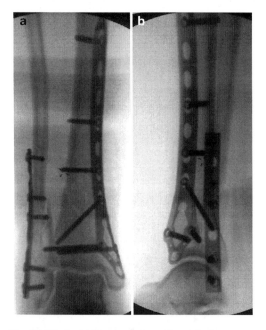

Fig. 24.11 (**a**, **b**) Intraoperative radiograph demonstrating alternate fixation pattern in an osteoporotic patient – note the longer plate and additional screws for supplemental stability

Anterior/Anterolateral Plating of the Distal Tibia

Submuscular anterior or anterolateral plating is primarily used for proximal fixation in simple two-part intraarticular fractures, in which the articular

and deep peroneal nerve, which typically course just lateral to the extensor hallucis longus tendon, are identified and protected throughout the procedure. A transverse arthrotomy is completed for full visualization of the intraarticular surface; further proximal dissection is completed in extraperiosteal fashion. The articular fragments are reduced anatomically under direct vision, provisionally stabilized with 1.6-mm Kirschner wires, and the reduction is verified fluoroscopically.

The provisionally selected anterior plate is then confirmed under fluoroscopy for adequacy of length, and passed in submuscular fashion, specifically avoiding the adjacent neurovascular bundle. A small stab incision is made at the proximal tip of the plate for manipulation where necessary until the plate is appropriately positioned. Cortical lag screws are placed through the plate distally for stabilization of a coronal plane fracture line; lag screws may alternatively be placed outside the plate for a sagittally oriented fracture line. Additional cortical screws are then placed – in general, three to four screws within the distal fragment should provide sufficient stability.

Stabilization of the proximal fragment is then completed through separate stab incisions over the respective screw holes. Because of the underlying tibialis anterior muscle, the stab incisions are made just lateral to the tibial crest to allow lateral retraction of the tibialis anterior muscle, and tend to be slightly longer than those used for medial plating.

Following stabilization and final fluoroscopic images, a deep drain is placed exiting proximally, and the extensor retinaculum is meticulously repaired. The remainder of the incision is closed in routine, layered fashion. We prefer interrupted 3–0 nylon suture for the skin layer, using the modified Allgöwer-Donati technique.

Anterolateral Approach

A 6-cm incision is made overlying the ankle joint just lateral to the extensor digitorum longus and peroneus tertius tendons. The superficial peroneal nerve is identified and gently mobilized laterally, and deep dissection continues through the extensor

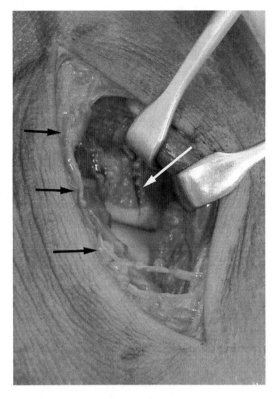

Fig. 24.13 Anterolateral approach – the peroneus tertius muscle is retracted medially. Note the superficial peroneal nerve (*black arrows*) and the intraarticular fracture line (*white arrow*)

retinaculum. The adjacent anterior tibial/dorsalis pedis artery and deep peroneal nerve, which typically course between the extensor hallucis longus and extensor digitorum longus tendons, are protected throughout the procedure. A transverse arthrotomy is completed for full visualization of the intraarticular surface; further proximal dissection is completed in extraperiosteal fashion (Fig. 24.13). A 4.5-mm Schanz pin may be temporarily placed in the lateral (nonarticular) talar neck for intraarticular distraction where necessary. The remainder of the procedure is completed as described for the anterior approach.

Locked Plates Versus Nonlocked Plates

The development of locked plating technology has been a major advance in the management of lower extremity fractures, and particularly in the distal tibia. The advantages of locked plating over conventional plating include increased overall construct stability, increased resistance to bending stresses, and decreased screw cutout and failure. Locked plates, however, are inherently more bulky, which may increase the risk of wound complications, as well as hardware prominence. Additionally, because of the increased stiffness of the plate, there is generally limited ability to compress comminuted metaphyseal fragments through the plate, even with initial nonlocking, cortical lag screws.

Although there are no specific guidelines as to absolute indications for locked plating, as a general rule, locked plating should be considered for fractures with significant metaphyseal comminution, whereby the locked implant bridges the comminuted segment to maintain axial length; fractures in patients with osteopenia, osteoporosis, or other significant medical comorbidities in which poor screw purchase would be otherwise anticipated.

Alternatively, a combination of locking and nonlocking screws may be utilized, creating a so-called hybrid construct. In this instance, the non-locking screws are first placed, either in lag fashion to stabilize secondary fracture lines, or in neutral mode to reduce the plate to bone. Locking screws are used thereafter, preventing toggle and potential cutout at the bone-implant interface. In this manner, some degree of micromotion and bone elasticity is permitted, thereby allowing endosteal bony callous formation.

Postoperative Protocol

After routine wound closure, the involved limb is placed in a protective splint for 10–14 days to allow incisional healing. The patient is then converted to a venous compression stocking and fracture boot, and early progression of motion is initiated to facilitate functional limb recovery. Advancement of weightbearing is variable depending on the individual fracture pattern and overall stability of the fixation construct, and ranges from 8 to 12 weeks postoperatively.

Results and Complications

Krettek et al. [4] first described the use of percutaneous plating in the management of distal femur and proximal tibia fractures. Subsequent authors have reported percutaneous applications for fractures of the distal tibia, primarily medial plating, using a variety of implants [5–13].

Helfet et al. [5] treated 20 complex distal tibia and pilon fractures with delayed percutaneous medial plating using precontoured ½ semitubular plates and screws, and reported no hardware failures or significant wound complications. All fractures healed and all patients in their series had good functional results.

Oh et al. [7] managed 21 extraarticular or minimal intraarticular distal tibia fractures with acute percutaneous medial plating with precontoured LC-DC plates and screws. There were no wound complications and all fractures healed without incident. Three patients had slight residual ankle stiffness, while all others regained full ankle range of motion. Similarly, Francois et al. [8] reported good results with indirect reduction and percutaneous medial plating in ten distal tibia and plafond fractures. There were no wound complications and all fractures ultimately healed.

Khoury et al. [9] treated 24 distal tibia fractures with percutaneous medial plating using a variety of plates ranging from 3.5-mm and 4.5-mm reconstruction plates to 3.5-mm and 4.5-mm broad LC-DC plates. They too reported no deep infections and only one superficial infection, and all patients regained good ankle range of motion. All fractures healed at an average of 12 weeks postoperatively.

Collinge et al. [11] treated 17 high-energy distal tibia fractures, including 11 open injuries, with prebent 4.5-mm narrow LC-DC plates and large fragment screws. They reported three superficial wound infections, all related to external fixator pin sites, and one deep infection. All patients with closed injuries regained knee and ankle range of motion within 5° of motion of the contralateral limb, while ankle range of motion in those with open injuries averaged 10° of dorsiflexion and 20° of plantarflexion.

Percutaneous techniques are, however, technically demanding and thus strict attention to detail is necessary to prevent axial, rotational, and angular malalignment. Helfet et al. [5] had four fractures heal with significant malalignment – two with >5° of varus angulation, and two with >10° of recurvatum, although none required further surgery. Maffulli et al. [12] had seven angular malunions (7–10° of residual angular malalignment) out of 20 distal tibia fractures. Borg et al. [13] had two malunions requiring revision surgery, and Oh et al. [7] had one rotational malunion out of 21 distal tibia fractures. Khoury et al. [9] had four malunions – one with 8° of valgus angulation, one with 7° of varus angulation, and two with 4–5° of recurvatum – although none required further surgery. In both instances of coronal plane malalignment, there was significant metaphyseal comminution and a "soft" 3.5-mm reconstruction plate had been used, leading the authors to recommend use of "solid" LC-DC plates for those fractures with substantial metaphyseal comminution.

Because of the generally high-energy nature of these injuries, delayed union or nonunion may still develop despite these biologic techniques, particularly in those patients with open injuries or substantial bone loss. Collinge et al. [11] reported three delayed unions and three nonunions among their patients with open injuries, including four with significant bone loss. All six patients healed after revision surgery and bone grafting. Francois et al. [8] had two delayed unions in their series that required bone grafting and eventually healed. Borg et al. [13] had two delayed unions and two nonunions out of 21 closed distal tibia fractures.

Conclusions

Periarticular distal tibia fractures are complex, challenging fractures to effectively manage. Because of the inherently limited soft tissue envelope and vascularity in the distal tibial metaphysis, subcutaneous/submuscular plating is an attractive option for certain extraarticular and simple intraarticular fractures. These techniques allow restoration of axial, sagittal, and rotational alignment in a biologically friendly manner, thereby providing sufficient bony stability to facilitate early range of motion, uncomplicated fracture healing, and optimum return of function. Although larger, randomized series with longer-term follow-up are necessary, particularly with respect to locked implants, the current preliminary series suggest promising results with these techniques.

References

1. Borrelli J Jr, Prickett W, Song E, et al. Extraosseous blood supply of the tibia and the effects of different plating techniques: a human cadaveric study. J Orthop Trauma 2002;16:691–95
2. Orthopaedic Trauma Association committee for coding and Classification: Fracture and dislocation compendium. J Orthop Trauma 1996;10(Suppl 1):51–5
3. Sanders R. Intra-articular fractures of the calcaneus: present state of the art. J Orthop Trauma 1992;6:252–65
4. Krettek C, Schandelmaier P, Tscherne H. Neue entwicklungen bei der stabilisierung dia- und metaphysarer frakturen der langen rohrenknocken. Orthopade 1997;26:408–21
5. Helfet DL, Shonnard PY, Levine D, et al. Minimally invasive plate osteosynthesis of distal fractures of the tibia. Injury 1997;28 (Suppl 1):SA-42–8
6. Helfet DL, Suk M. Minimally invasive percutaneous plate osteosynthesis of fractures of the distal tibia. Instr Course Lect 2004;53:471–5
7. Oh CW, Kyung HS, Park IH, et al. Distal tibia metaphyseal fractures treated by percutaneous plate osteosynthesis. Clin Orthop Relat Res 2003;408:286–91
8. Francois J, Vandeputte G, Verheyden F, et al. Percutaneous plate fixation of fractures of the distal tibia. Acta Orthop Belg 2004;70:148–54
9. Khoury A, Liebergall M, London E, et al. Percutaneous plating of distal tibial fractures. Foot Ankle Int 2002;23:818–24
10. Collinge CA, Sanders RW. Percutaneous plating in the lower extremity. J Am Acad Ortho Surg 2000;8:211–6
11. Collinge C, Sanders R, Dipasquale T. Treatment of complex tibial periarticular fractures using percutaneous techniques. Clin Orthop Relat Res 2000;375:69–77
12. Maffulli N, Toms AD, McMurtie A, et al. Percutaneous plating of distal tibial fractures. Int Orthop 2004;28:159–62
13. Borg T, Larsson S, Lidsjo U. Percutaneous plating of distal tibial fractures: preliminary results in 21 patients. Injury 2004;35:608–14

Round Table Discussion of MIS of the Foot and Ankle

25

Mark Easley, Nicola Maffulli, Steven L. Shapiro,
Juha Jaakkola, S. Robert Rozbruch,
Bradley M. Lamm, and Martinus Richter

Mark Easley: I have invited several of the contributing authors to participate in a roundtable discussion of minimally invasive surgery (MIS) for the foot and ankle. I am pleased to share the thoughts and expertise of Juha Jaakkola, Brad Lamm, Nicola Maffulli, Martinus Richter, Robert Rozbruch, and Steve Shapiro. While all of our contributing authors provide valuable insights to MIS in their respective chapters, I anticipate that this roundtable discussion will provide the reader with an important overview of current concepts in MIS as they pertain to the management of foot and ankle disorders.

N. Maffulli (✉)
Centre for Sports and Exercise Medicine, Barts and the London School of Medicine and Dentistry, Queen Mary University of London, London, UK

S.L. Shapiro
Savannah Orthopaedic Foot and Ankle Center, Savannah, GA, USA

J. Jaakkola
Southeastern Orthopedic Center, Savannah, GA, USA

S.R. Rozbruch
Limb Lengthening and Deformity Service, Hospital for Special Surgery, Weill Medical College of Cornell University, New York, NY, USA

B.M. Lamm
International Center for Limb Lengthening, Rubin Institute for Advanced Orthopedics, Sinai Hospital of Baltimore, Baltimore, MD, USA

M. Richter
Chirurgische Klinik, Klinikum Coburg, Coburg, Germany

While several techniques for the management of foot and ankle pathology have traditionally been performed with limited incisions, for example fixation of fifth metatarsal fractures, the concept of minimally invasive surgery for the foot and ankle has only recently gained appreciable attention. In my opinion, the evolution of MIS for the foot and ankle lags behind that for the knee, hip, spine, shoulder, and trauma surgery. Nicola, what is your view of the apparent lag of MIS in foot and ankle surgery?

Nicola Maffulli: From the beginning, the foot and ankle has been the "Cinderella subspeciality," often drawing from the advances in other subspecialities for its development. Thus, in my mind, it is not surprising that MIS for the foot and ankle is only recently emerging. MIS techniques for the foot and ankle simply have not been developed for the majority of foot and ankle procedures. Moreover, similar to the timeline for advances in other subspecialities, most foot and ankle surgeons favor traditional and/or extensile exposures, leaving the development of less invasive techniques to a group of select pioneers.

Mark Easley: So, with that said, Steve, you have used several minimally invasive techniques for years with great success. While you are a dedicated academician, you are in private practice. In your mind, what are the major advantages to MIS for foot and ankle surgery?

Steve Shapiro: Besides the obvious advantage of improved cosmesis (not to be underestimated when patients recommend a surgeon to their friend), it has been my experience that MIS affords a more rapid recovery and often the advantage of more precise and focused surgery. I performed traditional approaches to the foot and ankle for years, but have not looked back since employing MIS techniques. By and large, less invasive access reliably permits a more rapid return to normal activities, without compromising functional outcome. For example, while plantar fascia release and Morton's neuroma excision are relatively minor foot and ankle procedures, traditional approaches may still lead to delayed wound healing and delayed weightbearing due to soft tissue dissection. When performed endoscopically, recovery is greatly accelerated. Furthermore, the endoscope provides a much greater detail of the pathology that, in my hands, leads to greater precision.

Mark Easley: Juha, you have adopted a minimally invasive approach to several foot and ankle procedures, some performed with the aid of arthroscopy. Where do you see advantages of arthroscopy in managing foot and ankle disorders traditionally treated with extensile exposures?

Juha Jaakkola: My experience is best explained with my approach to the surgical management of displaced, intraarticular calcaneus fractures. Traditionally I utilized an extensile exposure that affords full visualization of the lateral calcaneus and, with mobilization of the fragments, adequate visualization to achieve an anatomic reduction, albeit with considerable reliance on intraoperative fluoroscopy. Despite the extensile approach, I was rarely ever able to visualize the entire posterior calcaneal articular facet. Using the arthroscopically assisted technique, I am able, in most cases, to better visualize the articular reduction of the posterior facet than with the traditional extensile approach. In my opinion, like for acetabular fractures or other intraarticular fractures, outcome of calcaneal fractures is probably heavily dependent on a congruent articular reduction.

Mark Easley: Any downsides?

Juha Jaakkola: Well, not necessarily a downside, but timing becomes more of an issue for arthroscopically assisted management of displaced calcaneal fractures. Since the approach is limited, comprehensive mobilization of fracture fragments is not possible with the MIS technique as it is with the extensile approach. Therefore, I must perform the arthroscopically assisted technique within the first 3–4 days, much like those surgeons who use external fixation in the management of displaced calcaneus fractures. Otherwise, the fracture fragments begin to bind and reduction without an extensile approach is not feasible.

Mark Easley: Should we categorize arthroscopically and endoscopically assisted surgeries as MIS?

Steve Shapiro: Absolutely! Physiologically, there is not a lot of soft tissue coverage about the foot and ankle, so often traditional approaches are not very extensive. To make the incisions even smaller, like MIS for TKA or THA, may not be plausible. Endoscopically and arthroscopically assisted techniques comprise a considerable number of procedures that define MIS of the foot and ankle.

Mark Easley: Rob, Juha mentioned external fixation. You are establishing yourself as a leader in the field of external fixation for the management of complex deformity of the foot and ankle. How does external fixation factor into MIS for foot and ankle disorders?

Robert Rozbruch: Mark, thank you for your confidence in my abilities! I am very fortunate that my institution provides me with the resources to utilize external fixation to treat foot and ankle pathology. It has been a particularly rewarding experience for me. Initially I practiced orthopedics with traditional techniques but acquired further training with several masters of external fixation. Since I have been able to apply the principles they taught me to foot and ankle deformity, I now favor external fixation over internal fixation when the indications permit. Here are some of my observations:

The use of external fixation helps promote MIS of the foot and ankle in two ways. First, the bony fixation is established through stab wounds avoiding soft tissue dissection needed for plate fixation. Second, correction of deformity is accomplished with a percutaneous osteotomy and the use of acute and/or gradual correction. This avoids the need for large exposures needed for closing wedge osteotomies and plate fixation.

Mark Easley: Any appreciable advantages in postoperative management?

Robert Rozbruch: No question. The external fixation techniques are very practical. In my hands, less exposure is less traumatic to the soft tissues and results in less postoperative pain and quicker bony healing compared with traditional extensile exposures. The use of circular external fixation is especially helpful at gaining stable fixation of the foot needed for complex ankle fusion. Moreover, the frames generally afford adequate stability to allow the patient to fully weight-bear on the operated extremity postoperatively.

Mark Easley: Brad, you also tend to favor external fixation in the management of complex foot and ankle deformity. In your practice, have principles of external fixation afforded a more minimally invasive approach compared with conventional open techniques?

Brad Lamm: Rob and I have had many occasions to share ideas, and I agree with Rob's observations. Prior to the use of external fixation in the foot and ankle, large deformities were generally corrected acutely, necessitating extensile exposures that often increased the risk for complications. With external fixation, I can now correct large deformities gradually without the need for extensile surgical exposures. As Rob mentioned, I view techniques of external fixation as minimally invasive procedures (despite the large frame construct), since the fixation (pins/wires) are placed percutaneously. When external fixation is combined with the MIS techniques of joint arthrodesis, osteotomy, and/or soft tissue releases, in my opinion, surgical outcome can be optimized and the complication rate remains low.

With respect to trauma, the combination of external fixation and MIS techniques limit soft tissue/periosteal stripping, potentially improving healing rates over conventional techniques of open reduction and internal fixation. While I recognize that percutaneous plating techniques may achieve the same goal of preserving blood supply to the fractures, external fixation confers one very important advantage! Minimally invasive plate osteosynthesis requires an anatomic reduction at the time of surgery. In contrast, while I attempt the same with external fixation, I have the luxury of making subtle adjustments postoperatively to optimize reduction and alignment, adjustments not possible with internal fixation.

Mark Easley: Some MIS techniques appear driven by technology. We are very fortunate to have a contribution by Martinus Richter, a pioneer in computer-assisted surgery (CAS) for the foot and ankle. Martinus, in your experience, what advantages does navigation provide in the evolution of MIS for the management of foot and ankle disorders?

Martinus Richter: Navigation, or more appropriately, CAS is helpful in complex three-dimensional corrections or reduction, and in closed placement of drills and/or screw positioning. I am convinced by my own experience in managing complex hindfoot and midfoot deformities that the improved accuracy afforded by CAS may lead to improved clinical outcomes compared with those reported using conventional techniques. Whereas CAS is too complex and time consuming for cases that are accurately and easily performed by the experienced surgeon, CAS provides superior guidance for procedures with limited visualization. Naturally, this advantage afforded by CAS is especially useful in MIS.

Mark Easley: Currently, the applications of CAS for the foot and ankle are few. Martinus, what developments do you anticipate for CAS in the foot and ankle, particularly with respect to MIS?

Martinus Richter: For the future, the integration of the different computerized systems will improve the handling and clinical feasibility of CAS technology. An integration of preoperative pedography, planning software, CAS, intraoperative three-dimensional imaging (ISO-C-3D™, ARCADIS™) and Intraoperative Pedography (IP) in one Integrated Computer System for

Operative Procedures (ICOP) will be possible. Within this kind of ICOP, the preoperative computerized planning will be able to include preoperative radiographic, CT, MRI, and pedography data. The preoperative computerized planning result will be transferred to the CAS device. Intraoperative two-dimensional (C-arm) or three-dimensional (ISO-C-3D) imaging will allow registration-free CAS and will be matched with preoperative CT and or MRI scans. The CAS system will be guided by biomechanical assessment with IP that allows not only morphological but also biomechanical based CAS. The intraoperative three-dimensional imaging (ISO-C-3D) data and the IP-data will be matched with the data from the planning software to allow immediate improvements of reduction, correction, and or drilling/implant position in the same procedure.

While this seems terribly complex, I envision that this integration will ultimately be manageable for most foot and ankle surgeons, just like most drivers can now make use of the navigation systems in their cars. Two decades ago, many people doubted that we would have practical applications for navigation systems in our vehicles. Today most manufactures offer navigation options. While navigation is rarely used for short and easy routes, they are used effectively for long and difficult journeys. Similarly, computerized methods of improved intraoperative imaging, guidance, and biomechanical assessment will help to realize the planned operative result. We will have these systems (ISO-C-3D, CAS, IP) available in a few years, but they will not be used in the easy standard case but for difficult and complex procedures. I anticipate that even the most complex procedures may be performed with very precise, focused interventions requiring very limited exposures and soft tissue dissection. In other words, with this technology, MIS will be a reality in the management of complex foot and ankle disorders.

Mark Easley: Finally, what about CAS and MIS in managing foot and ankle trauma?

Martinus Richter: The problem with MIS in foot and ankle trauma is limited visualization. In my hands, the use of computer-based visualization, i.e., intraoperative three-dimensional imaging (ISO-C-3D™, ARCADIS™) is advantageous

compared with conventional two-dimensional imaging. ISO-C-3D is most helpful in closed procedures and in providing information that is cannot be obtained with direct visualization or using a C-arm. With this technology, MIS can be effectively utilized without an increased risk of malreduction or inappropriate implant placement.

Mark Easley: Nicola, you have adopted and even developed several MIS techniques for the treatment of foot and ankle problems. I have no doubt that you are a believer in the techniques. However, would you please conclude our roundtable discussion with your views of the shortcomings of MIS in the foot and ankle.

Nicola Maffulli: Mark, I will continue to use MIS techniques for the foot and ankle and I will continue to channel some of my energies to improving and developing MIS for the foot and ankle. As I see it, there has been little or no scientific research in MIS for the foot and ankle. It is well and good to devise what appears to be a great technique, and to operate on many patients, who may be grateful to the surgeon, and surprised to find that they can return to work and normal activities in little time. However, very little has been published in peer-reviewed journals on the outcome of these procedures, and, to my knowledge, no research has compared traditional with less invasive procedures. We should channel our efforts to make sure that we do not lose sight of the fact that we wish that our patients are served well in the long term, not just that we are very clever with our saws, drills, and scalpels. I suspect that the only way in which these new techniques will become part of our armamentarium is to prove that they are indeed comparable with the traditional ones. Indications and patient selection for MIS techniques still need to be defined. Newer is not always better, and, for the time being, a technical advance is not necessarily a clinically relevant one. I look forward to prospective, randomized investigations comparing traditional and MIS techniques in the management of foot and ankle pathology necessitating surgical intervention.

Mark Easley: I thank all of you for participating in this roundtable discussion and for contributing to this section on MIS of the foot and ankle.

Computer Navigation in the Foot and Ankle Surgery

Martinus Richter

Foot and ankle surgery at the end of the twentieth century was characterized by the use of sophisticated computerized preoperative and postoperative diagnostic and planning procedures [1–3]. However, intraoperative computerized tools that assist the surgeon during his or her struggle for the planned optimal operative result are missing. This results in an intraoperative "black box" without optimal visualization, guidance, and biomechanical assessment [2]. The future will be characterized by breaking up this intraoperative "black box." We will have more intraoperative tools to achieve the planned result [2, 3]. Intraoperative three-dimensional (3D) imaging (ISO-C-3D), computer-assisted surgery (CAS), and intraoperative pedography (IP) are three possible innovations to realize the planned procedure intraoperatively [3]. These devices might be especially helpful for minimally invasive surgery.

These novel methods are in clinical use at our institution for further development. This chapter especially analyzes the feasibility and potential clinical benefit of navigation for foot and ankle surgery. Because ISO-C-3D and IP are two other innovations that are closely connected to navigation, these two methods are also described.

M. Richter (✉)
Chirurgische Klinik, Klinikum Coburg,
Coburg, Germany
e-mail: martinus.richter@klinikum-coburg.de

Intraoperative Three-Dimensional Imaging

In foot and ankle trauma care, malposition of extraosseous or intraarticular screws and gaps or steps in joint lines frequently remain undiscovered when using intraoperative fluoroscopy, and are only recognized on postoperative computed tomography (CT) scans [4]. Earlier preclinical studies showed that evaluation of reduction and implant position with a new C-arm-based 3D imaging device (ISO-C-3D) is better than with plain films or a C-arm alone and comparable to CT scans [5–9].

ISO-C-3D (Siemens AG, Germany) is a motorized C-arm that provides fluoroscopic images during a 190° orbital rotation computing a 119-mm data cube (Fig. 26.1a). From these 3D data sets, two-dimensional (2D) and multiplanar reconstructions can be obtained on the screen of the device without delay (Fig. 26.1b). For scanning, the situs is draped with a sterile plastic bag that is pulled over the legs and the table.

Study Results

A prospective consecutive clinical study was performed in a level one trauma center [10]. The aim of the study was to evaluate the feasibility and benefit of the intraoperative use of the ISO-C-3D for foot and ankle trauma care in this special environment. The hypothesis was that the ISO-C-3D

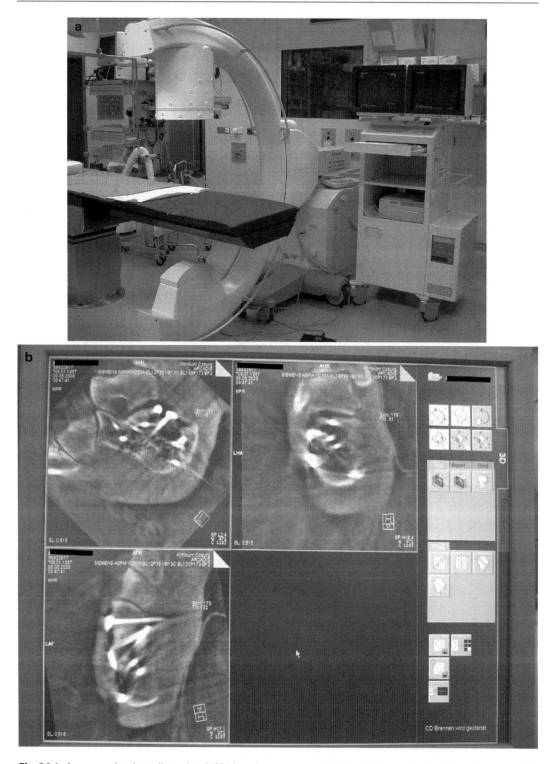

Fig. 26.1 Intraoperative three-dimensional (3D) imaging (*ISO-C-3D*). ISO-C-3D device in the operating room and carbon fracture table (**a**). *Monitor view* of an ISO-C-3D device showing multiplanar reformations of a calcaneus after open reduction and internal fixation with a plate and screws (**b**). *Top left* parasagittal reformation; *top right* coronal reformation; *bottom left* axial/horizontal reformation. The reformation planes can be chosen by the surgeon in any orientation compared with a CT scan

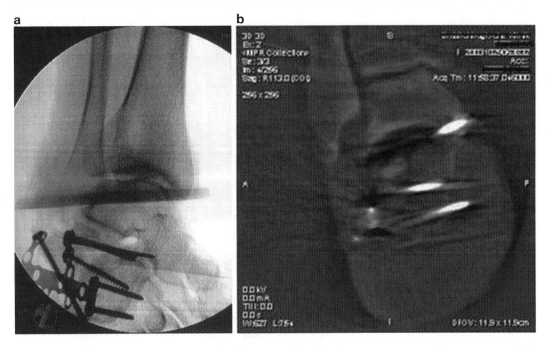

Fig. 26.2 Intraoperative 3D imaging (ISO-C-3D). Calcaneus fracture after open reduction and internal fixation with plate and screws. After evaluation with a C-arm including Broden's view (**a**), a correct reduction and implant position was confirmed by the surgeon. The ISO-C-3D scan showed a screw penetrating the posterior facet medially (**b**), and the screw position was corrected during the same procedure

could detect failures of reduction or implant position that had not been detected with a conventional C-arm in a considerable percentage of cases.

Patients with foot and ankle trauma or reconstruction surgery who were treated in the Trauma Department of the Hannover Medical School between July 1, 2003 and June 30, 2005 were considered for inclusion in the study. Before the use of the device, the reduction and implant position had to judged to be correct by the surgeon using a conventional C-arm. The patients were placed either on a special metal-free carbon table or on a standard table. Time spent, changes after use of the ISO-C-3D, and surgeons' ratings (visual analog scale [VAS], 0–10 points) were recorded. The surgeons' ratings for image quality for the carbon table and the standard table were compared (*t* test, significance level 0.05). The surgeons' ratings for image quality for the carbon table and the standard table were compared (*t* test, significance level 0.05).

One hundred and one patients/cases (no bilateral ISO-C-3D use) were included (Fractures: pilon, $n=15$; Weber-C ankles, $n=12$; isolated dorsal Volkmann, $n=3$; talus, $n=7$; calcaneus, $n=32$;

navicular, $n=2$; cuboid, $n=2$; Lisfranc fracture-dislocation, $n=8$; ankle/hindfoot arthrodesis with or without correction, $n=4/16$). Carbon table was use in 80 cases (79%) and a standard table in 21 cases (21%). The operation was interrupted for 430 s on average (range, 300–700 s); 100 s on average for preparation, 120 s on average for the ISO-C-3D scan, and 210 s on average for evaluation of the images by the surgeon. In 39% (39 of 101) of the cases, the reduction ($n=16$, 16%) and/or implant position ($n=30$, 30%) was corrected after ISO-C-3D scan during the same procedure. The ratings of the eight surgeons involved were 9.2 (range, 5.2–10) for feasibility, 9.5 (range, 6.1–10) for accuracy, and 8.2 (range, 4.5–10) for clinical benefit. The image quality was rated 9.1 (range, 8.0–10) for the carbon tables, and 8.7 (range, 7.0–10) for the standard tables (difference rating carbon table vs. standard table, *t* test, $p>0.05$). The image quality was rated 9.1 (range, 8.0–10) for the carbon tables, and 8.7 (range, 7.0–10) for the standard tables (difference rating carbon table vs. standard table, *t* test, not significant). Figure 26.2 shows a clinical example.

In this study, in almost 40% of cases, reduction and/or implant position was corrected after ISO-C-3D scan at the same procedure. The radiation contamination is comparable to a standard CT scan and corresponds to 39 s fluoroscopy time with a modern digital C-arm. The image quality with a carbon table is not better than with a standard table. Consequently, the use of a carbon table is not necessary for ISO-C-3D scan at the foot region.

In conclusion, the intraoperative 3D visualization with the ISO-C-3D can provide important information in foot and ankle trauma care that cannot be obtained from plain films or C-arm alone [11]. The use is not considerably time consuming. The ISO-C-3D is extremely useful in evaluating reduction and/or implant position intraoperatively and can replace a postoperative CT scan.

Computer-Assisted Surgery

CT-Based Computer-Assisted Surgery

The accuracy of the reduction in hindfoot and midfoot fractures and fracture-dislocations correlates with the clinical result [12–20]. The same is true for the correction of hindfoot and midfoot [19, 21–29]. However, an accurate correction or reduction with the conventional C-arm-based procedure is challenging [19, 30, 31]. CT-based CAS has become a valuable tool for the correction and reduction in other body regions [32–53]. Especially a more exact reduction could be achieved [32, 34, 38–40, 43–47, 49, 52, 54–57]. CT-based CAS may also be useful for the correction of hindfoot and midfoot deformities and for the reduction in hindfoot or midfoot fractures and fracture-dislocations, although it has not been used in the foot region so far [58].

Study Results

The purpose of an experimental study at our institution was to compare CT-based CAS assisted correction of hindfoot and midfoot deformities with C-arm-based correction [59]. Sawbone

(Pacific Research Laboratories, Vashon, WA, USA) specimen models "Large Left Foot/Ankle," "Large Left Foot/Ankle with Equinus Deformity," "Large Left Foot/Ankle with Calcaneus Malunion," and "Large Left Foot/Ankle with Equinovarus Deformity" were used. A CT scan of each deformity specimen model ($n=3$) was performed. The goal of the correction was to transform the shape of the pathology specimen models into the shape of the normal specimen model. Two methods were used for the correction: (a) conventional C-arm-based correction and (b) CAS-based (CT based, Surgigate™, Medivision, Oberdorf, Switzerland & Northern Digital Inc., Waterloo, Ontario, Canada) correction. Five specimens of each deformity model were corrected with each method. Standardized osteotomies were performed before the correction when necessary (in models with calcaneus malunion and equinovarus). The surgeon's direct view to the specimens was disabled by drapes. During the correction procedure, the visualization of the specimen was exclusively provided by the image of the C-arm or the CAS device. Retention was performed with 1.8-mm titanium K-wires. The following parameters were registered: time needed for entire procedure and different steps of the procedure, time of fluoroscopy, foot length, length and height of the longitudinal arch, calcaneus inclination, hindfoot angle for all models ($n=30$), and additionally Boehler's angle and the calcaneus length for the "calcaneus malunion" specimen models ($n=10$). The shape of the corrected specimens was graded as normal, nearly normal, abnormal, or severely abnormal. The parameters of the two correction method groups (CAS vs. C-arm) were statistically compared (t test, c^2 test). According to the specimen measurements, the differences between the corrected specimen models and the normal specimen model were also compared.

The shape was graded as normal in all specimens ($n=15$) in the CAS group, and in eight of the specimens in the C-arm group (other grades in C-arm group: nearly normal, $n=6$; abnormal, $n=1$; c^2 test, $p=0.05$). The time needed for the procedure was longer in the CAS group, and the fluoroscopy time was shorter in the CAS group than in the C-arm group (mean values and range shown, t test utilized):

- Time for the entire procedure, CAS, 782 s (range, 450–1,020 s), C-arm, 410 s (range, 210–600 s), $p<0.001$
- Fluoroscopy time, CAS, 0 s, C-arm, 11 s (range, 8–19 s), $p<0.001$

In three cases in the CAS group, the system crashed and was restarted (the times for the entire procedure in these cases were 1,000, 1,010, and 1,020 s).

The measurement *differences* between the corrected specimens and the normal specimen model were as follows (mean values and standard deviation shown, t test utilized): foot length, CAS, -1.7 ± 1.9 mm, C-arm, -4.1 ± 3.8 mm, $p=0.03$; length of longitudinal arch, CAS, -0.9 ± 0.9 mm, C-arm, -5.6 ± 4.9 mm, $p=0.001$; height of longitudinal arch, CAS, -0.1 ± 0.5 mm, C-arm, 1.7 ± 4.3 mm, $p=0.14$; calcaneus inclination, CAS, $0.1\pm1.4°$, C-arm, $2.7\pm4.8°$, $p=0.05$; calcaneus length, CAS, -0.5 ± 0.4 mm, C-arm, -2.8 ± 1.3 mm, $p=0.005$; Boehler's angle, CAS, $0.4\pm1.1°$, C-arm, $4.1\pm8.6°$, $p=0.37$.

When further analyzing the correction in the different pathology specimen models, the highest differences (lowest t values) between the CAS group and the C-arm group were observed in "calcaneus malunion" specimen model, followed by the "equinus deformity" and the "equinovarus deformity" specimen models.

In conclusion, in an experimental setting, CT-based CAS provided higher accuracy for the correction of hindfoot and midfoot deformities than C-arm-based correction [59].

The reasons for the double time needed with CT-based CAS in comparison with the C-arm-based method are the requirements of the data transfer of the DICOM data of the preoperative CT scan to the CAS device and especially the very time consuming matching process during the registration procedure. The main problems with the matching are based on the difficult bony architecture of the foot with 28 bones and more than 30 joints. Due to these anatomic conditions, the foot does not regularly maintain its complete integrity and position during the preoperative CT

and the registration. This makes the registration in the foot much more difficult than in other body regions like the spine or the pelvis with lesser and larger bones and joints [36, 38, 47, 58, 60].

In the clinical application of CT-based CAS at the foot, the problems with the registration will still increase, although the soft tissue coverage is favorable thin. When the registration was finally finished, the CT-based CAS as used in our study was more accurate and even easier and faster than the conventional C-arm, but the problems with the registration will prevent broad clinical use. Fortunately, while this experimental study was planned and performed, two CAS methods without registration were introduced, the C-arm-based CAS and the ISO-3-D-based CAS. These CAS methods without registration are especially interesting for the foot region. Clinical studies must show whether these registration-free methods can achieve high accuracy like CT-based CAS in real operations, and if this leads to better clinical results.

ISO-C-3D-Based Computer-Assisted Surgery

In our institution, ISO-C-3D-based CAS was co-developed and first used for retrograde drillings in osteochondral defects of the talus [61]. The goal in osteochondral defects of the talus in stages I and II, according to Berndt and Harty, is revascularization of the lesion [62]. A debridement of the chondral part is required if symptomatic [63, 64]. This debridement is limited to loose cartilage or cartilage with poor quality [63–65].

Subchondral drilling of the lesion allows revascularization. Retrograde drilling leaves the chondral surface intact and is therefore advantageous compared with antegrade drilling [66]. Arthroscopically guided drilling is limited to those lesions that could be arthroscopically identified [65]. In the remaining cases, open procedures are justified [67]. Based on these principles, CT-based CAS-guided retrograde drilling of osteochondral lesions has been described with promising results as a new technique [66, 68]. CT- and fluoroscopy-based navigation systems in current use are limited in their flexibility [59, 61]. The drawbacks of fluoroscopy are lack of 3D imaging intraoperatively. CT-based navigation still requires intraoperative cumbersome registration, extra preoperative planning, and imaging with further technical resources.

In addition to the current method of arthroscopic evaluation and treatment, we also introduce an alternative technique of using ISO-C-3D-based CAS-guided retrograde drilling of lesions.

Study Results

All patients with symptomatic osteochondrosis dissecans stadium I and II, according to Berndt and Harty, of the talus between June 1, 2003 and July 31, 2003 were included in a follow-up study. Exclusion criteria were a higher stadium or if the device was not available for the study because it was also being used for procedures other than foot and ankle. The patients were treated with ISO-C-3D-based navigated retrograde drilling. Time spent, accuracy, problems, and surgeons' rating (VAS, 0–10 points) were recorded and analyzed. The accuracy of the drillings were assessed by the intraoperative 3D imaging device (ISO-C-3D™). Clinical and radiological follow-ups

were performed using the following scores: VAS foot and ankle (VAS FA) and SF36 (standardized on a possible 100-point maximum scale for better comparison with the VAS FA).

Technical Background

An ISO-C-3D (description above, Fig. 26.1) is connected to a navigation system (Surgigate™, Medivision, Oberdorf, Switzerland & Northern Digital Inc.). After fixation of a dynamic reference basis (DRB) to the bone (Fig. 26.3a), an ISO-C-3D scan follows (Fig. 26.4b). The data are transferred to the navigation system. The starting point and end point, and direction and length of the drilling is planned on the screen of the navigation system using the standard software. A trajectory for the drilling is placed in the virtual bone on the screen. The drilling is performed with a modified navigated electrical power drilling machine (Powerdrive, Synthes Inc., Bochum, Germany, Fig. 26.3a, b). The direction and length of the drilling is shown on the monitor of the navigation device. Standard fluoroscopy is not needed during the entire procedure.

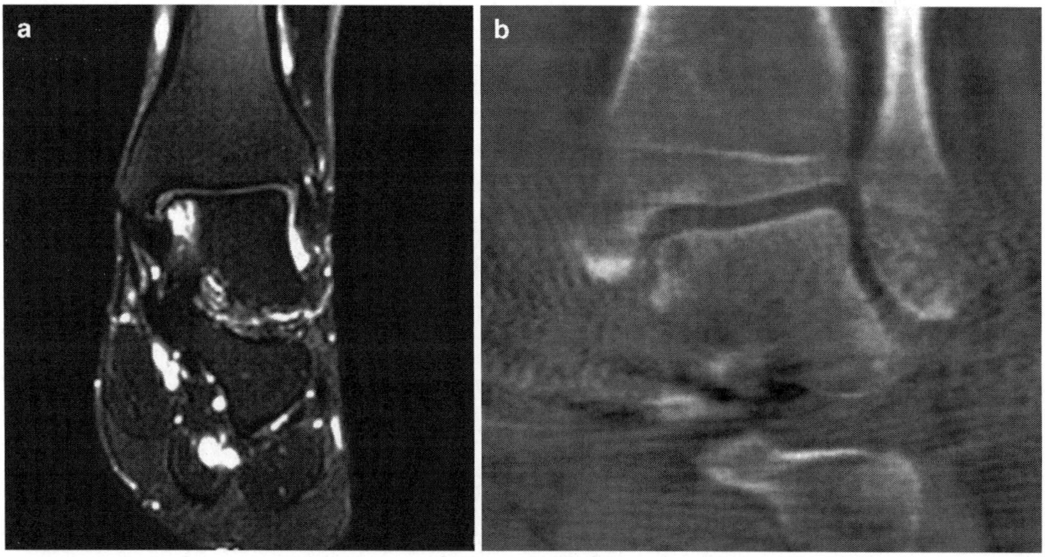

Fig. 26.3 ISO-C-3D-based computer-assisted surgery (*CAS*). ISO-C-3D-based CAS-guided retrograde drilling in osteochondrosis dissecans tali. MRI image (**a**) and ISO-C-3D image from data transferred to the navigation system (**b**) of an osteochondrosis dissecans tali (Hepple/Winson stadium II)

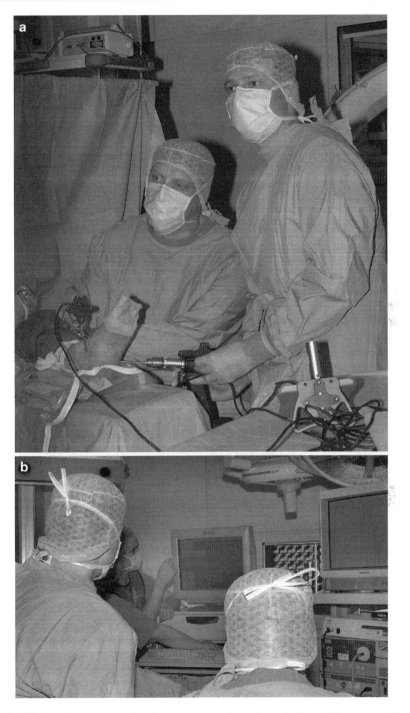

Fig. 26.4 ISO-C-3D-based computer-assisted surgery (*CAS*). ISO-C-3D-based CAS-guided retrograde drilling in osteochondrosis dissecans tali. Retrograde drilling with starting point at the lateral talar process (**a**) and visualization on the screen of the CAS device in real time (**b**)

Ten patients ($n=6$ at lateral talar shoulder; $n=4$ at medial talar shoulder) were treated with ISO-C-3D-based CAS-guided retrograde drilling. The time needed for preparation, including the placement of the DRB, scanning time, and preparation of the trajectories was 580 s (range, 500–750 s). All drillings were in the correct positions (deviation from planned position less than 2° and 2 mm). No surgery-related complication, in particular, no infection occurred. The surgeons' ratings were: feasibility, VAS 9 (range, 7.3–10); accuracy 8.5 (range, 5.8–10); and clinical benefit 8.5 (range, 5.7–10). The time of follow-up was 18 months (range, 12–28 months). Nine patients could be included in the follow-up study. One patient required OATS after initial clinical improvement, and had to be excluded. The VAS FA was 92 (range, 86–98), and the SF36 was 89 (range, 79–97). The different score categories averaged as follows:

- Pain: VAS FA, 85 (range, 69–100); SF36, 87 (range, 80–100)
- Function: VAS FA, 94 (range, 88–99); SF36, 96 (range, 83–100)
- Other complaints: VAS FA, 96 (range, 87–99); SF36, 85 (range, 67–93)

The ISO-C-3D-based CAS worked without problems in the described cases. However, the handling of the system is very complex. During the developing process, the systems was very trouble-prone due to computer control failures.

The introduced system was reliable and in frequent use at our department for surgical procedures in different body regions. The advantages of the introduced technique are an actual and almost real-time ISO-C-3D for the use of navigation without the need for anatomical registration and an immediate intraoperative control of surgical treatment [2]. Our results reveal that ISO-C-3D-based CAS-guided retrograde drilling is an alternative to arthroscopically guided or open drilling for osteochondral lesions of the talus. To date, we use the same ISO-C-3D, but a different navigation device that is easier to use (VectorVision™, BrainLAB Inc., Kirchheim-Heimstetten, Germany; for description, see below). The tremendous device costs for the ISO-C-3D-based CAS will prevent standard use for retrograde drilling in osteochondral lesions of the talus alone, despite the advantages. However, the ISO-C-3D-based CAS is also useful for other body regions such as the spine and pelvis. Furthermore, the ISO-C-3D alone is a valuable tool for intraoperative 3D visualization, as described above. Radiation protection for the patient and personnel is another essential topic. The radiation of an ISO-C-3D-based CAS-guided drilling procedure is, of course, higher compared with arthroscopically based drilling. However, the ISO-C-3D-based CAS procedures produce less radiation than all conventional C-arm-based procedures and CT-based CAS.

C-Arm-Based Computer-Assisted Surgery

As described above, CAS is considered to be useful for the correction of hindfoot and midfoot deformities and for the reduction in hindfoot or midfoot fractures and fracture-dislocations [59]. CT-based CAS provided high accuracy in an experimental setting, but the very cumbersome obligatory registration process prevented clinical use [59]. A registration-free C-arm-based CAS-guided correction was fortunately developed and studied at our institution.

Study Results

Patients with posttraumatic deformities of the ankle or subtalar joint with deformity (malalignment) were included in a prospective clinical follow-up study. C-arm-based CAS-guided arthrodeses with correction of the deformity were performed. Time spent, accuracy, problems, surgeons' rating (VAS, 0–10 points), and follow-up (VAS FA, American Orthopaedic Foot and Ankle Society Hindfoot Score [AOFAS], SF36) were analyzed. The accuracy of the corrections was assessed by a new C-arm-based 3D imaging device (ISO-C-3D).

Technical Background

A navigation system with wireless DRBs was used (VectorVision™, BrainLAB Inc.). The system was connected with a modified C-arm

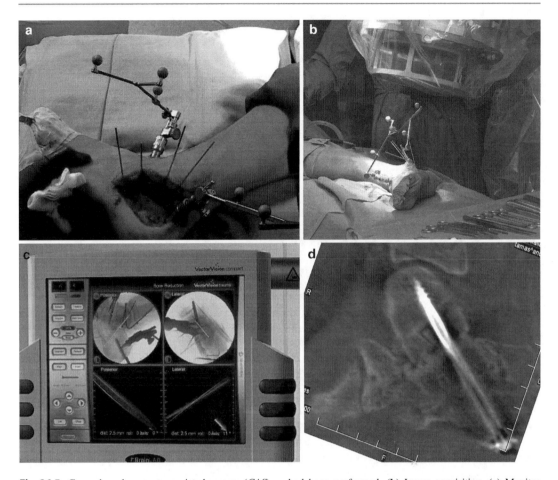

Fig. 26.5 C-arm-based computer-assisted surgery (*CAS*). C-arm-based CAS-guided correction of hindfoot deformity after malunited calcaneus fracture with flattening of the longitudinal arch and the Boehler's angle (0°), and hindfoot varus (10°). A correction arthrodesis of the subtalar joint with elevation of the longitudinal arch (planned Boehler's angle 30°) and correction of the varus was indicated. (**a**) The DRBs were fixed to the talar neck and to the posterior process of the calcaneus. Image acquisition and verification had been performed. (**b**) Image acquisition. (**c**) Monitor view during the navigation process. (**d**) Intraoperative imaging with ISO-C-3D (Siemens, Germany) after correction and screw fixation with bone blocks in the subtalar joint. The achieved supposed Boehler's angle was 30°. For the measurement of the Boehler's angle, the formerly posterior edge of the posterior facet was defined as the point located at the middle, i.e., the half height of the posterior rim of the posterior bone block

(Exposcope™, Instrumentarium Imaging Ziehm Inc., Nuremberg, Germany; Fig. 26.5a). One DRB was fixed to each of the two bones or fragments that had been planned for correction in relation to each other. With the C-arm, anteroposterior and lateral digital radiographic images were obtained, and the data were transferred to the navigation device. Then the correction was performed. During the correction, the angle motion and translational motion between the bones or fragments in all degrees of freedom were displayed on the screen of the navigation system (Fig. 26.5a). Furthermore, virtual radiographs with the moving bones or fragments were displayed on the screen. The C-arm was not used during the correction process. After correction, retention was performed with 2.0-mm K-wires. Then the accuracy of the correction was checked with C-arm and intraoperative 3D imaging with ISO-C-3D (Siemens Inc., Germany). Finally, screw fixation followed. The insertion of the screws was also C-arm-based CAS guided (data not shown).

Twelve patients were included (ankle correction arthrodesis, $n = 3$; subtalar correction arthrodesis, $n = 6$; combined ankle/subtalar joint correction arthrodesis, $n = 2$; Lisfranc correction arthrodesis, $n = 1$). The time needed for preparation, scanning time, and preparation on the screen for the correction was 500 s (range, 400–900 s). The correction process took 45 s (range, 30–60 s). All planned angles and translations were exactly achieved as planned before (deviation from planned correction less than $\pm 2°$ for angles or ± 2 mm for translations). Three surgeons were involved. Feasibility by VAS was 9.5 (range, 9–10); accuracy was 9.8 (range, 9.5–10); and clinical benefit was 9 (range, 8–10). Ten (83%) patients completed follow-up after 14 months (range, 6–27 months). All arthrodeses were fused at follow-up. The corrected angles and translations at follow-up (analyzed on radiographs) did not differ significantly from those measured intraoperatively (see above; t test, $p > 0.05$). The VAS FA averaged 47 (range, 25–81); the AOFAS Hindfoot Score, 57 (range, 40–64); and the SF36, 54 (range, 34–80). The different score categories averaged as follows: pain: VAS FA 47 (range, 14–85), SF36 46 (range, 11–93); function: VAS FA 41 (range, 14–85), SF36 45 (range, 8–85); and other complaints: VAS FA 52 (range, 19–83), SF36 70 (range, 55–84).

The feasibility of the introduced method was favorable. The time spent was less than 10 min for preparation. The correction process is very fast and extremely accurate, especially regarding the problems with the conventional C-arm-based correction. In our experience, the correction without CAS guidance needs more time because the necessary frequent C-arm controlling. Furthermore, it is much more difficult, not only because of the difficult visualization, but also because the very demanding correction process with 3D motion of two different fragments in relation to each other.

In conclusion, C-arm-based CAS-guided correction of posttraumatic deformities of the ankle and hindfoot region is feasible and provides very high accuracy and a faster correction process

[2, 69]. The significance of the introduced method is high in these cases because the improved accuracy may lead to an improved clinical outcome [19, 21–29, 58].

Intraoperative Pedography

For any kind of reduction or correction at the foot and ankle, an immediate biomechanical assessment of the reduction result would be desirable [19, 21–29]. This is especially true for a CAS-guided reduction or correction, which is supposed to be more accurate than a conventional reduction [2, 61]. The reduction or correction control is normally performed with a C-arm or an ISO-C-3D, if available [2, 10, 59]. Analyzing the position of the bones radiographically allows conclusions about the biomechanics of the foot [19, 70]. However, pedography is considered to be more effective for the analysis of the biomechanics of the foot [71]. So far, pedography for biomechanical assessment was only available during clinical follow-up [2]. An IP would be useful for immediate intraoperative biomechanical assessment [2].

Study Results

A new device was developed to perform IP. A feasibility study was first performed [72]. Then a study for validation followed to compare the introduced method with standard dynamic pedography [73]. Finally, a prospective consecutive randomized multicenter study is in progress to analyze the clinical benefit of IP.

For an intraoperative introduction of standardized forces to the foot sole, a device named Kraftsimulator Intraoperative Pedographie (KIOP, manufactured by the Workshop of the Hannover Medical School, Hannover, Germany; registered design no. 202004007755.8 by the German Patent Office, Munich, Germany, Figs. 26.6a, b and 26.7) was developed. The pedographic measurement is performed with a custom-made mat with capacitive

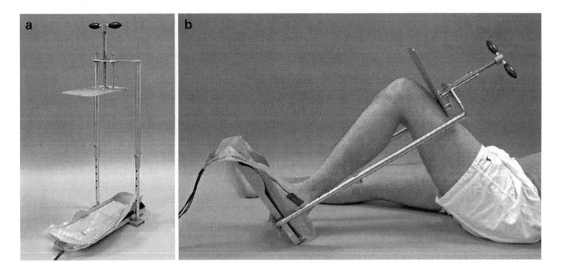

Fig. 26.6 Intraoperative pedography (*IP*). The newly developed device for intraoperative force introduction (*KIOP*). The custom-made mat for force registration (PLIANCETM, Novel, Inc.) is covered intraoperatively with a sterile plastic bag and is placed on the KIOP, as also shown in Fig. 26.7. The size of the mat is 16×32 cm. The mat includes 32×32 sensors with a sensor size of 0.5×1 cm. Figure 26.7 shows a scheme of the modus for IP

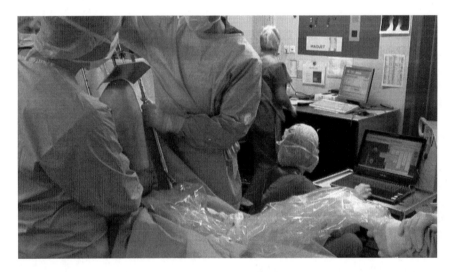

Fig. 26.7 Intraoperative pedography (*IP*). IP during a correction arthrodesis at the talonavicular joint (performed during a feasibility prestudy); 400 N comparable to half body weight was applied. The force measurements were displayed in real time on the screen of the pedography system. During the IP, KIOP is entirely sterile and the force measurement mat (PLIANCE™, Novel Inc.) is covered by a sterile plastic bag

sensors (PLIANCE™, Novel Inc., Munich, Germany). The system allows real-time pedography and comparison with the contralateral side. The measurements were performed in the neutral ankle position. In this neutral ankle position, the influence of the missing muscle action in the anesthetized patient is considered to be minimal because the electromyelogram (EMG) in awake standing individuals with a comparable ankle position is silent [74–76].

Validation Study

The validation was performed in two steps:

Step 1 was a comparison of standard dynamic pedography (three trials, walking, third step; and three trials, mid stance force pattern), static in the standing position (three trials), and pedography with KIOP in healthy volunteers (three trials; total force, 400 N). For dynamic pedography and pedography in the standing position, a standard platform (EMED™, Novel Inc.) was used.

Step 2 was a comparison of pedography in the standing position, pedography with KIOP in non-anesthetized and anesthetized patients (three trials; total force, 400 N). Patients with operative procedures performed at the knee or distal to the knee were excluded. Only patients with general or spinal anesthesia were included.

Additionally, a qualitative analysis was performed for both steps (Fig. 26.8a, b). The analysis was focused on the force distribution and not on the force values. The relation of the forces of different regions; the hindfoot, midfoot, and forefoot (first metatarsal, second to fourth metatarsal, fifth metatarsal), and medial vs. lateral were compared. The different measurement and qualitative analyses were compared (t test, one-way analysis of variance [ANOVA]).

The results of the validation process were as follows. In step 1, 30 individuals were included (age, 26.1 ± 8.6 years; sex, male:female $= 24{:}6$). In step 2, 30 individuals were included (age, 55.3 ± 30.3 years; sex, male:female $= 24{:}6$). No statistically significant differences were found in either step between the methods, nor between the methods of step 1 and 2 (t test and ANOVA, $p > 0.05$).Clinical Prospective Study.

Sixteen patients were included until March 15, 2006 (ankle correction arthrodesis, $n=2$; subtalar joint correction arthrodesis, $n=4$; correction arthrodesis midfoot, $n=4$; correction forefoot, $n=4$; Lisfranc fracture-dislocation). Nine patients were randomized for the use of IP, whereas four patients had no intraoperative measurement. The mean preoperative scores were as follows: AOFAS, 51.6 ± 22.6; VAS FA, 45.2 ± 14.4; and SF36, 47.3 ± 21.4. No score differences between the two groups occurred (t test, $p > 0.05$). The mean interruption of operative procedure for the IP was 323 ± 32 s. In four (44%) of the nine patients, changes were made after IP during the same operative procedure (correction modified, $n=3$; screw tightened, $n=1$). The follow-up has not been completed so far.

In conclusion, IP is feasible and valid because no statistical significant differences were found between the measurements of the introduced method for IP in anesthetized individuals and the standard dynamic and static pedography. In the future, dynamic IP with registration of the entire foot sole is planned for an even more sophisticated biomechanical assessment [2, 72, 73]. During clinical use, in 50% of the cases, a modification of the surgical correction was made after IP in the same surgical procedure. A follow-up of these patients has to be completed to show whether these changes improve the clinical outcome. In any case, IP was able to detect insufficient biomechanical behavior of the foot and it may lead to modifications in the same procedure, instead of after pedography in the office weeks or months later [2, 72, 73].

What Do We Need When?

The perfect surgeon who does not make any mistakes without any guidance does not need any of the introduced systems. However, the surgical staff involved in foot and ankle surgery consists of experienced surgeons as well as interns, residents, and fellows in training. In times of increasing legal pressure regarding working hours, the acquisition of surgical experience is harder. Tools for improved intraoperative imaging (ISO-C-3D), guidance (CAS), or biomechanical assessment (IP) may help the surgeon in training to achieve the planned result with less experience [3].

Iso-c-3d

ISO-C-3D is most helpful in closed procedures and/or when axial reformations provide information that is not possible to obtain with a C-arm or

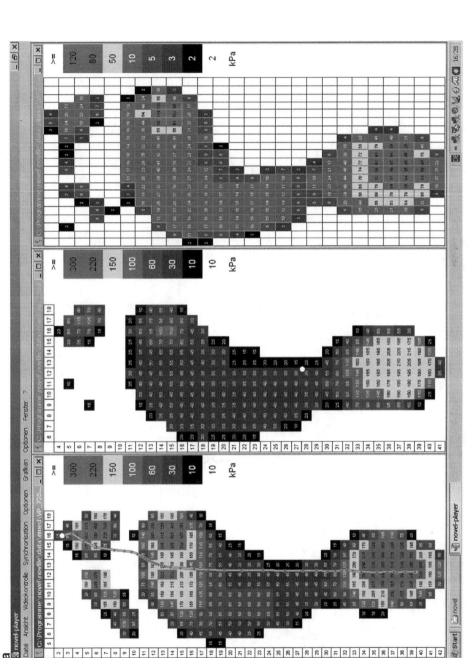

Fig. 26.8 Intraoperative pedography (*IP*). Images from the qualitative analysis of the validation process of IP. (**a**) Step 1: awake volunteer - *left* pedography with KIOP; *middle* static pedography in standing position; *right* standard dynamic pedography. For dynamic pedography and pedography in the standing position, a standard platform (EMED Novel Inc.) was used. (**b**) Step 2: non-anesthetized/anesthetized patient – *left* pedography with KIOP in a non-anesthetized individual; *middle* pedography in the standing position; *right* IP in an anesthetized individual

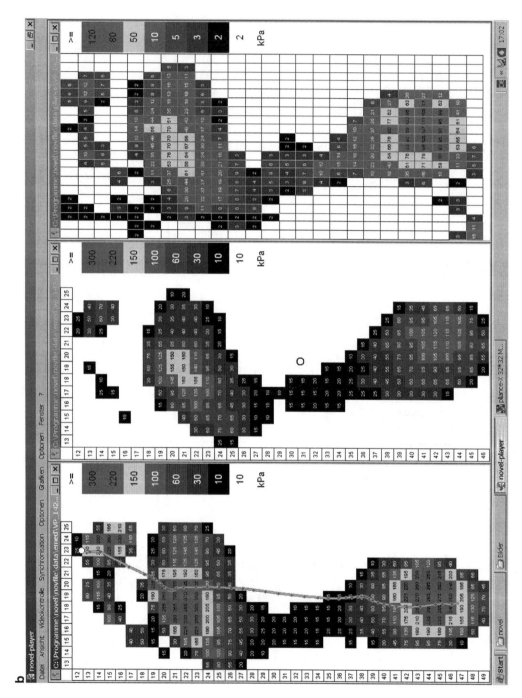

Fig. 26.8 (continued)

with direct visualization [10]. Weber-C fractures and calcaneus fractures are examples for these special situations. The ISO-C-3D is less helpful when easy visualization with a C-arm or under direct vision is possible, as, for example, in Weber-B fractures during open reduction and internal fixation.

Computer-Assisted Surgery

CAS is helpful in complex 3D corrections or reduction, and in closed placement of drillings and/or screw positioning [2, 59]. The significance of the introduced CAS methods is high in those cases because the improved accuracy may lead to an improved clinical outcome like complex corrections in the hindfoot and midfoot deformities [19, 21–29]. CAS is too complex and time consuming for cases that are accurately and easily performed by the experienced surgeon.

Intraoperative Pedography

IP will be useful for cases in which biomechanical assessment may lead to an immediate improvement of the achieved surgical result [2, 72, 73]. The same cases that are currently analyzed with clinical preoperative or postoperative pedography will potentially profit from IP. The surgeon's experience is also crucial for the use of IP, because experienced surgeons who do not use pedography in their office may also not use it intraoperatively. IP as introduced was made possible by the newly developed device for intraoperative force introduction (KIOP).

Integrated Computer System for Operative Procedures

For the future, the integration of the different computerized systems will improve the handling and clinical feasibility. An integration of preoperative pedography, planning software, CAS, ISO-C-3D, and IP in one integrated computer system for operative procedures (ICOP) will be favorable. Within this kind of ICOP, the preoperative computerized planning will be able to include preoperative radiographic, CT, magnetic resonance imaging (MRI), and pedography data. The preoperative computerized planning result will be transferred to the CAS device. Intraoperative 2D (C-arm) or 3D (ISO-C-3D) imaging will allow registration-free CAS and will be matched with preoperative CT and or MRI images. The CAS-system will be guided by biomechanical assessment with IP that allows not only morphological but also biomechanical-based CAS. The ISO-C-3D data and the IP data will be matched with the data from the planning software to allow immediate improvements of reduction, correction, and or drilling/implant position in the same procedure [3].

In conclusion, in the future, computerized methods for improved intraoperative imaging, guidance, and biomechanical assessment will help to realize the planned operative result [3].

The development will be similar to navigation systems in the car. Two decades ago, many people doubted that we need these systems. Today almost everybody has a system, but, of course, no one uses them for short and easy routes; rather, they are used for long and difficult journeys. Similarly, we will have these systems (ISO-C-3D, CAS, IP) available in a few years, but they will not be used in the easy standard case but for difficult and complex procedures. The costs of these systems are high, but the increased outcome will decrease the overall costs for the medical system [3].

Acknowledgments The author thanks Christian Krettek, MD, FRACS, Director of Trauma, Stefan Zech, MD, Jens Geerling, MD, Michael Frink, MD, Tobias Huefner, MD, Daniel Kendoff, MD, Musa Citak, MD, Nicolas Vanin, Patricia Droste, Claudia Schultz-Blum, Alke Bretzke, Carolina Böse, Angelika Heinrich, and Vital Karch, Trauma Department, Hannover Medical School, Hannover Germany for their valuable contribution in carrying out the surgical procedures and the handling of the introduced technical devices.

References

1. Dahlen C, Zwipp H. [Computer-assisted surgical planning. 3-D software for the PC]. Unfallchirurg 2001;104(6):466–479.
2. Richter M. Foot and Ankle Surgery: Today and in the Future. In: 5th Congress of the European Foot and

Ankle Society (EFAS), Montpellier, 29 April–01 May 2004, Abstracts, 2004.

3. Richter M. Computer based systems in foot and ankle surgery at the beginning of the 21st century. Fuss Sprungg 2006;4(1):59–71.

4. Euler E, Wirth S, Linsenmaier U, Mutschler W, Pfeifer KJ, Hebecker A. [Comparative study of the quality of C-arm based 3D imaging of the talus]. Unfallchirurg 2001;104(9):839–846.

5. Kotsianos D, Rock C, Euler E, Wirth S, Linsenmaier U, Brandl R et al. [3-D imaging with a mobile surgical image enhancement equipment (ISO-C-3D). Initial examples of fracture diagnosis of peripheral joints in comparison with spiral CT and conventional radiography]. Unfallchirurg 2001;104(9):834–838.

6. Kotsianos D, Rock C, Wirth S, Linsenmaier U, Brandl R, Fischer T et al. [Detection of tibial condylar fractures using 3D imaging with a mobile image amplifier (Siemens ISO-C-3D): comparison with plain films and spiral CT]. Rofo Fortschr Geb Rontgenstr Neuen Bildgeb Verfahr 2002;174(1):82–87.

7. Kotsianos D, Wirth S, Fischer T, Euler E, Rock C, Linsenmaier U et al. 3D imaging with an isocentric mobile C-arm comparison of image quality with spiral CT. Eur Radiol 2004;14(9):1590–1595.

8. Rock C, Kotsianos D, Linsenmaier U, Fischer T, Brandl R, Vill F et al. [Studies on image quality, high contrast resolution and dose for the axial skeleton and limbs with a new, dedicated CT system (ISO-C-3D)]. Rofo Fortschr Geb Rontgenstr Neuen Bildgeb Verfahr 2002;174(2):170–176.

9. Rock C, Linsenmaier U, Brandl R, Kotsianos D, Wirth S, Kaltschmidt R et al. [Introduction of a new mobile C-arm/CT combination equipment (ISO-C-3D). Initial results of 3-D sectional imaging]. Unfallchirurg 2001;104(9):827–833.

10. Richter M, Geerling J, Zech S, Goesling T, Krettek C. Intraoperative three-dimensional imaging with a motorized mobile C-arm (SIREMOBIL ISO-C-3D) in foot and ankle trauma care: a preliminary report. J Orthop Trauma 2005;19(4):259–266.

11. Richter M, Geerling J, Kendoff D, Hufner T, Krettek C. Intraoperative 3-D Imaging with a Mobile Image Amplifier (ISO-C 3D) in Foot and Ankle Trauma Care. In: American Orthopaedic Foot and Ankle Society, 19th Annual Summer Meeting, Final Program 78, 2003.

12. Adelaar RS. The treatment of complex fractures of the talus. Orthop Clin North Am 1989;20(4):691–707.

13. Amon K. Luxationsfraktur der kuneonavikularen Gelenklinie. Klinik, Pathomechanismus und Therapiekonzept einer sehr seltenen Fussverletzung. Unfallchirurg 1990;93(9):431–434.

14. Brutscher R. Frakturen und Luxationen des Mittel- und Vorfusses. Orthopäde 1991;20(1):67–75.

15. Hansen STJ. Functional reconstruction of the foot and ankle. Philadelphia, PA: Lippincott Williams & Wilkins, 2000.

16. Hildebrand KA, Buckley RE, Mohtadi NG, Faris P. Functional outcome measures after displaced intra-articular calcaneal fractures. J Bone Joint Surg Br 1996;78(1):119–123.

17. Richter M, Wippermann B, Krettek C, Schratt E, Hufner T, Thermann H. Fractures and fracture dislocations of the midfoot - occurrence, causes and long-term results. Foot Ankle Int 2001;22(5):392–398.

18. Suren EG, Zwipp H. Luxationsfrakturen im Chopart- und Lisfranc-Gelenk. Unfallchirurg 1989;92(3): 130–139.

19. Zwipp H. Chirurgie des Fusses, 1st edn. Berlin Heidelberg New York: Springer, 1994.

20. Zwipp H, Dahlen C, Randt T, Gavlik JM. Komplextrauma des Fusses. Orthopäde 1997;26(12): 1046–1056.

21. Adelaar RS, Kyles MK. Surgical correction of resistant talipes equinovarus: observations and analysis – preliminary report. Foot Ankle 1981;2(3):126–137.

22. Coetzee JC, Hansen ST. Surgical management of severe deformity resulting from posterior tibial tendon dysfunction. Foot Ankle Int 2001;22(12):944–949.

23. Koczewski P, Shadi M, Napiontek M. Foot lengthening using the Ilizarov device: the transverse tarsal joint resection versus osteotomy. J Pediatr Orthop B 2002;11(1):68–72.

24. Marti RK, de Heus JA, Roolker W, Poolman RW, Besselaar PP. Subtalar arthrodesis with correction of deformity after fractures of the os calcis. J Bone Joint Surg Br 1999;81(4):611–616.

25. Mosier-LaClair S, Pomeroy G, Manoli A. Operative treatment of the difficult stage 2 adult acquired flatfoot deformity. Foot Ankle Clin 2001;6(1):95–119.

26. Sammarco GJ, Conti SF. Surgical treatment of neuroarthropathic foot deformity. Foot Ankle Int 1998;19(2):102–109.

27. Stephens HM, Walling AK, Solmen JD, Tankson CJ. Subtalar repositional arthrodesis for adult acquired flatfoot. Clin Orthop Relat Res 1999 Aug; (365):69–73.

28. Toolan BC, Sangeorzan BJ, Hansen ST Jr. Complex reconstruction for the treatment of dorsolateral peritalar subluxation of the foot. Early results after distraction arthrodesis of the calcaneocuboid joint in conjunction with stabilization of, and transfer of the flexor digitorum longus tendon to, the midfoot to treat acquired pes planovalgus in adults. J Bone Joint Surg Am 1999;81(11):1545–1560.

29. Wei SY, Sullivan RJ, Davidson RS. Talonavicular arthrodesis for residual midfoot deformities of a previously corrected clubfoot. Foot Ankle Int 2000;21(6):482–485.

30. Bailey EJ, Waggoner SM, Albert MJ, Hutton WC. Intraarticular calcaneus fractures: a biomechanical comparison or two fixation methods. J Orthop Trauma 1997;11(1):34–37.

31. Trnka HJ, Easley ME, Lam PW, Anderson CD, Schon LC, Myerson MS. Subtalar distraction bone block arthrodesis. J Bone Joint Surg Br 2001;83(6):849–854.

32. Bargar WL, Bauer A, Borner M. Primary and revision total hip replacement using the Robodoc system. Clin Orthop Relat Res 1998 Sep; (354):82–91.

33. Claes J, Koekelkoren E, Wuyts FL, Claes GM, Van Den HL, Van De Heyning PH. Accuracy of computer navigation in ear, nose, throat surgery: the influence of matching strategy. Arch Otolaryngol Head Neck Surg 2000;126(12):1462–1466.

34. Delp SL, Stulberg SD, Davies B, Picard F, Leitner F. Computer assisted knee replacement. Clin Orthop Relat Res 1998 Sep; (354):49–56.

35. DiGioia AM III, Jaramaz B, Colgan BD. Computer assisted orthopaedic surgery. Image guided and robotic assistive technologies. Clin Orthop Relat Res 1998 Sep; (354):8–16.

36. DiGioia AM III, Jaramaz B, Plakseychuk AY, Moody JE Jr, Nikou C, Labarca RS et al. Comparison of a mechanical acetabular alignment guide with computer placement of the socket. J Arthroplasty 2002;17(3): 359–364.

37. Hassfeld S, Muhling J. Navigation in maxillofacial and craniofacial surgery. Comput Aided Surg 1998;3(4):183–187.

38. Jaramaz B, DiGioia AM III, Blackwell M, Nikou C. Computer assisted measurement of cup placement in total hip replacement. Clin Orthop Relat Res 1998 Sep; (354):70–81.

39. Kamimura M, Ebara S, Itoh H, Tateiwa Y, Kinoshita T, Takaoka K. Accurate pedicle screw insertion under the control of a computer-assisted image guiding system: laboratory test and clinical study. J Orthop Sci 1999;4(3):197–206.

40. Kato A, Yoshimine T, Hayakawa TM et al. [Computer assisted neurosurgery: development of a frameless and armless navigation system (CNS navigator)]. No Shinkei Geka 1991;19(2):137–142.

41. Kerschbaumer F. ["Numerical imaging, operation planning, simulation, navigation, robotics". Do the means determine the end? (editorial)]. Orthopade 2000;29(7):597–598.

42. Klos TV, Banks SA, Habets RJ, Cook FF. Sagittal plane imaging parameters for computer-assisted fluoroscopic anterior cruciate ligament reconstruction. Comput Aided Surg 2000;5(1):28–34.

43. Klos TV, Habets RJ, Banks AZ, Banks SA, Devilee RJ, Cook FF. Computer assistance in arthroscopic anterior cruciate ligament reconstruction. Clin Orthop Relat Res 1998 Sep; (354):65–69.

44. Laine T, Lund T, Ylikoski M, Lohikoski J, Schlenzka D. Accuracy of pedicle screw insertion with and without computer assistance: a randomised controlled clinical study in 100 consecutive patients. Eur Spine J 2000;9(3):235–240.

45. Langlotz F, Bachler R, Berlemann U, Nolte LP, Ganz R. Computer assistance for pelvic osteotomies. Clin Orthop Relat Res 1998 Sep; (354):92–102.

46. Merloz P, Tonetti J, Cinquin P, Lavallee S, Troccaz J, Pittet L. [Computer-assisted surgery: automated screw placement in the vertebral pedicle]. Chirurgie 1998;123(5):482–490.

47. Merloz P, Tonetti J, Pittet L, Coulomb M, Lavallee S, Troccaz J et al. Computer-assisted spine surgery. Comput Aided Surg 1998;3(6):297–305.

48. Ploder O, Wagner A, Enislidis G, Ewers R. [Computer-assisted intraoperative visualization of dental implants. Augmented reality in medicine]. Radiologe 1995; 35(9):569–572.

49. Radermacher K, Portheine F, Anton M, Zimolong A, Kaspers G, Rau G et al. Computer assisted orthopaedic surgery with image based individual templates. Clin Orthop Relat Res 1998 Sep; (354):28–38.

50. Schlenzka D, Laine T, Lund T. Computer-assisted spine surgery. Eur Spine J 2000;9(Suppl 1):S57–S64.

51. Tonetti J, Carrat L, Blendea S, Merloz P, Troccaz J, Lavallee S et al. Clinical results of percutaneous pelvic surgery. Computer assisted surgery using ultrasound compared to standard fluoroscopy. Comput Aided Surg 2001;6(4):204–211.

52. Tonetti J, Carrat L, Lavallee S, Pittet L, Merloz P, Chirossel JP. Percutaneous iliosacral screw placement using image guided techniques. Clin Orthop Relat Res 1998 Sep; (354):103–110.

53. Weihe S, Wehmoller M, Schliephake H, Hassfeld S, Tschakaloff A, Raczkowsky J et al. Synthesis of CAD/CAM, robotics and biomaterial implant fabrication: single-step reconstruction in computer aided frontotemporal bone resection. Int J Oral Maxillofac Surg 2000;29(5):384–388.

54. Birkfellner W, Huber K, Larson A, Hanson D, Diemling M, Homolka P et al. A modular software system for computer-aided surgery and its first application in oral implantology. IEEE Trans Med Imaging 2000;19(6):616–620.

55. Schiffers N, Schkommodau E, Portheine F, Radermacher K, Staudte HW. [Planning and performance of orthopedic surgery with the help of individual templates]. Orthopade 2000;29(7):636–640.

56. Schlenzka D, Laine T, Lund T. [Computer-assisted spine surgery: principles, technique, results and perspectives]. Orthopade 2000;29(7):658–669.

57. Thoma W, Schreiber S, Hovy L. [Computer-assisted implant positioning in knee endoprosthetics. Kinematic analysis for optimization of surgical technique]. Orthopade 2000;29(7):614–626.

58. Bechtold JE, Powless SH. The application of computer graphics in foot and ankle surgical planning and reconstruction. Clin Podiatr Med Surg 1993;10(3): 551–562.

59. Richter M. Experimental comparison between computer assisted surgery (CAS) based and C-Arm based correction of hind- and midfoot deformities. Osteo Trauma Care 2003;11:29–34.

60. Foley KT, Smith MM. Image-guided spine surgery. Neurosurg Clin N Am 1996;7(2):171–186.

61. Richter M, Geerling J, Zech S, Krettek C. ISO-C-3D based computer assisted surgery (CAS) guided retrograde drilling in a osteochondrosis dissecans of the talus: a case report. Foot 2005;15(2):107–113.

62. Berndt AL., Harty M. Transchondral fractures (osteochondritis dissecans) of the talus. Am J Orthop 1959;41-A:988–1020.

63. Alexander AH, Lichtman DM. Surgical treatment of transchondral talar-dome fractures (osteochondritis

dissecans). Long-term follow-up. J Bone Joint Surg Am 1980;62(4):646–652.

64. Tol JL, Struijs PA, Bossuyt PM, Verhagen RA, van Dijk CN. Treatment strategies in osteochondral defects of the talar dome: a systematic review. Foot Ankle Int 2000;21(2):119–126.

65. Taranow WS, Bisignani GA, Towers JD, Conti SF. Retrograde drilling of osteochondral lesions of the medial talar dome. Foot Ankle Int 1999;20(8):474–480.

66. Fink C, Rosenberger RE, Bale RJ, Rieger M, Hackl W, Benedetto KP et al. Computer-assisted retrograde drilling of osteochondral lesions of the talus. Orthopade 2001;30(1):59–65.

67. Seil R, Rupp S, Pape D, Dienst M, Kohn D. [Approach to open treatment of osteochondral lesions of the talus]. Orthopade 2001;30(1):47–52.

68. Rosenberger RE, Bale RJ, Fink C, Rieger M, Reichkendler M, Hackl W et al. [Computer-assisted drilling of the lower extremity. Technique and indications]. Unfallchirurg 2002;105(4):353–358.

69. Richter M, Geerling J, Frink M, Zech S, Knobloch K, Dammann F et al. Computer assisted surgery based (CAS) based correction of posttraumatic ankle and hindfoot deformities - preliminary results. Foot Ankle Surg 2006;12:113–119.

70. Zwipp H. Biomechanik der Sprunggelenke. Unfallchirurg 1989;92(3):98–102.

71. Rosenbaum D, Becker HP, Sterk J, Gerngross H, Claes L. Functional evaluation of the 10-year outcome after modified Evans repair for chronic ankle instability. Foot Ankle Int 1997;18(12):765–771.

72. Richter M, Frink M, Zech S, Droste P, Knobloch K, Krettek C. Technique for intraoperative use of pedography. Tech Foot Ankle 2006;5(2):88–100.

73. Richter M, Frink M, Zech S, Vanin N, Geerling J, Droste P et al. Intraoperative pedography - a new validated method for intra operative biomechanical assessment. Foot Ankle Int 2006;27(10):833–842.

74. Duranti R, Galletti R, Pantaleo T. Electromyographic observations in patients with foot pain syndromes. Am J Phys Med 1985;64(6):295–304.

75. Kawakami O, Sudoh H, Watanabe S. Effects of linear movements on upright standing position. Environ Med 1996;40(2):193–196.

76. Trepman E, Gellman RE, Solomon R, Murthy KR, Micheli LJ, De Luca CJ. Electromyographic analysis of standing posture and demi-plie in ballet and modern dancers. Med Sci Sports Exerc 1994;26(6):771–782.

Index

G.R. Scuderi and A.J. Tria (eds.), *Minimally Invasive Surgery in Orthopedics: Foot and Ankle Handbook*,   221
DOI 10.1007/978-1-4614-0893-2, © Springer Science+Business Media, LLC 2012